**Heart Disease
in Paediatrics**

POSTGRADUATE PAEDIATRICS SERIES

under the General Editorship of

JOHN APLEY
C.B.E., M.D., B.S., F.R.C.P., J.P.

Consultant Paediatrician, United Bristol Hospitals and Bath Clinical Area; Lecturer in Diseases of Children, University of Bristol

Heart Disease
in Paediatrics
Second Edition

S. C. JORDAN
MD, FRCP

Consultant Cardiologist
Bristol Royal Hospital for Sick Children

and

OLIVE SCOTT
MD, FRCP

Consultant Paediatric Cardiologist
Leeds Regional Thoracic Centre
Killingbeck Hospital, Leeds

Butterworths
London Boston Sydney Wellington Durban Toronto

First published 1973
Second edition 1981

© Butterworth & Co. (Publishers) Ltd. 1981

> **British Library Cataloguing in Publication Data**
>
> *Jordan, S. C.*
> *Heart disease in paediatrics—2nd ed.–*
> (Postgraduate paediatrics series)
> 1. Paediatric cardiology
> I. Title   II. Scott, Olive   III. Series
> 618.912′2   RJ421
>
> ISBN 0–407–19941–1

Typeset by CCC, in Great Britain by William Clowes (Beccles) Limited, Beccles and London
Printed in England by Mackays of Chatham.

Contents

SECTION III.   SPECIAL PROBLEMS

Preface

Since the first edition of this book in 1973, paediatric cardiology has expanded and developed rapidly. More consultant paediatric cardiologists have been appointed and centres are being developed throughout the country to ensure that all children with heart disease may benefit from advances in investigation and treatment. There have been an increasing number of meetings to share knowledge and the first World Congress of Paediatric Cardiology in 1980 established the speciality in its own right.

The purpose of this book has not changed but it has been completely revised and brought up to date. One important new development has been the use of non-invasive investigations and this new edition has a section on echocardiography and its value is indicated when individual lesions are discussed. The use of ambulatory electrocardiographic monitoring in the study and treatment of arrhythmias is also discussed.

There is a new chapter on the advances in cardiac surgery in which the various operations (many of them eponymous) are defined and the use of new materials and prostheses discussed.

Early diagnosis and early referral of newborn infants has improved the outlook for many of them and there are details of the best way of managing these babies in the special chapter on the newborn infant.

The aim for the future must be to correct anatomical abnormalities sufficiently early to keep the function of the heart as normal as possible enabling children not only to survive operation but to lead truly normal lives.

S.C.J.
O.S.

Preface to the First Edition

This book does not aim to be a comprehensive work on all aspects of paediatric cardiology. It is intended for the paediatrician and others who look after children to use as an introduction to paediatric cardiology and to provide up-to-date knowledge of the methods of diagnosis and treatment, particularly of congenital heart disease. The approach is essentially a practical one. It indicates to what extent the clinical signs and symptoms, assisted by radiological and electrocardiographic findings, can indicate the diagnosis, and when further investigation by cardiac catheterization and angiography will be required.

The two authors, one a paediatrician with cardiological training and one a cardiologist with special experience in paediatric cardiology, have slightly different views on some of the subjects, so that the text has been a result of the two approaches. In a book of this size it has not been possible or desirable to discuss in detail some of the more controversial aspects of paediatric cardiology, and indeed views on such topics as early corrective surgery in infancy are changing rapidly at the moment. This should not deter the paediatrician, as the same principles apply with regard to referral of patients for further investigation and treatment.

Few paediatricians will be directly concerned with cardiac catheterization, but decisions regarding surgery are frequently influenced by the results of this investigation and a section has therefore been included on the technique and interpretation.

One of the most striking changes in paediatric cardiology in recent years has been the increasing interest in the management of the newborn infant with heart disease and a special chapter has been included, which presents a scheme to simplify diagnosis in this difficult group of patients.

S.C.J.
O.S.

GENERAL CARDIOLOGY

CHAPTER 1

Incidence and Aetiology of Congenital Heart Disease

INCIDENCE

Congenital heart disease is the commonest single group of congenital abnormalities, accounting for about 30 per cent of the total. The incidence is about 8/1000 live births. There are eight common lesions which account for 85 per cent of all cases. They are ventricular septal defect, patent ductus arteriosus, atrial septal defect, pulmonary valve stenosis, aortic stenosis, coarctation of the aorta, tetralogy of Fallot and transposition of the great arteries. The remaining 15 per cent is made up of a variety of more rare and complex lesions.

Congenital heart disease as a whole occurs with equal frequency in males and females, but some lesions such as aortic stenosis, coarctation of the aorta, transposition of the great arteries and tetralogy of Fallot are more common in males whereas patent ductus arteriosus and atrial septal defect are more common in females. About 13 per cent of patients who have one congenital heart defect will have an additional cardiac defect. Between 10 and 15 per cent of patients with cardiac defects will have another *non*-cardiac deformity (Campbell, 1965).

Recurrence in family

The risks of a sibling being affected by congenital heart disease is between 2 and 4 per cent. There is a high degree of concordance in that the sibling usually has the same lesion or one of its components

3

(e.g. pulmonary stenosis or ventricular septal defect occurs in siblings of patients with tetralogy of Fallot). The studies of Nora, McGill and McNamara (1970) give recurrences in siblings (*Table 1.1*). Now that children with congenital heart disease survive to have children

TABLE 1.1

Proportion of siblings and offspring of index patients with congenital heart disease who were also affected

	Per cent risks to siblings	Per cent risks to offspring
Patent ductus arteriosus	3.4	4.3
Ventricular septal defect	4.4	4.0
Atrial septal defect	3.2	2.5
Pulmonary stenosis	2.9	3.6
Coarctation of aorta	1.8	2.7
Transposition of the great arteries	1.9	—
Tetralogy of Fallot	2.7	4.2
Aortic stenosis		3.9

of their own, it is important to know the risks of their children being affected. Nora and Nora (1976) have determined these (*Table 1.2*). Again the majority of children had the same lesion as the affected parent. The results of this study are within the range one would expect in multifactorial inheritance. The recurrence rate is worrying but the data is still insufficient for us to know whether there will be an absolute increase in affected children. Nora's data suggests that individuals with congenital heart disease marry later and restrict their families more than the population as a whole. If another member of the family has congenital heart disease, recurrence rates increase two or threefold (Nora and Nora, 1978).

Recently Child and Dennis (1977) have calculated the sibling recurrence risk of endocardial fibroelastosis to be 5.4 per cent and hypoplastic left heart to be only 0.5 per cent.

Parents who have had one child with congenital heart disease should if they wish be advised by a genetic counsellor.

AETIOLOGY

The first question parents ask when they realize their child has a heart defect is 'what caused it?' Unfortunately we are still unable to answer this question precisely in the majority of patients.

Inheritance

A few families are reported in which a defect, especially atrial septal defect, follows a dominant pattern of inheritance.

Chromosomal abnormalities

Some chromosomal abnormalities are associated with congenital heart disease (*Table 1.2*) but these account for about 5 per cent of patients with congenital heart disease. The cardiovascular abnormality in Turner's syndrome is most commonly coarctation of the

TABLE 1.2

Incidence of congenital heart disease in children with chromosomal abnormalities

Chromosome abnormality	Name of syndrome	Incidence of CHD (%)	Type of defect
Partial deletion of 5	Cri du chat	50	VSD
21 Trisomy	Mongolism (Down's syndrome)	60	A-V defects VSD: ASD: Fallot
18 Trisomy	—	90	VSD; PDA; single umbilical artery; DORV; coarctation
13 Trisomy	—	90	VSD; ASD; single umbilical artery; dextrocardia
XO	Turner's syndrome	40	Coarctation, AS

CHD Congenital heart disease	PDA	Patent ductus arteriosus
VSD Ventricular septal defect	DORV	Double outlet right ventricle
A-V Atrioventricular defect	AS	Aortic stenosis
ASD Atrial septal defect		

aorta but in the XX and XY phenotype (Noonan's syndrome) pulmonary stenosis with dysplastic pulmonary valve and hypertrophic cardiomyopathy occur. About two-thirds of patients with Down's syndrome have heart lesions and the majority have atrioventricular defects. Tetralogy of Fallot, patent ductus arteriosus, atrial septal defect and ventricular septal defects also occur.

Multifactorial inheritance

The most readily acceptable theory for the genetic basis of congenital heart disease is the multifactorial hypothesis. The hypothesis suggests that the genetic material concerned with the normal development of the heart is carried on a number of genes and that abnormalities of these genes may not in themselves be enough to cause cardiac abnormalities, but in the presence of other environmental factors the genes predispose to the occurrence of such defects. In other words there is a genetic susceptibility to develop congenital heart disease if the appropriate environmental hazard occurs.

Environmental factors

Maternal vitamin deficiency (Wilson and Warkany, 1949; Smithells, 1977) may cause cardiac defects. In 1 per cent of congenital heart disease cases rubella in the first trimester is associated with patent ductus arteriosus, ventricular septal defect, tetralogy of Fallot and peripheral pulmonary stenosis. Drugs taken during pregnancy are being increasingly suspected since thalidomide was found to be associated with peripheral pulmonary stenosis. Phenytoin is associated with an increased incidence of heart disease and warfarin is teratogenic. Pregnancy testing drugs are also under suspicion.

Congenital heart block is commonly seen in infants of mothers who have systemic lupus erythematosis. There is an increased incidence of congenital heart disease in infants of mothers who have diabetes. Smoking in the mother is associated with a higher incidence of congenital heart disease, and alcoholism produces abnormal babies half of whom have heart lesions, most commonly septal defects.

REFERENCES

Campbell, M. (1965). Causes of malformations of the heart. *Br. med. J.* **2**, 895
Child, Anne H. and Dennis, N. R. (1977). The genetics of congenital heart disease. *Birth Defects: Original Article Series.* **Volume XIII. No. 3A,** 85–91
Nora, J. J., McGill, C. W. and McNamara, D. G. (1970). Empiric recurrence risks in common and uncommon congenital heart lesions. *Teratology* 3, 325–329
Nora, J. J. and Nora, A. H. (1976). *Circulation.* **53.**4, 701–702
Nora, J. J. and Nora, A. H. (1978). *Genetics and Counseling in Cardiovascular Disease.* Springfield: Charles C. Thomas
Smithells, R. S. (1977). Maternal nutrition in early pregnancy. *Brit. J. Nutr.* **38**, 497–506
Wilson, J. G. and Warkany, J. (1949) Aortic arch and other anomalies in offspring of vitamin A deficient rats. *Brit. J. Nutr.* **38**, 497–506

The Fetal Circulation and the Changes at Birth in Relation to Congenital Heart Disease

THE FETAL CIRCULATION

To appreciate the haemodynamic effects of congenital heart lesions, there must be clear understanding of the fetal circulation and the changes which take place after birth to establish the normal, independent circulation. These changes influence the circulation in normal infants but are of profound importance in infants with congenital heart disease. *A congenital heart lesion is not a static condition; changes continue to take place throughout the patient's life, but the most significant of these occur at birth.*

In the fetus, blood comes from the placenta via the umbilical vein and is relatively well oxygenated ($Po_2 = 30$ mmHg). Half of this blood passes through the liver and the remainder bypasses the liver through the ductus venosus and continues up the inferior vena cava, which receives blood leaving the liver by the hepatic veins and blood returning from the lower half of the body of the fetus. Most of the inferior vena caval blood passes through the foramen ovale to the left atrium and so to the left ventricle, ascending aorta and coronary circulation. This ensures that blood of a high Po_2 enters the cerebral and coronary circulations. A small amount of inferior vena caval blood passes through the tricuspid valve into the right ventricle. Blood returning from the head and neck of the fetus enters the right atrium by the superior vena cava, is joined by coronary sinus blood and then enters the right ventricle and pulmonary artery (*Figure 2.1*). In the fetus only about 15 per cent of the right ventricular blood enters the lungs, and the rest passes through the ductus arteriosus into the descending aorta where it is joined by blood from the ascending aorta. In the fetus the ductus arteriosus is as large as the aorta itself and pressures in the pulmonary artery and aorta are equal.

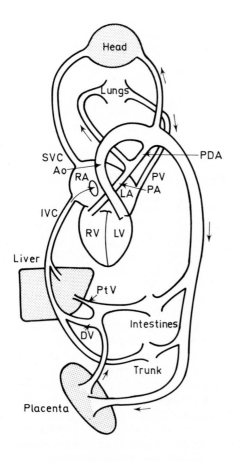

Figure 2.1. The fetal circulation. Ao: aorta; DV: ductus venosus; IVC: inferior vena cava; LA: left atrium; LV: left ventricle; PtV: portal vein; PV: pulmonary vein; RA: right atrium; RV: right ventricle; PA: pulmonary artery; PDA: patent ductus arteriosus; SVC: superior vena cava

In the fetus there is a high pulmonary vascular resistance and the muscular pulmonary arteries are constricted and have a thick medial muscular layer.

After birth the following changes take place.

1. The pulmonary vascular resistance falls and the pulmonary blood flow increases.
2. The systemic vascular resistance rises.
3. The patent ductus arteriosus closes.
4. The foramen ovale closes.
5. The ductus venosus closes.

The initial fall in pulmonary vascular resistance at birth is associated with expansion of the lungs with air. The pulmonary arterial vasoconstriction ceases and there may be active dilatation of the vessels. The greatest fall in the pulmonary artery pressure takes place in the *first two to three days of life* and then there is a more gradual fall to normal adult levels by *two weeks of life* (Rudolph, 1970). The medial muscle layer of the small pulmonary arteries thins out in the first few days of life as these vessels dilate, and thereafter the histological changes in the pulmonary vessels follow the fall in the pulmonary artery pressure.

Once the low resistance placental circulation is removed at birth, the systemic resistance rises. While the ductus remains open, there is a preferential flow through it from the aorta to the lungs. In turn the pulmonary venous return is increased and there is increased flow to the left atrium and left ventricle. The ductus closes functionally within 10–15 hours of birth, so any flow through it lasts a relatively short time. If there is hypoxia of the fetal blood for any reason (for example, pulmonary disease) it will cause a rise in pulmonary artery pressure and favour a right-to-left shunt through the ductus. The administration of 100 per cent oxygen causes the ductus to constrict. In normal mature infants the ductus closes permanently within two or three weeks of birth. The histological changes have been well described by Gittenberger-de-Groot (1979).

The foramen ovale closes functionally at birth. A shunt through it from the right atrium to the left may occur if the pulmonary artery and right ventricular pressures rise in response to hypoxia. Occasionally, a left-to-right shunt through the foramen may persist for some months if the flap covering it does not seal completely.

The importance of changes in the circulation after birth in relation to congenital heart disease has been clearly shown by Rudolph (1970).

EFFECT OF CONGENITAL HEART DEFECTS ON CHANGES IN THE CIRCULATION AT BIRTH

Large communication between pulmonary and systemic circulations

Since the pulmonary vascular resistance falls rapidly in the first two or three days of life, it would be expected that a large communication between the pulmonary and systemic circulations, such as patent ductus arteriosus, ventricular septal defect and aortopulmonary window, would exert its greatest effect in the first few days of life, due to a preferential flow of blood from the high resistance systemic circulation to the low resistance pulmonary circulation. This does not in fact happen.

It seems that when a large communication exists, the rate of fall of pulmonary vascular resistance proceeds more slowly; this delays the onset of symptoms and helps the circulation to adapt to the defect more gradually. The postnatal changes in the main pulmonary artery and its branches may also play a part in maintaining the pulmonary artery pressure at a higher level for a longer period. There is frequently a pressure drop between the main pulmonary artery and its branches, suggesting some stenosis, but as the infant grows this pressure difference disappears (Rudolph, 1970). All these lesions tend to produce left ventricular failure due to the high pulmonary flow which in turn leads to an increased pulmonary venous return and high left atrial pressure. The symptoms and signs of left ventricular failure in left-to-right shunts are rarely seen before 3–4 weeks of age. If lung disease is present, the left-to-right shunt may decrease because of the rise in pulmonary artery pressure and a right-to-left shunt through these defects may occur.

Heart lesions dependent on ductal patency

If the oxygenation of aterial blood after birth is inadequate the closure of the ductus may be delayed or prevented. The incidence of patent ductus arteriosus in individuals born and living at high altitude is greater than those born at sea level. In some congenital heart defects, babies can only survive if the ductus arteriosus remains patent. Such defects are, severe tetralogy of Fallot with marked hypoplasia of the outflow tract to the lungs; pulmonary atresia; critical pulmonary stenosis; aortic atresia and critical aortic stenosis; severe coarctation of the aorta.

Even though the normal constriction of the ductus depends on a rise in arterial oxygen concentration, the duct still constricts after birth in hypoxic babies and this may happen suddenly. The risks of palliative surgery in these babies have been high mainly because of severe hypoxaemia and acidosis. Oxygenation in these babies can be improved dramatically by infusing prostaglandin E1 or E2. Initially this was infused into the aorta opposite the ductus arteriosus (Sharpe and Larsson, 1975) but it is also effective when given intravenously (Olley, 1975). In heart lesions where there is interruption of the aortic arch or severe coarctation of the aorta, the ductus arteriosus may supply blood to the descending aorta and lower part of the body. If the duct closes there is a reduced systemic flow and tissue hypoxia with metabolic acidosis results. Again prostaglandins are effective in dilating the ductus and improving the state of the child before surgery (*see* p. 173).

Persistent patency of the ductus arteriosus in premature infants

In the premature infant there is delay in closure of the ductus and about 50 per cent of infants under 1500 grams in weight have patency of the ductus. The incidence is higher when there is associated hyaline membrane disease. In the premature infant there is a rapid fall in pulmonary vascular resistance which favours a left-to-right shunt. Cardiac failure commonly occurs if the duct is open in premature infants. If the infant can tolerate the heart failure and the latter responds to medical treatment, then the duct will eventually close – it rarely remains open for more than three months (Rudolph, 1977; Hallidie-Smith and Girling, 1971). The situation has changed now that more premature infants survive with ventilatory support (*see* p. 70).

Obstruction of flow into or from the left ventricle (mitral atresia; aortic atresia; coarctation of aorta)

When there is severe obstruction to flow of blood from the left ventricle, the pressure in it rises and this results in a high left atrial pressure. The valvular action of the foramen ovale may then be overcome and it remains widely open with a resultant left-to-right shunt at atrial level. This left-to-right shunt, however, may be beneficial by reducing the left atrial pressure and lessening the severity of pulmonary oedema. Similarly, in mitral atresia the left atrial pressure rises and an open foramen ovale may be the only means by which pulmonary venous blood may enter the right side of the heart.

Obstruction of flow from the right atrium or right ventricle (tricuspid atresia; pulmonary atresia with intact ventricular septum)

The only way in which blood can reach the left side of the heart is by the open foramen ovale. A high right atrial pressure favours the foramen remaining open. Similarly, in total anomalous pulmonary venous drainage, the foramen ovale must remain open to permit blood to reach the left side of the heart.

Transposition of the great arteries

An open foramen ovale and a patent ductus arteriosus may be the only routes by which blood can shunt from the systemic to the pulmonary circulation and vice versa in transposition of the great arteries. If the left atrial pressure rises the foramen may close despite its patency being essential for life. Enlargement of the foramen ovale or the creation of an atrial septal defect has been effective in prolonging life in this lesion.

Total anomalous pulmonary venous drainage to the portal vein

The ductus venosus usually closes at birth but may remain open when the pulmonary veins all drain into the portal vein, thus making a free passage of blood into the interior vena cava without going through the liver. When the ductus venosus closes, however, the blood in the anomalous vein has to pass through a high resistance circuit in the liver, the pressure in the anomalous pulmonary vein rises and pulmonary oedema results.

REFERENCES

Gittenberger-de-Groot, A. (1979). Ductus arteriosus – histological observations in paediatric cardiology Vol. 2. In *Heart Disease in the Newborn*, Eds. M. J. Godman and R. M. Marquis. London: Churchill Livingstone

Hallidie-Smith, K. A. and Girling, D. J. (1971). Persistent ductus arteriosus in ill and premature babies. *Archs Dis. Childh.* **46**, 246

Olley, P. M. (1975). Non-surgical palliation of congenital heart malformations. *New Engl. J. Med.* **292**, 1292–1294

Rudolph, A. M. (1970). The changes in the circulation after birth. *Circulation* **41**, 343

Rudolph, A. M. (1977). In *Paediatric Cardiology*. Eds R. H. Anderson and E. A. Shinebourne. Vol. 47, pp. 409–412. London: Churchill Livingstone

Sharpe, G. L. and Larsson, K. S. (1975). Studies on closure of the ductus arteriosus: *in vivo* effect of prostaglandins. *Prostaglandins* **9**, 704–707

CHAPTER 3

Normal Haemodynamics: The Generation of Heart Sounds and Murmurs

NORMAL HAEMODYNAMICS

It is important for the reader to be familiar with the normal physiology of the heart before he studies the abnormal.

The heart can be considered as two pumps connected in series by two systems of vessels. The pressure generated by the right ventricle drives the blood through the pulmonary circuit and the pressure generated by the left ventricle drives the blood through the systemic circuit.

In a normal heart the resistance to flow of blood imposed by the pulmonary circuit is low, but the resistance imposed by the systemic circuit, as soon as the adaptation following birth occurs, is much higher, being about ten times greater than the pulmonary resistance. The resistance in the systemic circuit varies under differing physiological conditions and during exercise it falls when the muscle vessels dilate to allow a greater flow of blood through them. The pulmonary resistance shows little variation except when there is hypoxia or acidaemia, both of which cause it to increase.

Cardiac output

The output of blood from the right and left ventricles must be the same in a healthy heart; this is simply termed the 'cardiac output' and is expressed in litres/minute. According to Starling's 'law of the heart', the force generated by the muscle fibres is a function of their resting length. In practice, the resting length depends upon the degree of filling of the ventricles, so that increased filling of the heart results in increased cardiac output. The contractile properties of the heart can be increased by drugs such as digoxin and isoprenaline and are reduced in heart failure.

Normal pressures and oxygen saturations

The normal resting values in childhood are shown in *Figure 3.1*. The state of the patient must be stable throughout the period of

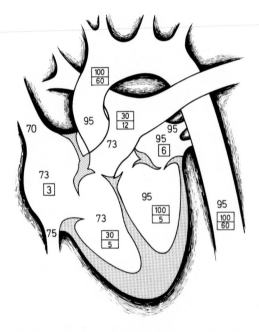

Figure 3.1. Normal values. Pressure in mmHg, within squares; percentage oxygen saturations, unsquared

measurement. There is a variation in the oxygen values in the right atrium depending on the exact site of sampling. The figures given are average ones. If a sample is taken in the atrium near the mouth of the coronary sinus the value is low; if the sample is rather low down in the inferior vena cava the oxygen saturation may be high because it contains blood from the renal veins which have a high oxygen saturation. There must be a rise of 10 per cent, eg from 65 per cent to 75 per cent saturation in two sets of samples between the superior vena cava and the right atrium for it to be significant of a left-to-right shunt. A rise of 5 per cent between the right atrial and right ventricular samples indicates a shunt at ventricular level and a rise of 3 per cent between right ventricle and pulmonary artery indicates a left-to-right shunt at pulmonary artery level.

It must be appreciated, however, that a lot of selective streaming of blood occurs in the heart and more than one set of samples may be required. Furthermore, the findings at catheterization should always be considered along with the clinical, radiological and electrocardiographic findings, otherwise mistakes in diagnosis will be made.

NORMAL HEART SOUNDS

Four heart sounds occur in the cardiac cycle. There is still argument as to their cause but accepted explanations are as follows.

The first sound is produced by closure of the atrioventricular valves, mainly the mitral valve.

The second sound is due to the closing of the semilunar valves. There are two components of this sound; the first is due to closure of the aortic valve and the second to closure of the pulmonary valve. They are normally separated by 0.02–0.03 seconds. Normally, the splitting of this sound increases in inspiration, at which time there is greater filling of the right ventricle and the closure of the pulmonary valve is slightly delayed.

The third sound is due to rapid filling of the ventricles during diastole. It is heard in one-fifth of all normal children.

The fourth sound is the result of atrial contraction which causes a brief increase in flow into the left ventricle. It occurs just before the first sound.

ABNORMAL SOUNDS

The first sound is loud in children when they are nervous and excited or in the presence of anaemia or pyrexia. It is loud in mitral stenosis, when it is preceded by a presystolic murmur.

The second sound. An abnormally wide split occurs in atrial septal defect when the right ventricle is overfilled with blood and pulmonary valve closure is further delayed. The splitting is 'fixed'; that is, it does not vary with respiration. This is because the two atria are functioning as one, and respiration has the same effect on both the pulmonary and the systemic circuits. In pulmonary stenosis there is wide splitting of the second sound asociated with delay in emptying of the right ventricle, while the second element of the sound is soft.

When the resistance in the pulmonary circuit is the same as in the systemic circuit then the aortic and pulmonary valves close at the same time and a loud, single second sound is heard.

In aortic stenosis the aortic closure sound is delayed and splitting of the second sound is closer, or it may be single. In severe aortic stenosis the aortic closure may occur after pulmonary closure and splitting then increases during expiration (reversed or paradoxical splitting). This also occurs in diseases of the myocardium such as cardiomyopathy.

Ejection clicks occur in aortic valve stenosis and in pulmonary valve stenosis. There is some argument whether the click is associated with the dilatation of the artery beyond the narrowing or whether it is produced by the sudden restriction of the upward movement of the dome-shaped stenotic valve. Certainly the time of its occurrence is related to the severity of the stenosis. The more severe the stenosis, the nearer is the ejection click to the first sound. Ejection clicks may also be heard when there is a large dilated aorta in tetralogy of Fallot, coarctation of the aorta, persistent truncus arteriosus or a dilated pulmonary artery as in pulmonary hypertension.

Mid- or late systolic clicks come from the mitral valve and are due to a sudden backward prolapse of one or both cusps during systole. Sometimes the clicks are multiple and frequently there is also a late systolic murmur. Rarely similar clicks are produced by a floppy tricuspid valve.

HEART MURMURS

Murmurs may be innocent or organic. Organic heart murmurs occur when blood flows through an abnormal valve or an abnormal orifice in the heart or between the great vessels. They may occur between the first and second sounds, when they are systolic, or between the second and first sounds, when they are diastolic.

The loudness of a murmur depends both on the gradient through which the blood travels and on the amount of blood flowing through the hole or orifice. A large amount of blood flowing through a moderate sized ventricular septal defect with a big pressure difference between the two ventricles will make a louder noise than either a very small defect with little blood flow or a very large defect where the pressures in the two ventricles are similar.

Systolic murmurs

Systolic murmurs have been classified by Leatham (1958) as follows:

1. Ejection systolic murmurs, caused by forward flow of blood through a normal or diseased semilunar valve, aortic or mitral.
2. Regurgitant murmurs, caused by retrograde flow of blood through an incompetent atrioventricular valve or through a ventricular septal defect.

Ejection murmurs show a diamond-shaped pattern on the phonocardiogram and end before the onset of the second sound. They are heard in aortic stenosis and pulmonary stenosis when blood is flowing though a narrowed orifice. A similar though softer type of murmur occurs when there is an increased flow of blood through a normal semilunar valve, as occurs through the pulmonary valve in artrial septal defect. Murmurs due to aortic stenosis are rather shorter than those due to pulmonary stenosis.

Regurgitant murmurs usually last throughout systole (pansystolic) and are plateau-shaped on the phonocardiogram. In an uncomplicated ventricular septal defect there is a gradient between the left and right ventricles throughout systole. In free mitral regurgitation there is a gradient between the left ventricle and left atrium throughout systole. Early systolic murmurs are heard in very small ventricular septal defects; late systolic murmurs in very mild mitral regurgitation.

Diastolic murmurs

Diastolic murmurs occur when the semilunar valves are incompetent, when the atrioventricular valves are narrowed, or when they are normal but there is an increased volume of blood flow through them. The murmur of aortic regurgitation has a high pitch and is soft and often difficult to hear. It is best heard down the left sternal edge when the patient sits forward and holds his breath in expiration. The murmur of pulmonary incompetence associated with a high pulmonary artery pressure (Graham Steell murmur) is indistinguishable from it. The murmur of pulmonary incompetence when there is a low pulmonary artery pressure is lower pitched.

The diastolic murmurs of mitral stenosis are low pitched and rumbling, and best heard when the patient turns on his left side. The murmur due to increased flow through the mitral valve with ventricular septal defects and patent ductus arteriosus is short and low pitched. The diastolic murmur due to increased flow through the tricuspid valve is softer, increases with inspiration and is best heard in the erect posture after exercise. It is heard rather sooner after the second sound than the mitral diastolic flow murmur.

Continuous murmurs

Continuous murmurs are heard when blood flows between two parts of the circulation with a gradient in diastole and systole. The usual cause is a patent ductus arteriosus (*see* p. 65).

The various types of murmur are illustrated diagrammatically in *Figure 3.2*.

INNOCENT MURMURS

The terms 'benign', 'functional' and 'physiological' are also used to describe innocent murmurs. 'Innocent' seems the most satisfactory term because it is best understood by the child or his parents. The term is used to describe murmurs which occur in patients who have no abnormality of the heart. It is very important that doctors appreciate the innocence of these murmurs and that parents are reassured that their child's heart is normal and the child himself is not unnecessarily restricted in his activities. If there is any doubt the child should be referred to a cardiologist.

The frequency with which innocent murmurs are heard varies, but they are often accentuated by factors which produce tachycardia – fever, excitement and exercise – and disappear when the heart rate slows. They often vary with respiration, disappearing with inspiration, and are affected by changes in posture. Innocent murmurs may occur in systole or be continuous. A diastolic murmur by itself is never innocent.

Three main types of innocent systolic murmur are recognized in childhood.

Vibratory murmur

The character and pitch of the vibratory murmur are very like the buzzing of a bee. It is very short and occurs in mid-systole. It is less

19

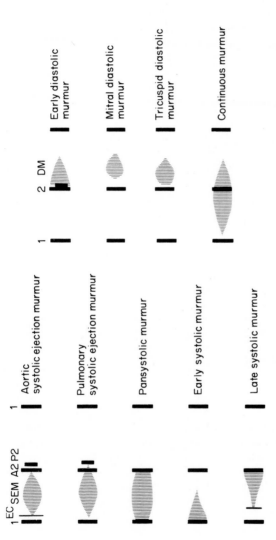

Figure 3.2. Types of murmur. 1: first sound; EC: ejection click; SEM: systolic ejection murmur; A2 and P2: aortic and pulmonary components of second heart sound; DM: diastolic murmur

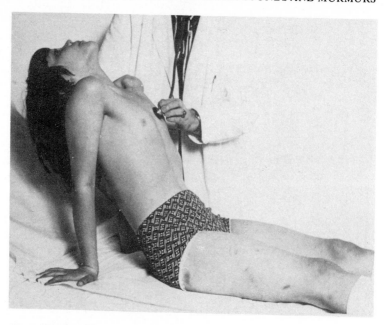

Figure 3.3. Vibratory systolic murmur is markedly reduced or disappears when patient sits up with neck extended

obvious when the patient sits up and extends his neck, and often disappears when he sits with his hands behind him and arches his back. It is commonest under the age of 10 years and usually disappears at puberty. (*Figure 3.3.*)

Pulmonary systolic murmur

The pulmonary systolic murmur is a soft blowing ejection systolic murmur occupying the early part of systole, heard in the second left interspace close to the sternum and conducted upwards to the infraclavicular region. The differential diagnosis is a mild degree of pulmonary stenosis, but the second sound is normally split when the murmur is innocent and the electrocardiogram and radiograph are quite normal. It is commonest in older children and adolescents.

Venous hum

A venous hum, due to blood cascading into the great veins, is a blowing, continuous murmur best heard in the supraclavicular fossa but often quite loud below the clavicles. The hum is abolished or greatly diminished when the internal jugular vein on the same side as the murmur is compressed, when the patient turns his head from the side to a midline position and when he lies down flat or performs the Valsalva manoeuvre.

BLOOD PRESSURE

Blood pressure measurement in children has in the past been difficult and often inaccurate. It is often difficult to hear the Korotkoff sounds in children but now they can be sensed with an ultrasonic Doppler device giving a clear sharp signal indicating the systolic pressure. The other problem has been precise knowledge about the correct width and length of the cuff. Steinfeld *et al.* (1978) have done much to clarify this. They conclude that the cuff bladder should be as follows:

1. *Width*. This should cover two-thirds of the upper arm. It is best to apply a cuff as wide as possible.
2. *Length*. The bladder should completely encircle the upper arm; overlap does not matter.

It is important to have a variety of lengths and widths of cuff on a paediatric ward so that the appropriate size can be fitted to each patient. It is still difficult to measure the diastolic pressure indirectly. It may be that the newly developed method using the oscillometric principle will give accurate diastolic and mean arterial pressures and be particularly valuable in premature infants.

If sophisticated equipment is not available the flush method gives a reading which is lower than the true systolic pressure but is useful for comparing the pressure in the arms and legs. The cuff is applied in the usual way and then, after wrapping a crepe bandage firmly round the hand and forearm, the cuff is inflated above the expected systolic pressure and the bandage removed. The skin will appear blanched. The sphygmomanometer pressure is then lowered 5 mmHg at a time, slowly, and the skin observed. A reading is made when the skin shows a pink flush. This pressure represents a point a little below the true systolic pressure. (*See* p. 339 for normal values.)

REFERENCES

Steinfeld L., Dimich I., Reder R., Cohen M. and Alexander H. (1978). Sphygmo-manometry in the pediatric patient. *J. Pediat.* **92**, 934.

CHAPTER 4

Cardiac Investigations

RADIOLOGY

A radiograph of the heart and lungs in congenital heart disease is only of value if the film fulfils strict criteria.

1. It must be straight.
2. It must be taken during full inspiration.
3. It must be of the correct penetration for accurate assessment of the vascularity of the lungs.

A posteroanterior film should be taken initially and lateral or oblique views can then be added as indicated. In children over six months of age the posteroanterior film is taken with the patient erect at a tube distance of 6 feet. In children under six months of age the film is taken with the patient lying down and is an anteroposterior one with a tube distance of 5 feet.

Heart size and shape

The size of the heart is best estimated by measuring the cardiothoracic diameter, that is, the ratio of the transverse diameter of the heart to the greatest *internal* diameter of the chest. A line is drawn down the centre of the film and the distance from this central line to the furthest point on the right heart border, added to the distance from the central line to the furthest point on the left heart border, gives the transverse cardiac diameter (*Figure 4.1*). If the cardiothoracic ratio is less than 0.5, the heart is not enlarged overall.

The heart chambers and great vessels should than be assessed. The reader must be familiar with the normal heart before he can assess the abnormal. The right heart border is made up of the superior vena cava above, and the right atrium below, and the inferior vena cava is seen below the right atrium (*Figure 4.2*). On the

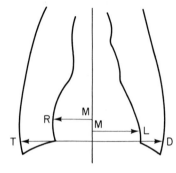

Figure 4.1. Measurement of cardiothoracic ratio. The cardiac diameter is the sum of M–R and M–L, the distances of the right and left cardiac borders from the midline. The thoracic diameter (TD) is the greatest diameter inside the ribs

left heart border the aorta, pulmonary artery and left ventricular outlines are seen. The main pulmonary artery is straight or slightly convex. The left atrial appendage lies below the pulmonary artery but normally merges imperceptibly with the left ventricular border.

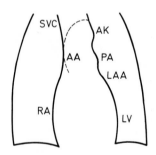

Figure 4.2. Normal cardiac silhouette. AA: ascending aorta; AK: aortic knuckle; LAA: left atrial appendage; LV: left ventricle; RA: right atrium: SVC: superior vena cava

Details about the enlargement of the heart chambers and great vessels are given under individual lesions and a table of common heart shapes in infancy is given on pages 246–247. *Figure 4.3* shows the enlargement of various structures for comparison one with another. In the posteroanterior film, when there is enlargement of the right ventricle the cardiac apex is tilted upwards and has a small radius of curvature; when the left ventricle is enlarged the apex points downwards and has a larger radius. The size of the ventricles cannot be assessed accurately, however, in a posteroanterior film

24

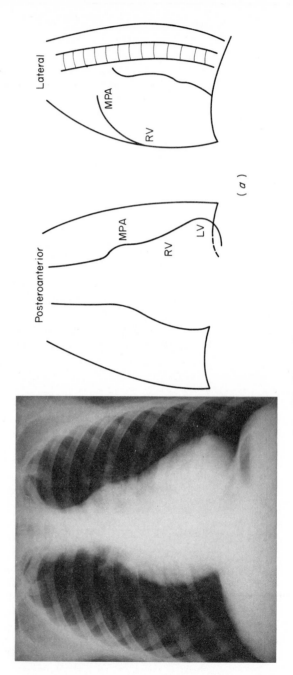

Figure 4.3a. See caption on facing page

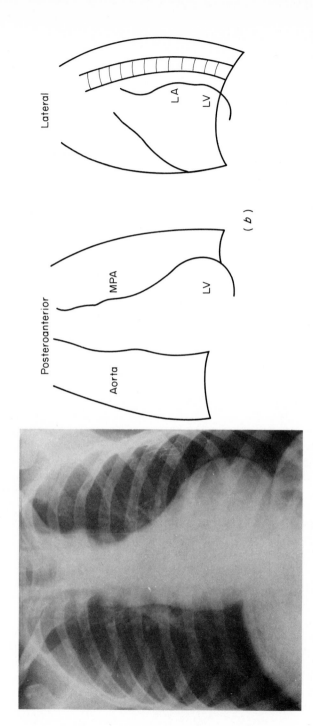

Figure 4.3a, b. Radiological signs of ventricular enlargement, with line drawings in posteroanterior and lateral projections. LA: left atrium; MPA: main pulmonary artery; RV: right ventricle; LV: left ventricle; Ao: aorta. (*a*) **Right ventricular enlargement (severe pulmonary stenosis).** (*b*) **Left ventricular enlargement (aortic stenosis and coarctation)**

and a lateral film is necessary for this. An enlarged right ventricle is seen bulging anteriorly. An enlarged left ventricle bulges posteriorly over the vertebral bodies.

Vascularity of the lungs

An assessment of lung vascularity is of great importance in the diagnosis of congenital heart disease. When it is increased, there must be a left-to-right shunt, resulting in an excessive flow of blood to the lungs. When it is decreased, there must be some obstruction to the flow of blood into the lungs.

The hilar vessels should be noted on the right and left sides. The left hilum is more difficult to assess because of the overlying pulmonary trunk. The pulmonary arteries branch like a tree, producing a definite vascular pattern. The assessment of minor changes in pulmonary vascularity is difficult and it may only be possible to say that the vascularity is *not* increased or *not* decreased— comments which nevertheless are helpful in diagnosis when used in conjunction with clinical findings and electrocardiograms.

Bronchial arteries

The bronchial arteries frequently enlarge in congenital heart lesions, particularly when there is a diminished flow to the lungs by the normal route through the pulmonary artery. These vessels, however, do not show the free, tree-like branching of pulmonary arteries and appear as more uniform 'blobs' throughout the lungs. The bronchial supply is sometimes excessive and the lung fields appear well vascularized without a prominent pulmonary artery being seen. We can then infer that there is severe pulmonary stenosis or atresia.

Pulmonary venous congestion

Differentiation of pulmonary venous congestion from increased pulmonary vascularity is important. In the former the lungs have a hazy appearance and the shadowing is diffuse, the hilar shadows are prominent but indistinct and smudgy. It is seen in lesions causing obstruction to flow on the left side of the heart. Such obstruction may be at any level from the pulmonary veins to the aorta.

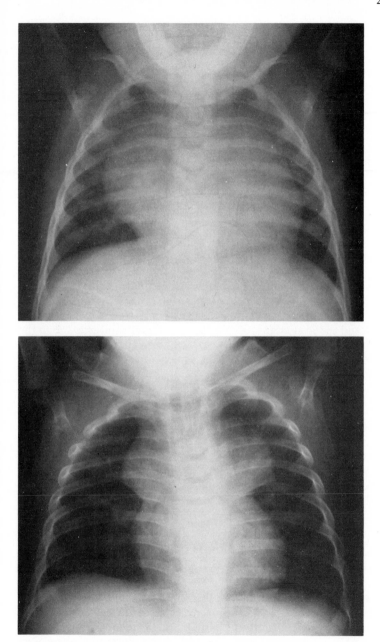

Figure 4.4. Variations in thymic enlargement in infancy

Enlargement of the thymus gland

In infancy a large thymus often makes interpretation of the heart shape difficult. The thymus can assume many guises. There may be a broad pedicle, or a sail-shaped shadow or an apparently large globular heart (*Figure 4.4*). A lateral view often helps by showing that the shadow is in the upper anterior mediastinum but sometimes it merges with the heart shadow and one cannot be certain that it is the thymus from radiographic evidence alone. The absence of symptoms and signs of congenital heart disease, however, and the normal electrocardiogram support the opinion that the thymus gland is enlarged and repeat radiography some six or twelve months later shows that the shadow has become smaller or disappeared.

Abdominal viscera

The upper part of the abdomen is visible on the chest radiograph and the observer should note the position of the stomach and liver. The gas bubble of the stomach is usually clearly visible on the left side and the liver edge is seen running obliquely upwards and to the left. In dextrocardia the stomach may be on the right side, and in cases associated with cyanosis and asplenia the horizontal border of a midline liver may be noted.

Skeletal structures

The vertebrae and ribs should be examined carefully. Rib notching may be seen in children with coarctation and, rarely, from enlarged collateral pulmonary arteries in pulmonary atresia. Slipper vertebrae and hemivertebrae are sometimes seen as associated congenital abnormalities.

Fluoroscopy

Fluoroscopy is rarely used now in the diagnosis of congenital heart disease. The increased radiation involved and the marginal help it gives make it unjustifiable, except occasionally in identifying paracardiac shadows such as pericardial cysts or pericardial effusions.

Barium swallow

Occasionally, a barium swallow is used to confirm left atrial enlargement and to show the presence of coarctation of the aorta, aberrant arteries or a vascular ring.

ELECTROCARDIOGRAPHY

Special training and experience are required to produce good electrocardiograms from restless infants and children. In infants it is easier to make the recording when the child is taking a feed or sucking a dummy and they are often happier sitting on their mother's knee than lying on a couch. Technicians need time to win the child's confidence.

Direct-writing machines are the most practical. The paper should be at least 5 cm wide and it is useful to be able to record at 50 mm/second as well as 25 mm/second. Movements are common in infants and deflect the tracing off the paper, so a machine with an automatic self-centring device is valuable.

Electrode positions

The epidermis in infants and children is thin and skin resistances are lower than in adults. It is sufficient to wipe the skin with a dry swab and apply a little jelly before positioning the electrode. The limb electrodes may be placed on the upper arms or thighs rather than wrists and ankles if it is more convenient. In children it is necessary to record further leads from the right chest, V_3R or V_4R, in addition to the usual precordial leads. If they are not recorded, right ventricular hypertrophy and atrial hypertrophy may be missed. The standard and unipolar limb leads are the same as in adults. If the patient has dextrocardia then leads V_6R to V_1 must be recorded.

Recording

Records are made at a paper speed of 25 mm/second and the machine must be standardized so that a current of 1 mV produces a deflection of 10 mm. (Each small square on the paper is 1 mm².) If the QRS complexes are tall, the standardization can be halved so that 1 mV produces a deflection of 5 mm and the trace can then be accommodated on the paper.

Interpretation

Electrocardiograms are often bewildering to paediatricians and yet they are of great help in the diagnosis of congenital heart disease. In a few lesions such as tricuspid atresia and endocardial cushion defects they are diagnostic. In conditions such as ventricular septal defects, the electrocardiogram gives useful information about the haemodynamic state, and in lesions like pulmonary stenosis it is valuable in assessing the severity of the lesion and the need for further investigation. The more the electrocardiogram is studied the greater help it may be, but it is proposed here to summarize the findings which will help the paediatrician most in making the diagnosis, assessing its severity and deciding when to refer the patient to a cardiologist. An electrocardiogram should always be performed when the patient is first seen. Changes in the electrocardiogram as the patient grows may be very valuable in making decisions about investigations with a view to surgery or in supporting the impression that the lesion is improving with growth, as may happen sometimes in ventricular septal defect.

Deflections of the electrocardiogram (*Figure 4.5*)

The P wave

P waves in children and infants are of shorter duration than in adults, and the initial (right atrial) and terminal (left atrial)

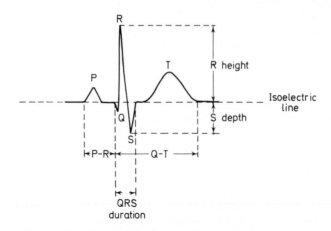

Figure 4.5. Measurement from the electrocardiogram. Note that the P–R interval is measured from the start of the P wave to the start of the QRS complex, the Q–T interval from the start of QRS to the end of T

components are less well separated. The P wave duration in infancy is between 0.04 and 0.07 seconds and gradually increases with age to between 0.06 and 0.1 seconds in adolescence. The tallest P waves are usually seen in standard lead 2, V_4R and V_1, and 2.5 mm (0.25 mV) is the upper limit of normal.

Atrial hypertrophy

Right atrial hypertrophy produces spiked P waves over 2.5 mm in leads 2 and V_1 or V_4R. In infancy left and right atrial hypertrophy may be difficult to distinguish, but in leads V_4R and V_1 left atrial hypertrophy may produce a large negative component to the P wave (*Figure 4.6*). Right atrial hypertrophy is seen in severe pulmonary stenosis, pulmonary atresia and tricuspid atresia. Left atrial hypertrophy is seen with mitral valve disease, left ventricular obstruction and primary myocardial disease affecting the left ventricle.

Besides demonstrating left and right atrial hypertrophy, the P waves may show an abnormal pattern, indicating that the atria are being activated by an anomalous pacemaker.

The QRS complex

The duration of the normal QRS complex is between 0.06 and 0.08 seconds and varies little with actual age within the paediatric span. Prolongation of the QRS duration may be due to ventricular hypertrophy, bundle branch block (or lesser degrees of intraventricular conduction delay), electrolyte abnormalities (high serum potassium), metabolic diseases (hypothyroidism) or drugs (digitalis).

The Q wave is due to depolarization of the interventricular septum (from the left side of the heart to the right). In children, Q waves are normally present in leads 2, 3, AVF, V_5 and V_6. Large Q waves occur in these leads when there is hypertrophy of the septum in left ventricular hypertrophy or biventricular hypertrophy. Q waves in other leads are rare in childhood but may occur with anomalous coronary arteries, hypertrophic obstructive cardiomyopathy and L-transposition of the great arteries. In the latter condition the ventricular septum is depolarized in a direction opposite to normal and Q waves occur in leads V_4R and V_1 instead of V_5 and V_6. The normal Q wave usually measures between 2 and 3 mm, and values greater than 4 mm are abnormal.

R and S waves. The sizes of the R and S waves in the various leads of the electrocardiogram are determined by the thickness of the ventricular wall. Detection of early right or left ventricular hypertrophy is accomplished by recognizing that these voltages lie

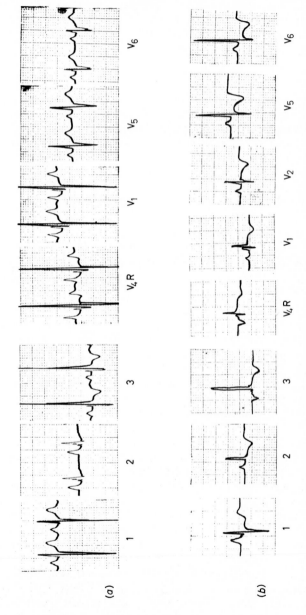

Figure 4.6. (a) Right and (b) left atrial hypertrophy. Note that the shape of the P wave in leads 1 and 2 is similar in both tracings and also that the deep, wide, negative P wave of left atrial hypertrophy seen in V_4R would have been missed if this lead had been omitted. Tracing (a) from a 10-year-old boy with severe Fallot's tetralogy; tracing (b) from a 12-year-old girl with congestive cardiomyopathy

33

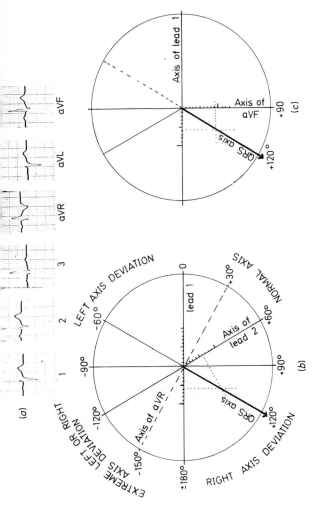

Figure 4.7. Calculation of the QRS axis (in the frontal plane), (*b*) Using leads 1 and 2. **Measure the height of R in lead 1 (2 mm) and subtract the depth of S (8 mm). Plot the answer (−6) along the axis of lead 1, which is horizontal (0 degrees). In lead 2, R − S = 9 − 3 = +6 which is plotted on the axis of lead 2, which is at 60 degrees.** Drop perpendiculars from these axes and the line from the origin through the intersection is the electrical axis. (*c*) The same calculation, using aVF instead of lead 2. This has the advantage that it is at right-angles to lead 1, but the result of R − S (10 − 3 = 7) has to be multiplied by a factor, 1.3, to allow for the fact that a VF is an augmented unipolar lead and not, like lead 1, a bipolar lead. (A rough method is to look for a lead where R and S are nearly equal, in this case a VR. The axis will be at right-angles to the axis of that lead, and it will be clear from examining one other lead in which direction it points)

outside the normal range for the patient's age (*Table 4.1*). More precise data on percentiles for various QRS measurements based on computer analysis of data are available. (Davignon *et al.*, 1980.)

QRS axis

The electrical axis of the heart is the direction of the maximum electrical force during depolarization. Its approximate value can be derived from the QRS complexes in two or more leads. The usual method is to employ leads 1 and 2, but an easier method uses lead 1 and aVF (*Figure 4.7*). The normal QRS axis at birth averages +135 degrees (+60 to +180 degrees) and changes gradually to +60 (+10 to +100 degrees) at 1 year and more slowly to +65 (+30 to +90 degrees) at 10 years. Right axis deviation is usually due to right ventricular hypertrophy, but left axis deviation is usually not due to left ventricular hypertrophy but to some interference with the conduction tissue in the left ventricle (as in ventricular septal defects or atrioventricular canal defects). The reason for the paradox is that whereas the free wall of the right ventricle lies to the right of the left ventricle, the free wall of the left ventricle lies posteriorly. Left axis deviation is a feature of endocardial cushion defects and of tricuspid atresia.

Unless otherwise specified the electrical axis is that in the frontal plane, and is derived from the standard or unipolar leads. Using the chest leads (usually V_2 and V_5) it is possible similarly to calculate the horizontal plane axis. Usually the transition zone between right and left ventricles, where there are equal R and S waves, is at lead V_3.

TABLE 4.1
Normal voltages (mm = 1/10 mV) in precordial leads

	V_4R R	V_1 R	V_1 S	V_5 R	V_6 R	V_6 S
Birth	8 (4–12)	12 (5–20)	10 (0–20)	9 (2–20)	5 (1–13)	6 (0–15)
6 months	5 (2–7)	11 (3–17)	10 (1–25)	20 (10–28)	14 (5–25)	3 (0–10)
1 year	4 (0–7)	9 (2–16)	10 (1–12)	20 (5–30)	14 (5–25)	3 (0–7)
10 years	2.5 (0–6)	5 (1–12)	10 (1–25)	20 (5–40)	16 (5–30)	2 (0–5)

Figures in parentheses indicate the normal range.

Clockwise rotation is indicated by an S wave greater than R in V_4 and anticlockwise rotation by an R wave greater than S in V_2. Clockwise rotation is caused by enlargement of the right atrium or right ventricle. Anticlockwise rotation is seldom seen alone, and, if it is, usually represents a change in over-all position of the heart (as in collapse of the right lower lobe, or left pneumothorax).

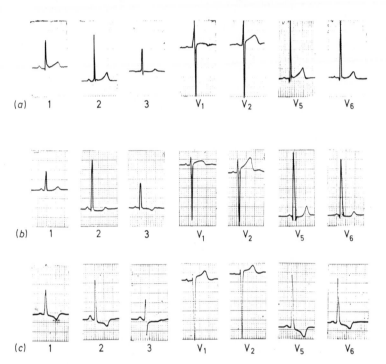

Figure 4.8. Left ventricular hypertrophy: (*a*) mild; (*b*) moderate; (*c*) severe. All three tracings are from patients with aortic stenosis

Criteria of left ventricular hypertrophy (LVH) (*Figure 4.8*)

1. Tall R waves in V_5 and V_6 and deep S waves in V_1. Figures for individual leads outside normal limits for age, or the sum of S in V_1 and R in V_5 or V_6 (whichever is the larger) of more than 40 mm (over 1 year) or more than 30 mm under 1 year (mild LVH). (When the main bulk of the left ventricle lies posteriorly, deep S waves are seen in V_1 but V_5 and V_6 do not show large R waves. When the left ventricle lies more anteriorly and to the left,

R in V_5 and V_6 is tall, but S in V_1 not so deep. The use of the sum of S in V_1 and R in V_5 or V_6 to some extent overcomes the effect of variations in position.)

2. Any of the criteria in (1) plus either prolongation of QRS duration beyond normal limits for age, or flattening of T waves in V_5 and V_6 (moderate LVH).

3. Criteria of (1) and (2) plus T wave inversion in V_5 and V_6 (severe LVH). Left bundle branch block may also occur with severe left ventricular hypertrophy, but this is rare in childhood.

Left ventricular hypertrophy occurs in aortic stenosis and aortic regurgitation, coarctation of the aorta, moderate sized ventricular septal defect, patent ductus and mitral regurgitation. It is also seen in systemic hypertension, and in both congestive and obstructive cardiomyopathy.

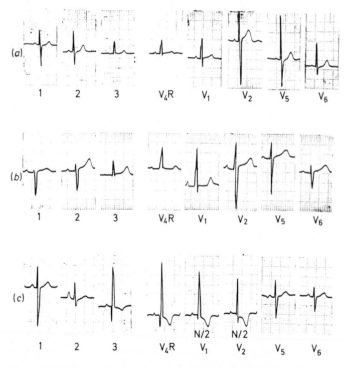

Figure 4.9. Right ventricular hypertrophy: (*a*) mild; (*b*) moderate; (*c*) severe. All three tracings are from patients with pulmonary stenosis of different degrees

Criteria of right ventricular hypertrophy (RVH) (*Figure 4.9*)

1. Frontal plane QRS axis to right of normal limits for age *or* R waves in V_4R or V_1 greater than normal *or* (over the age of 12 months) R wave greater than S in V_1.
2. S in V_6 greater than normal for age (15 mm in first week, 10 mm from 1 to 24 weeks, 7 mm from 6 to 12 months, 5 mm above 1 year).
3. Large R waves in V_4R or V_1 plus prolongation of QRS duration (moderate RVH), usually with reduced R waves in V_5 or V_6.
4. Upright T waves in V_4R and V_1 after the age of 3 days, with R wave greater than S in V_1 (moderate RVH).
5. Tall R waves in V_4R and V_1 widening of QRS beyond 0.09 seconds and deep T wave inversion in V_4R and V_1 (severe RVH). In severe right ventricular hypertrophy the right ventricle frequently extends as far as V_5 or V_6. T wave inversion in these leads does not therefore indicate associated left ventricular hypertrophy.

In addition to these criteria, right ventricular hypertrophy may simulate right bundle branch block. The distinction is difficult without resource to vectorcardiography. Pre-excitation (Wolff–Parkinson–White syndrome) may simulate right ventricular hypertrophy.

Right ventricular hypertrophy occurs in pulmonary stenosis and pulmonary hypertension, in Fallot's tetralogy and in transposition of the great arteries.

Biventricular hypertrophy (*Figure 4.10*)

Moderate or severe hypertrophy of one ventricle usually results in an apparent diminution of the electrical activity of the other ventricle. For this reason coexisting hypertrophy of both ventricles is difficult to diagnose. The following criteria are the most helpful.

1. Tall R waves and deep S waves in leads V_3 and V_4 (total R+S over 50 mm at any age).
2. Left ventricular hypertrophy plus a wide or bifid R wave in V_4R or V_1 over 8 mm in height.
3. Right ventricular hypertrophy plus T wave inversion in V_{5-6} (T upright in V_{1-2}) or q waves 3 mm or more in V_{5-6}.
4. Criteria for right ventricular hypertrophy and left ventricular hypertrophy satisfied.

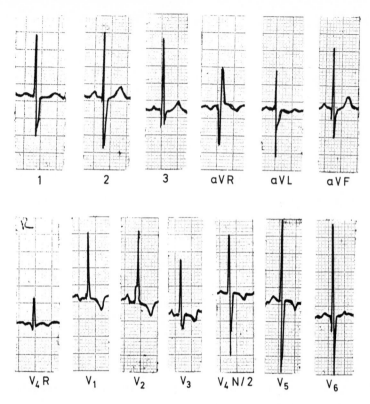

Figure 4.10. Biventricular hypertrophy. The R wave in V_1 is 18 mm, indicating right ventricular hypertrophy, but R in V_6 is 25 mm, which is just within normal limits. In V_4 (which is recorded at half normal sensitivity) RS measures 70 mm, indicating that there is biventricular hypertrophy. The q wave in V_6 is 5 mm, which is also suggestive. From a 3-year-old girl with a large ventricular septal defect and hyperdynamic pulmonary hypertension.

Suggestive features are also deep q waves in leads V_5 and V_6 (due to septal hypertrophy) and the presence of moderate or marked hypertrophy of one ventricle together with normal activity of the other.

Q–T interval

The Q–T interval is measured from the earliest portion of the QRS complex to the end of the T wave. It is affected both by heart rate and by age, being longest in older children with slow rates. The normal range is from 0.2 seconds at birth to 0.4 seconds in adolescence.

An increased Q–T interval is seen in myocarditis, hypothyroidism, hypothermia and hypocalcaemia; a short Q–T in hypokalaemia.

A long Q–T interval may be familial and sometimes associated with deafness (Lange–Nielsen syndrome). Sudden death may occur due to ventricular arrhythmias (pp. 305–306).

T waves

The normal T wave should measure about one-quarter to one-third of the magnitude of the R wave in leads with predominant R waves. After the first 3 days of life the T wave is inverted in V_4R and V_1 and usually inverted in V_2 and V_3 in early childhood. The age at which the T waves become upright in V_2 and V_3 varies from 5 to 15 years, and usually the T waves go through a biphasic or 'dimpled' pattern, rather than becoming flat, in the intermediate period. Inverted T waves are also seen normally in aVR and, when the heart is in a vertical position, in aVL. When the heart is horizontally inclined, T is also inverted in lead 3. Inverted T waves in other leads may be due to ventricular hypertrophy, myocardial disease, pericarditis and severe hypothyroidism. Flat T waves are seen in myocarditis and hypothyroidism. Abnormally tall T waves are seen in hyperkalaemia.

Specific electrocardiographic diagnosis

A few electrocardiographic patterns are suggestive of certain lesions.

Prolongation of the P–R interval suggests an endocardial cushion defect, or Ebstein's anomaly.

Right bundle branch block pattern suggests atrial septal defect. With right axis deviation, an ostium secundum defect is likely; with left axis deviation, an ostium primum. Right bundle branch block pattern with right atrial hypertrophy suggests Ebstein's anomaly.

Left axis deviation suggests an endocardial cushion defect or ventricular septal defect. Extreme left axis deviation (-90 to -150 degrees) suggests a large ventricular septal defect or origin of both great arteries from the right ventricle.

Right atrial hypertrophy and absence of right ventricular hypertrophy in cyanotic lesions suggests either tricuspid atresia or pulmonary atresia with intact ventricular septum. If there is left axis deviation in addition, tricuspid atresia is almost certain. If the axis lies between $+30$ and $+90$ degrees, pulmonary atresia with intact ventricular septum is likely. If the axis is beyond $+90$ degrees, tricuspid atresia with transposition is likely. A similar pattern is also seen with Fallot's tetralogy with an associated large atrial septal defect.

Absence of right ventricular hypertrophy in a patient who clinically has the Eisenmenger syndrome suggests a single ventricle of the 'double inflow left ventricle' type; that is, with a rudimentary right ventricle and transposed great arteries.

Deep T wave inversion in left ventricular leads (V_{5-6}) in a heart with no murmur suggests primary myocardial disease (endocardial fibroelastosis or cardiomyopathy). Deep Q waves, in the absence of ventricular hypertrophy, suggest hypertrophic obstructive cardiomyopathy or anomalous coronary artery.

ULTRASOUND CARDIOGRAPHY

Introduction

Ultrasound or echocardiography has proved a most useful non-invasive technique in paediatric cardiology, both for diagnosis and for following changes in the circulation occurring naturally or as a result of surgery. Being safe and painless, it can be repeated as often as necessary. Like other investigations its findings should be combined with clinical examination and other investigations but sometimes, as in hypertrophic cardiomyopathy, mitral valve prolapse or pericardial effusion, the echo is the most helpful investigation.

Apparatus and methods

The recording of ultrasound echoes from the heart requires a source of pulses of ultrasound energy, a receiver to convert these into an electrical signal (usually the two are combined), suitable electronics to amplify and process the signal, and a suitable recorder. Two methods of recording are used. In the first or M-mode (for motion) a continuous recording of the echoes obtained from one direction only is made. The transducer is moved and angled manually to record echoes from different parts of the heart including the four valves, aorta, two ventricles, interventricular septum and left atrium. The depth of any object from the transducer determines the delay between the transmitting and receiving of the echo and this delay is then reconverted by the recorder to give a 'depth' picture (*Figure 4.11a*). Since the depths of the various echoes can be measured accurately to about 0.5 mm this method is very good for quantitative estimations such as left ventricular wall thickness, but it does not allow demonstration of the relationship between various parts of the heart. In order to do so alternative methods of displaying

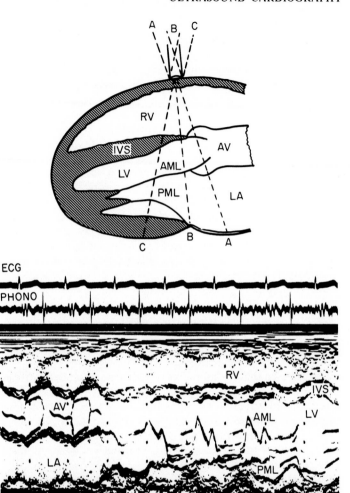

Figure 4.11. M-mode scan. As the transducer is angled from position A through B to C the corresponding parts of the heart are displayed. Lettering as in *Figure 4.12*

simultaneously echoes from different parts of the heart have been developed and these produce a two-dimensional picture of a section of the heart, either by using a series of transducers (a 'phased array') or by mechanically rotating the transducer through an arc ('sector scan'—*Figure 4.12*).

Figure 4.11 demonstrates the M-mode tracings obtained from different parts of the heart. *Figure 4.12* shows two-dimensional (sector scan) pictures from different orientations of the transducer. In addition to still photographs (usually obtained by a 'Polaroid' camera) moving pictures of the heart structures can be recorded either on videotape or on cine film.

Uses

Echocardiography is now done routinely on all patients before cardiac catheterization. It is valuable in diagnosing single ventricle, over-riding aorta, atretic valves, hypoplasia of the left heart, and truncus arteriosus. The exclusion or otherwise of these lesions before catheterization then shortens that procedure or makes it unnecessary. It is of particular value in diagnosing pericardial effusion and myocardial disease, and in following the progress of lesions before and after surgery and assessing the function of prosthetic valves.

CARDIAC CATHETERIZATION AND ANGIO-CARDIOGRAPHY

Indications

It must be stressed that not all patients with congenital heart disease require further investigation. If the diagnosis is certain, and the lesion is mild and surgery is not thought to be required, then cardiac catheterization is unnecessary. The only exception to this rule is when more precise information is desirable; for example, if a baby is being considered for adoption or when the patient wants to follow some strenuous occupation or activity.

Over the age of 1 year it is usually possible to make a reasonably accurate diagnosis from clinical examination, radiology and the electrocardiogram. Ultrasound cardiography is also used to supplement the clinical information. Cardiac catheterization is advised when operation is thought necessary and the investigation is performed near to the elective time for surgery. The investigation gives the surgeon precise information about the anatomy of the lesion and of the haemodynamics in the heart. It excludes any additional lesion which might otherwise have been overlooked. Many centres no longer investigate patients with simple ostium secundum defects, coarctation of the aorta and small patent ductus arteriosus.

It is in the newborn infant and young child with severe heart

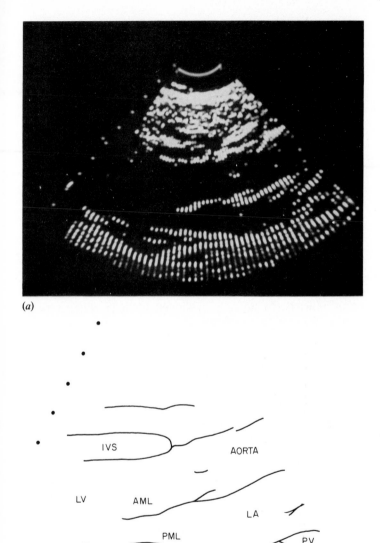

Figure 4.12. (*a*) Two-dimensional sector scan (cf. *Figure 4.11*). (*b*) is diagrammatic representation of scan showing aorta, left atrium (LA), left ventricle (LV), interventricular septum (IVS), anterior (AMS) and posterior (PML) mitral valve leaflets. A pulmonary vein (PV) can be identified. The dots on the left represent one centimetre depth

disease that cardiac catheterization and angiography have become not only essential but a matter of urgency. Advances in surgery and the use of cardiopulmonary bypass in infants enable an increasing number of infants to be helped surgically and make it essential to obtain an accurate diagnosis. In many of these sick infants more than one lesion is present and it is necessary for the surgeon to be aware of all the abnormalities before he can plan any operative procedure. It means that the most severely ill infants often need the most detailed studies to avoid incorrect management.

Repeat catheterization may be necessary in some patients, in particular to assess changes in pulmonary vascular resistance or changes in gradients across stenotic valves, or sometimes to assess the results of surgical treatment.

Risks

Since the procedure is a diagnostic one and carries a risk, parents should always be seen before the investigation and the hazards of catheterization should be fully explained to them. Their written permission for cardiac catheterization and angiography must, legally, be obtained.

The mortality rate in children over 4 months is less than 0.5 per cent but in newborn infants it is higher. In infants, special attention must be given to the prevention of hypothermia, disturbances of acid–base balance and blood loss and the investigation should be carried out as quickly as possible. This, and the need to recognize the significance of the findings while catheterization is in progress, requires an operator with expert skill and experience.

Complications

Arrhythmias during cardiac catheterization are usually transient and can be corrected by removing the catheter or stimulating the heart again with the catheter. Failing this, drugs or dc shock can be used. Although ventricular fibrillation is uncommon a defibrillator ready for instant use is essential.

Procedure

Patients for elective catheterization are admitted to the ward 24 hours before the procedure to ensure that there is no intercurrent infection and to determine whether there has been any change in the heart condition. Radiographs, electrocardiograms and echocardiograms can be performed where necessary before the catheter.

Sedation

The aim is to have the patient in a steady quiet state throughout the procedure. Feeds are withheld for 6 hours before the procedure. In infants under the age of 3 months no sedation is required and the infant will suck a dummy moistened with glycerine. The Toronto mixture

chlorpromazine	6.25 mg/ml
promethazine	6.25 mg/ml
pethidine	25.00 mg/ml

usually provides satisfactory sedation unless the procedure is prolonged. The dose is 1 ml/10 kg body weight (half this dose is used for cyanosed infants). Some centres prefer to use general anaesthesia with intubation and controlled ventilation in infants.

Electrocardiography

The electrocardiogram is recorded on an oscilloscope throughout the procedure.

Right heart catheterization

Almost all venous catheterizations are carried out from the femoral vein using a percutaneous technique. After cleansing the skin with iodine or chlorhexidine in spirit and covering the surrounding area with sterile towels, the femoral artery is palpated to give the position of the femoral vein. A small amount of local anaesthetic is infiltrated 1 cm below the skin crease and a small stab incision made. A suitable needle is then inserted into the femoral vein at an angle of about 45 degrees with the skin (a shallower angle is used in newborn infants) and a 0.25 or 0.35 mm flexible guide wire passed into the vein. The needle is withdrawn and a dilator and sheath (normally 5 or 6 French gauge) passed over the guide wire and into the vein. Different catheters can then be inserted for sampling and pressure measurement. New types of catheter which have a double lumen are available. One lumen communicates with a tiny balloon near the tip of the catheter which can be distended with CO_2 (Swan–Ganz catheter). This makes manipulation of the catheter much easier and it is particularly valuable for entering the pulmonary artery in transposition of the great arteries. There is a lower incidence of ectopic beats when they are used and myocardial staining is less frequent during angiography through a balloon catheter.

Left heart catheterization

In most infants and about 25 per cent of older children the foramen ovale is patent and the left atrium and left ventricle can be catheterized through it. Where the foramen ovale is closed the same route can be achieved by using a special long needle to puncture the atrial septum in the fossa ovalis where the wall is thin. A catheter can then be slid over the needle into the left atrium and left ventricle. Even the child size of needle and catheter make it difficult to achieve this in children under the age of 2 or 3 years, and then catheterization of the left heart is carried out by passing the catheter back from the axillary or femoral artery. It is usually possible to insert a catheter into the femoral artery by the Seldinger technique described for venous catheterization, but arterial spasm is a problem in small children and permanent occlusion of the artery may occur, although this is usually asymptomatic and does not lead to any longterm disability. An alternative approach is by a cut-down into the axillary artery, whose extensive collateral circulation makes occlusion less important.

Catheters

Catheters are made of nylon or Teflon and are covered with a radio-opaque material. Samples of blood can be withdrawn through the catheters which can also be attached to a manometer to record the intracardiac pressures. A Goodale–Lubin catheter which has an end hole and two side holes close to the tip is best used for taking samples from small hearts.

Oxygen content

The oxygen content of the blood sample is most commonly measured by a haemoreflector. This method may not give accurate absolute values but it is sufficiently precise to show significant changes in oxygen content in the chambers of the heart. The values obtained are used in calculating the amount of blood flowing through the defects (*see below*).

Intracardiac pressure

Intracardiac pressure waves are displayed throughout the procedure on an oscilloscope and a permanent record on paper can be made at any time. The wave forms indicate whether the catheter is in the atrium, ventricle or an artery and show any changes in pressure (for example, across a stenosed valve).

Dye-dilution curves

Tracer substances such as indocyanine green are injected into the heart and blood is continuously sampled through a cuvette and the concentration displayed on a recorder. Small shunts which may be overlooked by oximetry can be picked up. For example, if dye is injected into the right ventricle and this dye appears very early in a peripheral artery, it means there is a right-to-left shunt at or beyond ventricular level. If there is a left-to-right shunt the dye recirculates to the lungs and appears in a peripheral artery at the usual time, does not rise as high as normal and falls very slowly, giving a plateau-type curve. The dye curve can also be used to estimate blood flow and therefore cardiac output.

Angiography

Radio-opaque dye may be injected through the catheter to enter any chamber of the heart or its great vessels and its passage through the heart may be viewed in two planes. In the past, frontal and lateral views were taken, but increasing information is now obtained from oblique views. Ventricular septal defects are best seen in the left anterior oblique position to profile the septum. The branches of the pulmonary arteries are best seen with the patient tilted up from the supine position. Dyes are now safer and more injections can be made in different planes. The definition on cine films has continued to improve and this has now replaced still films.

Useful calculations from the data obtained at cardiac catheterization

In order to measure the amount of blood flowing in the pulmonary or systemic circulation, we must know the amount of oxygen the patient consumes per minute. This is difficult to measure in young children although some of the problems are being overcome. It is often assumed from tables when the surface area of the patient is known (*see* calculation A, *Table 4.2*).

TABLE 4.2

Calculations from the data obtained at cardiac catheterization

Calculation (A). Calculating according to the Fick principle:

Systemic blood flow (in litres/minute) written as

$$Qs = \frac{O_2 \text{ consumption, ml/min}}{O_2 \text{ content of systemic arterial blood} - O_2 \text{ content of mixed venous blood}}$$

Pulmonary blood flow (in litres/minute) written as

$$Qp = \frac{O_2 \text{ consumption, ml/min}}{O_2 \text{ content of pulmonary venous blood} - O_2 \text{ content of pulmonary arterial blood}}$$

Calculation (B)

$$\frac{\text{Pulmonary blood flow (Qp)}}{\text{Systemic blood flow (Qs)}} = \frac{\dfrac{O_2 \text{ consumption ml/min}}{\left(\begin{array}{c} O_2 \text{ content} \\ \text{pulm. venous blood} \end{array}\right) - \left(\begin{array}{c} O_2 \text{ content} \\ \text{pulm. art. blood} \end{array}\right)} \times \left(\begin{array}{c} O_2 \text{ content} \\ \text{syst. art. blood} \end{array}\right) - \left(\begin{array}{c} O_2 \text{ content} \\ \text{mixed syst. venous blood} \end{array}\right)}{O_2 \text{ consumption, ml/min}}$$

The O_2 consumption cancels, therefore:

$$\frac{Qp}{Qs} = \frac{O_2 \text{ content systemic arterial blood} - O_2 \text{ content mixed systemic venous blood}}{O_2 \text{ content pulmonary venous blood} - O_2 \text{ content pulmonary arterial blood}}$$

In a normal heart this ratio $\dfrac{Qp}{Qs}$ is $\dfrac{1}{1}$

When there is a left-to-right shunt $\dfrac{Qp}{Qs}$ is greater than 1

When there is a right-to-left shunt $\dfrac{Qp}{Qs}$ is less than 1

Cardiologists often express the size of shunts using this ratio

Calculation (C)

Pulmonary vascular resistance (PVR) = $\dfrac{\text{pulmonary artery mean pressure (PAP)} - \text{left atrial mean pressure (LAP)}}{\text{pulmonary blood flow}}$

i.e. $\text{PVR} = \dfrac{\text{PAP} - \text{LAP}}{\text{Qp}}$ units

The normal value is between 1 and 3 units for a patient with 1 m² body surface area

Systemic vascular resistance (SVR) = $\dfrac{\text{systemic arterial mean pressure (SAP)} - \text{right atrial mean pressure (RAP)}}{\text{systemic blood flow}}$

i.e. $\text{SVR} = \dfrac{\text{SAP} - \text{RAP}}{\text{Qs}}$ units

The normal value is between 10 and 20 units for a patient with 1 m² body surface area

$$\frac{\text{PVR}}{\text{SVR}} = \frac{\text{PAP} - \text{LAP}}{\text{Qp}} \times \frac{\text{Qs}}{\text{SAP} - \text{RAP}}$$

If these absolute blood flows cannot be measured because of difficulty in measuring O_2 consumption, it is valuable to relate the pulmonary blood flow to the systemic blood flow as a ratio (*see* calculation B, *Table 4.2*). Cardiologists often express the size of shunts using this ratio.

When Qp/Qs is more than 2:1, the left-to-right shunt is of a moderate size and surgery is usually advised if the pulmonary vascular resistance is not significantly raised. It is difficult to measure the absolute figure for pulmonary vascular resistance and fortunately this is now becoming less important because infants can now be operated on before pulmonary vascular disease develops. The ratio of the pulmonary to systemic resistance is of some value (calculation C).

BIBLIOGRAPHY

Cassels, D. E. and Ziegler, R. F. (Eds.) (1966). *Electrocardiography in Infants and Children.* New York: Grune and Stratton; London: Heinemann
Davignon, A., Rautaharju, P., Boisselle, E., Soumis, F., Mégélas, M. and Choquette, A. (1980). Normal ECG standards for infants and children. *Paediat. Cardiol.* **1**, 123
Liebman, J. (1968). In *Heart Disease in Infants, Children and Adolescents.* p. 183. Eds A. J. Moss and F. H. Adams. Baltimore: Williams and Williams
Scott, O. and Franklin, D. (1963). The electrocardiogram in the normal infant. *Br. Heart J.* **25**, 441

CHAPTER 5

Cardiac Surgery

Since over half of all children with congenital heart disease will have some form of operation, it is appropriate to consider some of the principles of cardiac surgery before proceeding to discuss individual lesions.

TYPES OF OPERATION

Surgery may be 'palliative', aiming mainly to relieve the patient's symptoms and prevent undesirable secondary effects of the lesion, or 'corrective', in which the surgeon tries to repair the lesions as completely as possible. Although the latter produces great benefits, it cannot always strictly be described as a complete cure.

Palliative operations

These are mainly used in young infants too small for corrective procedures or to help children when the lesion is not amenable to corrective surgery.

Systemic to pulmonary arterial shunts

These are designed to increase pulmonary blood flow in conditions associated with pulmonary oligaemia.

1. *Blalock–Taussig procedure* (*Figure 5.1*) in which the anastomosis is made between the subclavian artery and pulmonary artery on

the right or left side. If the subclavian artery is high up or the pulmonary artery very small a Gor-Tex tube can be inserted between these two vessels to make sure there is adequate flow to the pulmonary artery. This anastomosis is preferred because it is easily closed at the time of complete repair and rarely results in distortion of the pulmonary artery.

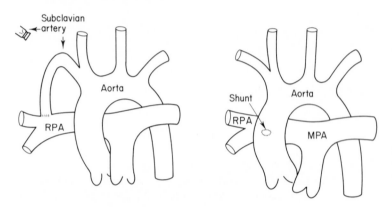

Figure 5.1. Blalock–Taussig (left) and Waterston's shunts. RPA: right pulmonary artery; MPA: main pulmonary artery.

2. *Waterston operation (Figure 5.1).* This is an anastomosis between the ascending aorta and right pulmonary artery. It is the only operation possible in newborn infants who have minute pulmonary arteries. It has the disadvantage that there is often kinking and narrowing of the pulmonary artery proximal to the shunt which needs patching at complete repair; furthermore the Waterston shunt is more difficult to close at the time of complete repair.
3. *Potts operation* – an anastomosis is made between the descending aorta and left pulmonary artery. It is seldom used now as it often produced pulmonary hypertension and it is difficult to close at the time of corrective surgery.
4. *Glenn operation (Figure 5.2)* in which the superior vena cava is anastomosed directly to the right pulmonary artery. It is rarely used now having been mainly superseded by the Fontan operation.
5. *Fontan operation (Figure 9.10,* p. 182). A conduit is inserted from the right atrium to the pulmonary artery. There is divided opinion as to whether a valve should be placed in the conduit, but a modified procedure is now in use in which a conduit is placed

from the right atrium to the right ventricle and the patient's own pulmonary valve is used. This demands a right ventricle and pulmonary valve of adequate size. The pulmonary resistance must be low and the pulmonary artery of reasonable size for anastomosis of the conduit. (*See under* Tricuspid atresia, p. 182.)

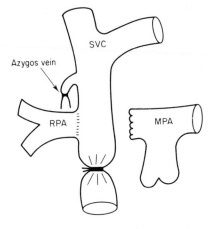

Figure 5.2. Glenn operation. The superior vena cava (SVC) is anastomosed to the right pulmonary artery

Banding of the pulmonary artery

Infants with complex abnormalities associated with high pulmonary blood flow and pulmonary artery pressures at or near systemic level may be helped by restricting the blood flow through the lungs. This is achieved by 'banding', that is tying a piece of tape around the pulmonary artery, tight enough to reduce the pressure beyond the band to about half that proximally. This also protects the infant's pulmonary arteries from the development of hypertensive pulmonary vascular disease.

This procedure was widely used to treat heart failure in infants with large ventricular septal defects, but has now been superseded by early surgical closure for these infants where symptoms cannot be controlled by medical therapy. It is still used when there are multiple ventricular septal defects and in complex lesions such as single ventricle and L-transposition associated with high pulmonary blood flow.

CLOSED INTRACARDIAC OPERATIONS

It is possible to open up a stenosed pulmonary valve, without the use of cardiopulmonary bypass, by inserting bougies through the right ventricular wall and breaking a way through the pulmonary valve. Now that cardiopulmonary bypass is a safe procedure, even in infancy, most surgeons prefer to carry out pulmonary valvotomy as an 'open-heart' procedure.

Mitral valvotomy can also be carried out as a closed procedure. A special dilator is inserted through a stab incision in the apex of the left ventricle and guided into the mitral orifice by a finger inserted through the left atrial appendage. This procedure is suitable for rheumatic mitral stenosis, which is still seen in childhood in some countries, but not for the more complex forms of obstruction.

OPEN-HEART SURGERY

Almost all operations on the heart itself require the surgeon to be able to arrest the heart action, drain it of blood and carry out the repair under direct vision. Simple occlusion of the return of blood to the right heart allows the surgeon only about two minutes and the same procedure with 'conventional' hypothermia (surface cooling to 32°C) only allows about 7–8 minutes, and these techniques are not suitable for operation in the left heart, due to the risk of systemic air embolism. Since cardiopulmonary bypass became safe, surgeons have abandoned these methods and use one of two techniques which allow much longer operating times.

Total cardiopulmonary bypass

Cannulae are inserted into the right atrium (or both venae cavae) and the venous blood sucked or allowed to drain into a heart lung machine (*Figure 5.3*) in which it is oxygenated and then returned to the aorta by a pump which is capable of producing flows and pressures comparable to those in the normal circulation. The aortic root is isolated and perfused separately with a cold (5°C) solution containing potassium which both arrests the heart action and also protects the myocardium. Provided that the myocardium is reperfused every 30–40 minutes with oxygenated blood, this procedure allows theoretically unlimited time for operation, but in practice haemolysis of the blood (by the oxygenerator, pump and sucker),

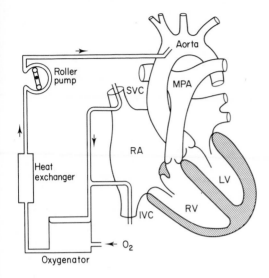

Figure 5.3. Total cardiopulmonary bypass

and non-perfusion of the lungs limit the safe period to about three hours, which is usually ample time for even complex repairs.

Profound hypothermia

Cooling the whole patient to 12–15°C allows the circulation to be stopped completely for up to 60 minutes. As the heart ceases to function adequately at temperatures below about 27°C an extracorporeal circulation is required, but it is still possible to use the patient's own lungs (*Figure 5.4*), although the technique is more complicated and most surgeons prefer to use the same circuit as for total cardiopulmonary bypass. In infants the initial cooling (to about 27°C) can be carried out by surface cooling, so shortening the period of bypass required.

The technique is particularly useful for infants and gives a much lower incidence of postoperative pulmonary problems, probably because the lungs are unperfused for a much shorter period.

Risks of open-heart surgery

It is still a popular misconception that cardiopulmonary bypass is intrinsically a risky procedure. In the hands of experienced teams,

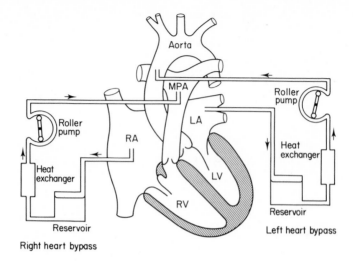

Figure 5.4. Profound hypothermia

using the technique regularly, deaths due to the procedure itself are virtually unknown, and the overall percentage risk attached to a straightforward intracardiac operation such as closure of atrial septal defect is very low—about 0.2 per cent. The morbidity is rather more important, particularly the possibility of brain damage owing to inadvertent introduction of air into the circulation, or to platelet emboli, which probably occurs in about 1 per cent of operations although it is usually minor and allows complete recovery.

Palliative or corrective surgery in infancy

Surgeons differ in their views, but there has been a steady trend towards earlier corrective operation. Whereas ten years ago only a few corrective intracardiac operations were performed, Turley, Tucker and Ebert (1980), reporting their surgical experience of 502 infants treated from 1975 to 1979, indicate that 84 per cent of operations were corrective, with an overall mortality of only 9 per cent. Only 5 per cent received palliative operations of the conventional types described above. Ten per cent had unconventional operations such as direct enlargement of the pulmonary outflow tract in pulmonary atresia.

Apart from a steadily reducing mortality, early corrective operation has other strong advantages. The improvement in the infant's condition is usually more dramatic and parents are spared the long wait between palliative and corrective operations. Furthermore, the earlier the heart muscle is relieved of the effects of the heart lesion—either diastolic overload, when there are large left-to-right shunts, or systolic overload, when there is obstruction to flow—then the more likely it is to return to normal as the child grows and the function of the heart is optimal. Cardiologists now aim not only to make the heart anatomically normal but functionally so as well.

Postoperative management

Following straightforward operations such as closure of VSD or ASD or pulmonary valvotomy most children required no special postoperative therapy, and are discharged home at about the tenth postoperative day. By six weeks after operation, almost all are back to school and normal activities.

Complex operations involving long periods of perfusion, and particularly those where a total correction is not possible, require intensive postoperative care, with artificial ventilation and often circulatory support with inotropic drugs such as dopamine. They stay longer in hospital—frequently for 3–6 weeks, and go home on treatment with diuretics and, often, digoxin. A longer period of convalescence is clearly required, but the patients are usually closely watched by the cardiac surgeon and paediatric cardiologist in Out-Patients, and treatment gradually reduced and discontinued. Very few patients need to take permanent therapy.

Postoperative complications

The immediate complications are dealt with in the postoperative intensive care unit, but it is important for those looking after the child subsequently to know what has occurred, for both physical and psychological reasons. Longterm ventilation may sometimes lead to tracheal or laryngeal stenosis as well as other pulmonary problems. Prolonged urinary catheterization may leave residual infection or phymosis. When there has been temporary postoperative heart block, the chances of a late recurrence are quite high. Prolonged stay in intensive care units is often associated with psychological problems for months, or even years, after physical recovery has occurred.

Equally important is the communication to physicians and other workers of statements made to the child and parents. It may have been considered wise at the time not to tell the parents about complications which were expected to be self-limiting, and a subsequent casual remark can produce feelings of insecurity and distrust.

Late results and complications of surgery

After successful surgery most children have a rapid period of growth and increased wellbeing; this is most striking in children who have previously had heart failure. Patients who have been cyanosed (tetralogy of Fallot) become pink immediately after surgery but the finger clubbing takes six to nine months to regress. It is important to remember that when a Blalock–Taussig shunt has been performed the arm pulses on the affected side will be absent or markedly reduced. This does not happen after a Waterston operation. A Horner's syndrome is not uncommon after a shunt operation in small children and resolves after 2–3 months.

Residual murmurs

After closure of patent ductus, ventricular septal defect or atrial septal defect, the heart sounds should be normal and there are no murmurs. In other operations loosely described as 'curative' residual murmurs are common. Following pulmonary valvotomy for pulmonary stenosis, a soft systolic murmur is heard and often an early diastolic murmur of pulmonary incompetence owing to failure of the valve to close completely after it has been cut. Such systolic and diastolic murmurs are often impressive after correction of tetralogy of Fallot when a patch has been used to widen the pulmonary valve ring. Aortic valvotomy is frequently followed by systolic and early diastolic murmurs for the same reasons. It is important to stress that the persistence of murmurs does not mean that the operation has been unsuccessful.

Chest X-ray

The heart size gradually returns to normal after repair of ventricular septal defects, atrial septal defects and closure of patent ductus arteriosus. Where a patch has been inserted, e.g. in the right ventricular outflow tract in repair of tetralogy of Fallot, the heart shadow will appear larger on the X-ray and there will be a bulge on the upper left heart border. Also, after a shunt procedure, the heart will increase in size and the lung fields show increased pulmonary blood flow.

ECG

This may actually look worse after a right ventriculotomy as there is usually a complete right bundle branch block pattern. This is not associated with any symptoms in childhood. If, however, some of the branches of the left bundle are severed and the distal part of the bundle of His is damaged, the patient also shows left axis deviation on the ECG, and is at risk of complete heart block when healing and fibrosis occur. Such patients usually have transient complete heart block in the immediate postoperative period. If the heart block recurs a pacemaker is required and the parents must be warned to report any episodes of syncope or dizziness. It is uncommon now for injury to the sinus node to occur following repair of atrial septal defects but the sinus node may be injured during the Mustard operation for transposition of the great arteries. Nodal rhythm may result and this may become very slow and periods of sinus arrest occur. Sudden death may follow if a pacemaker is not inserted. Ambulatory ECG monitoring will help in showing periods of marked slowing or sinus arrest.

Ventricular extrasystoles and ventricular tachycardia may occur postoperatively when there has been severe left or right ventricular hypertrophy preoperatively, or when either ventricle has been incised, particularly if there have been multiple operations. Ventricular tachycardia always needs treatment, occasional ventricular extrasystoles can be ignored, but multifocal ones, or those occurring in runs of two or more, should be treated as indicated in Chapter 17. This complication might be avoided by earlier operation and surgical techniques designed to minimize trauma to ventricular muscle, such as closing ventricular septal defects from the right atrium.

Infective endocarditis

This is possible following pulmonary or aortic valvotomy, repair of tetralogy of Fallot and most complex operations, but does not occur following successful repair of VSD, ASD or patent ductus. The need to prevent this complication is one of the best reasons for longterm follow-up in patients with susceptible lesions.

Late deterioration

Patients who have had complex operations, particularly those in whom conduits or valves have been inserted, may show gradual or sudden deterioration. Shrinkage of the intracardiac patch following Mustard's operation leads to pulmonary oedema, and degeneration of conduits, particularly those with heterograft valves, leads to gradually increasing cardiac failure. Even though it may be inconvenient for patients and parents, it is essential for the cardiac team to follow such patients carefully, and in most cases indefinitely (and if necessary to assess by postoperative catheters). We do not know for how long conduits and prosthetic valves will remain satisfactory and serial studies by echocardiography are valuable in following the patient's progress.

Patients who have had operations involving valve replacement or insertion of conduits early in life will certainly require operations as they outgrow their implanted prostheses. Additionally, artificial valves seem particularly prone to clotting in young children, even when anticoagulants are given, and reoperation may be required urgently.

A particular problem is posed by the teenager who has already had several palliative operations for a severe but correctable abnormality (for example pulmonary atresia with ventricular septal defect). When the pericardial and both pleural cavities have been entered with resultant vascular adhesions, the risks of operation may be so high as to outweigh the possible benefits of a corrective operation.

REFERENCES

Turley, K, Tucker, W. Y. and Ebert, P. A. (1980). *J. thorac. cardiovasc. Surg.* **79**, 194

CONGENITAL CARDIAC DEFECTS

In all congenital heart lesions there is a spectrum of severity from mild to severe and the treatment varies depending on the severity of the lesion.

Congenital heart disease is not a static condition; changes take place throughout the patient's life, sometimes for better, sometimes for worse. Treatment will therefore vary with the severity of the lesion at any given time.

The abnormal anatomy of the heart should be corrected early so that the function of the heart is as near normal as possible.

CHAPTER 6

Acyanotic Lesions with Left-to-Right Shunts

PATENT DUCTUS ARTERIOSUS

Definition

The ductus arteriosus, which *in utero* serves to divert blood from the lungs into the descending aorta, normally closes functionally within 10–15 hours of birth. Closure is brought about by constriction of specialized tissue, confined to the ductus, which is present from 25 weeks of intrauterine life and shows progressive maturation over the next 10–12 weeks: (Gittenberger de Groot, 1979).

Incidence

In mature infants, persistent patency of the ductus probably results from a primary anatomical defect of this specialized tissue in the ductal wall (Gittenberger-de-Groot, 1977). Such patients account for about 7 per cent of all congenital heart defects. Patency of the ductus in premature infants has increased as smaller babies survive (p. 70). Patency of the ductus arteriosus in association with other lesions such as pulmonary atresia is related to arterial hypoxaemia, and is dealt with under the respective primary lesion.

Natural history

The natural history is related to the size of the ductus and to the changes which occur in the pulmonary circulation after birth. If the ductus does not close during the first two weeks of life, spontaneous closure thereafter is rare, except in premature infants in whom spontaneous closure may occur up to three months after birth. Campbell (1968) calculated that, after infancy, only 0.6 per cent of all ducts would close spontaneously every year. By the age of 60 years about 20 per cent will have closed. In Cosh's series (1957) of 69 patients with patent ductus arteriosus, closure occurred in 4 at the following ages – 15, 23, 23 and 29 years. The ductus closed in only 1 of the 48 adults reviewed by Mark and Young (1965). The general prognosis for patients with a small ductus is good but a number deteriorate in the third or fourth decades (Campbell, 1955). As with so many congenital heart lesions the most dangerous periods are infancy and then the third and fourth decades. By the age of 45 years about 42 per cent of those untreated patients who survived infancy will have died (Campbell, 1968).

The possibility of bacterial endarteritis developing remains throughout life. In 1943 Keys and Shapiro reported that bacterial endarteritis was the cause of death in 42 per cent of patients over 17 years of age. Surgery and antibiotics have completely altered this situation. Out of 69 of Cosh's patients, 6 (9 per cent) developed bacterial endarteritis, 4 died before penicillin was available and 2 recovered after penicillin treatment. The incidence of complicating bacterial endarteritis now is probably 0.45 per cent per annum. It occurs on the intima of the pulmonary artery opposite the ductus arteriosus, so that pulmonary emboli are relatively common.

Heart failure may occur in infants who have a large ductus, but thereafter it is rare until adult life is reached.

In a few patients with large ducts, severe pulmonary hypertension occurs. When the pulmonary vascular resistance exceeds the systemic resistance, the flow of blood through the ductus is reversed and an Eisenmenger situation develops (p. 274).

Clinical presentation

The symptoms and signs depend on the size of the ductus and the presentation is therefore described separately for the small, medium and large ductus.

SMALL DUCTUS

The patient with a small ductus has no symptoms. He is pink and there is no dyspnoea. The heart is of normal size. The pulses and blood pressure are normal. There may occasionally be a thrill in the second left interspace and the classic continuous murmur is heard in the pulmonary area below the left clavicle. It is usually discovered during a routine medical examination. This small ductus may be confused with a venous hum but, whereas a venous hum disappears in the horizontal position, the continuous murmur of a ductus becomes louder. The radiograph and electrocardiogram are normal.

MEDIUM-SIZED DUCTUS

Symptoms of a medium-sized ductus may be present between the second and fifth months of life but are not severe. Feeding may be slower and chest infections more common but there is a reasonable

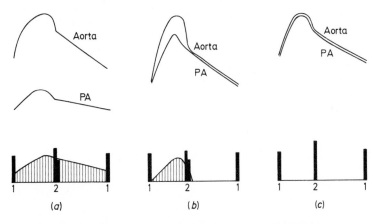

Figure 6.1. Relationship between intravascular pressures and murmurs in patent ductus arteriosus. (*a*) Small or moderate-sized ductus without rise in pulmonary artery pressure; there is a gradient throughout the cardiac cycle. (*b*) Large ductus with increased pulmonary vascular resistance but large left-to-right shunt; the gradient is only during systole when there is a large volume of blood ejected into the aorta. (*c*) With severe pulmonary hypertension with only a small left-to-right shunt or a right-to-left shunt there is no significant gradient. PA: pulmonary artery pressure. 1 and 2: first and second heart sounds

gain in weight. There may be excessive breathlessness on exercise and the child is more easily tired than his friends but is able to lead a fairly normal life.

The child's size and weight are usually below normal standards. He is never cyanosed, but has a slightly increased respiration rate at rest. The brachial and femoral pulses are collapsing in quality. The blood pressure shows a diastolic pressure that is lower than normal, the pulse pressure therefore being increased. There is moderate cardiac enlargement with overactivity of the heart, particularly the left ventricle, but there is some increase in the right ventricular activity also. A thrill is often felt in the first and second left interspaces. In the same area there is a loud continuous murmur. It must be appreciated that this murmur *continues* from systole into diastole through the second sound without any interruption. It increases towards the end of systole and fades away in diastole before the first sound (*Figure 6.1*). The murmur is produced by blood flowing through the ductus during both systole and diastole because the pressures in the aorta are higher than those in the pulmonary artery throughout the cardiac cycle. It is interesting to note the accuracy of the diagram of the murmur which Gibson drew in his article on the subject in 1900; it is the same as that recorded on the phonocardiogram today.

When the ductus is of a moderate size a separate mid-diastolic murmur may be heard at the apex, caused by the excessive flow of blood through a normal mitral valve.

The second sound in the pulmonary area is loud and closely split. A pulmonary ejection click may be heard.

Radiology

Radiology shows cardiac enlargement, particularly of the left ventricle. The pulmonary artery is of moderate size, the hilar vessels are moderately large and there is an increase in the vascularity of the lungs.

Electrocardiography

The electrocardiogram shows mainly increased left ventricular activity but there is some increase in the right ventricular activity also. The P wave in lead 2 is often broad, indicating increase in size of the left atrium.

Investigation is not usually necessary in this group. If the continuous murmur is lower down the left sternal edge, however, other causes of continuous murmurs must be excluded.

LARGE DUCTUS

Patients with a large ductus have severe symptoms and infants usually present with feeding problems and poor weight gain between the first and fourth months of life. The infant is breathless during feeds and may sweat profusely. He remains pink, however, and the pulses are collapsing or of full volume. The systolic thrill may not be present and only a systolic murmur may be heard in the second left interspace. The murmur does not extend into diastole because the diastolic pressures in the aorta and pulmonary artery are the same and no flow occurs through the ductus during diastole (*Figure 6.1*). A mid-diastolic murmur is usually heard at the apex due to excessive flow through the mitral valve. The second sound in the pulmonary area is loud and single.

Heart failure may occur, and is often associated with a respiratory infection. All these patients have a severe degree of pulmonary hypertension with the pulmonary pressure at or approaching systemic pressure. In some patients the large flow of blood through the ductus contributes to this pressure; when the ductal flow is cut off at operation there is an immediate fall in the pressure in the pulmonary artery and after operation the pulmonary artery pressure returns to normal (hyperdynamic pulmonary hypertension). In another group the high pressure in the pulmonary artery is due mainly to changes in the pulmonary arterioles which increase the pulmonary vascular resistance and so limit the flow through the ductus because the pulmonary vascular resistance is almost as high as the systemic (reactive pulmonary hypertension). In patients operated on under a year of age, however, the resistance is low and the pressure falls to normal following operation.

Radiology

Radiology shows marked enlargement of both ventricles, the pulmonary artery and its branches.

Electrocardiography

The electrocardiogram shows combined ventricular enlargement but the degree of left ventricular activity is greater than the right.

Cardiac catheterization

Cardiac catheterization is necessary because most patients with a large ductus do not have the classic continuous murmur. A step-up in oxygen saturation is detected in the pulmonary artery (*Figure 6.2*). The presence of a ductus is best confirmed by passing a catheter through it. The catheter always takes the same route through a ductus and enters the descending aorta (*Figure 6.3*). If the catheter enters either the ascending aorta or the arch it suggests that the defect is not a ductus but the much rarer aortopulmonary window. It is also important to confirm that there is sufficient flow through the ductus from the aorta to the pulmonary artery to make surgical closure safe.

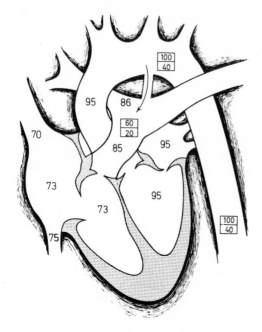

Figure 6.2. Patent ductus arteriosus. Pressures in
mmHg, within squares; percentage oxygen saturations,
unsquared

Treatment

Surgical closure of the uncomplicated ductus is recommended as
soon as the diagnosis is made, irrespective of the patient's age. Most
patients who are diagnosed in the first year of life have symptoms
and operation is required to relieve these. If there is a chest infection
or heart failure when the patient is first seen this should be treated
medically. In the majority of patients heart failure can be controlled.
It is only rarely that surgery has to be contemplated in the presence
of infection or heart failure but nevertheless under such conditions
it may be life-saving. The risk of operation in infancy is about 1 per
cent.

   In patients with no symptoms or few symptoms the mortality of
the operation in an established unit is less than 0.2 per cent.
Spontaneous closure is uncommon except in premature infants and
the number deteriorating in the third and fourth decades is a valid
reason for advising closure, apart from the risk of bacterial
endarteritis (Campbell, 1955). Young children tolerate the operation
well and can be discharged seven to ten days after the operation. The

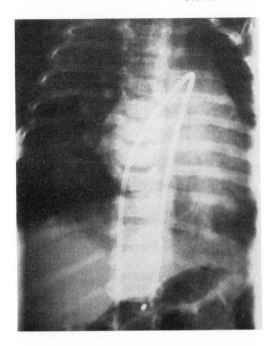

Figure 6.3. Catheter passed from main pulmonary artery
through the patent ductus into the descending aorta

ductus is usually ligated with two ligatures. The children can lead
normal lives after recovery from the operation and penicillin cover
for dental manipulations is no longer necessary.

The decision about recommending surgery for a patient with a
large ductus and pulmonary hypertension is often difficult. If there
are equal pressures in the aorta and pulmonary artery but only a
small left-to-right shunt, particularly in children over the age of
about two years, it is probable that there is already hypertensive
pulmonary vascular disease (*see* p. 91) and closure of the ductus is
unlikely to reverse this process. It is however important to check
that there are not other factors influencing the pulmonary vascular
resistance, such as left heart obstruction or hypoxia due to respiratory
problems. The latter consideration can be resolved by repeating the
pressure and saturation measurements while the patient breathes
100 per cent oxygen. Cases have been reported (Rudolph and co-
workers, 1958) in which the pressure does not fall and may continue
to rise after surgery. On the other hand, cases have also been reported
in which closure of the ductus has resulted in a fall in pulmonary

artery pressure even when there has been a small right-to-left shunt, as long as the left-to-right shunt is the greater. The risks of surgery rise to 5 per cent when the duct is large and there is severe pulmonary hypertension. Surgical division of the ductus is necessary when the duct is large.

In patients with severe pulmonary hypertension preoperatively a repeat cardiac catheterization two years following closure may be helpful in indicating the prognosis and determining whether restrictions on physical activity are required.

PERSISTENT PATENCY OF THE DUCTUS ARTERIOSUS IN PREMATURE INFANTS

Aetiology and incidence

Now that more very premature and low birthweight babies are being kept alive by assisted ventilation, there is an increased incidence of patent ductus arteriosus.

The ductus only obtains its specialized contractile tissue in the last three months of fetal life, and it is likely that the ductus remains patent for some time in all infants born before 30 weeks' gestation. As the infant becomes more mature, the ability of the ductus to close promptly and completely increases, and clinically recognizable patency becomes less common.

In premature babies the pulmonary arteries have a thin muscle coat and, when the ductus remains patent after birth, these can expand rapidly and allow a high pulmonary blood flow, so that breathlessness and heart failure develop more rapidly than in a fullterm infant in whom the ductus remains patent.

Cotton and Stahlmanetal (1978) estimated that 44 per cent of infants of less than 1500 g birthweight develop breathlessness and heart failure due to patent ductus arteriosus. As the ductus develops its contractile tissue it will tend to close, and patency beyond three months of age is rare (Rudolph, 1977, Hallidie-Smith and Girling, 1971).

Prostaglandins have been demonstrated in high concentrations in the area of the ductus and can be shown to play a part in maintaining the normal patency prior to delivery (Olley and Coceani, 1979). This discovery has led to the possibility of pharmacological manipulation of the ductus (Olley *et al.*, 1979).

Clinical examination

Symptoms usually occur 3–7 days after birth, but when the respiratory distress syndrome is present these may be obscured. The respiratory rate rises and lower costal and intercostal recession become apparent. The liver enlarges and the pulse volume is usually increased. There is a short systolic murmur in the pulmonary area and often a short diastolic murmur in the mitral area, although this is less obvious than in the mature infant. Chest X-rays show generalized enlargement of the heart, and it may be possible to see increased size of pulmonary vessels.

Diagnosis

Since, in a premature infant, patent ductus is the most likely cause of symptoms, it is usually possible to make a presumptive diagnosis on clinical grounds. Cardiac catheterization in a very small baby is generally regarded as too traumatic and unnecessary.

Echocardiography shows enlargement of the left atrium and a value 1.5 times higher than the aortic dimension indicates a large ductus. Echocardiography is useful in monitoring response to treatment and a reduction in size of the left atrium if the ductus is closing. A hyperoxia test is useful in excluding more complex congenital heart disease with a ductus-dependent pulmonary circulation (p. 240).

Treatment

Initially an attempt should be made to control the heart failure. Fluids are restricted to 150 ml/kg per day and sufficient oxygen given (usually 30 per cent is adequate) to prevent hypoxia which tends to keep the duct open. The haematocrit should be maintained at 0.4–0.45, if necessary by small blood transfusions. Hypoglycaemia and hypocalcaemia must be corrected. Digoxin (0.03 mg/kg over 24 hours i.m. followed by 0.01 mg/kg daily in 2 divided doses, orally) is given, and frusemide 1 mg/kg i.m. daily or twice daily.

Artificial closure of the ductus is indicated if heart failure is not promptly controlled, or if an artificially ventilated infant cannot be weaned off the ventilator. Three methods have been used.

Firstly a trial of oxygen therapy for 24 hours. An inspired concentration of about 40 per cent is used, which for this period is safe. There is little clear evidence as to how often this succeeds, but 50 per cent success is claimed.

Inhibition of prostaglandin activity by indomethacin is now well established, but the optimum dose is still disputed. Heymann, Rudolph and Silverman (1976) recommend a single dose of 0.3 mg/kg or two or more doses of 0.1 mg/kg. Alpert et al. (1979a) suggest using a 1 mg/ml solution in 0.2 M phosphate buffer at pH 7.2 giving 0.1–0.2 mg/kg orally or rectally. A second dose is given, if necessary, at 8–12 hours and a third at 18–24 hours. Higher doses are associated with acute renal failure (usually recoverable). Halliday, Hirata and Brady (1979) reported closure of the ductus in 24 out of 36 infants weighing less than 1500 g, the least successful group being those over 14 days of age. Alpert *et al.* (1979a) treated 50 infants (some with more than one dose) and 22 responded favourably. They found that oral and rectal administration were equally successful. Obeyesekere *et al.* (1980) found partial or complete closure in 12 of 16 premature infants, the 4 who failed to respond being all below 1000 g and 26 weeks' gestation.

Contra-indications to indomethacin include: poor urinary output, hyperbilirubinaemia or bleeding disorder, since the drug causes alteration in platelet function (Kocsis *et al.*, 1973). If indomethacin fails to close the ductus or improve symptoms significantly, surgical closure is indicated. This needs to be done with as little disturbance to the infant as possible, and many surgeons carry it out with assisted ventilation and local anaesthesia in the Special Care Unit. The 22 infants reported by Alpert (1979a) as failures of indomethacin therapy were all treated surgically with no deaths. Merritt *et al.* (1979) had 2 deaths in 26 patients treated surgically and 3 deaths in 26 treated with indomethacin.

It has become recognized that early closure of the ductus not only saves lives but also leads to a reduction in morbidity. Cotton *et al.* (1978) reported 38 premature infants with patent ductus treated without surgical or pharmacological intervention. Of these 11 died. Many of the survivors had persistent pulmonary complications attributable to prolonged artificial ventilation, and 5 had retrolental fibroplasia.

THE REVERSED DUCTUS

The term 'reversed ductus' refers to a patent ductus arteriosus associated with severe pulmonary hypertension in which there is a right-to-left shunt through the ductus. This is the Eisenmenger syndrome (Wood, 1958).

There seem to be two groups of cases. In one there is a high pulmonary vascular resistance from birth and, although initially there may be a left-to-right shunt, it is not of sufficient size to cause symptoms: any heart murmur is insignificant (*see Figure 6.1*) and heart disease usually remains undiagnosed for several years. In the second group there is initially a large left-to-right shunt in infancy and a high pulmonary vascular resistance develops as a secondary phenomenon. Although shunt reversal can occur in childhood, it is rare. If there is already reversal of flow when the child is first seen, it may be difficult to establish on historical grounds whether a significant left-to-right shunt was present in infancy. Cyanosis is usually not obvious and may be missed completely if the toes are not examined and their colour compared with the fingers. The right arm is usually still perfused with fully oxygenated blood. The left arm receives some of the desaturated blood coming through the ductus and the legs receive a greater quantity of desaturated blood. This means that when the reversal has been present for some time, there is clubbing of the toes, mild clubbing of the left hand but no clubbing of the right hand.

The clinical findings in these patients are those found in the Eisenmenger syndrome (*see* p. 274). Closure of the ductus is contra-indicated in this situation.

OTHER CAUSES OF CONTINUOUS MURMURS

Although the signs of a patent ductus arteriosus are usually characteristic and further investigation is not required, there are other lesions which give rise to continuous murmurs and may sometimes cause difficulty in diagnosis. The site of these murmurs is usually different from that of a patent ductus and they lack the characteristic 'systolic rattle' and the crescendo quality in systole so characteristic of a patent ductus.

Venous hum

The venous hum is caused by flow of blood in the large veins in the neck. It varies with the position of the neck, being loudest when the neck is extended. The hum can be abolished or minimized by firm pressure over the jugular veins or by turning the neck. It disappears when the patient lies flat.

Aortopulmonary window

Aortopulmonary window is a fistulous connection between the aorta and pulmonary artery close to their origins. It is usually associated with pulmonary hypertension and has to be differentiated from a large patent ductus with pulmonary hypertension. If it is small, however, there may be a continuous murmur which is heard lower down the left sternal edge than the classic ductus murmur and is very loud. It can be differentiated from a patent ductus by aortography, but it is relatively so rare (about 1 to every 100 ducts) that it is better to take the risk of finding it at thoracotomy. Recently a distal type of defect between the ascending aorta and the bifurcation of the pulmonary artery has also been described.

Coronary arteriovenous aneurysm

Coronary arteriovenous aneurysm is a fistula between a coronary artery (usually the right) and one of the chambers of the heart (usually on the right side). The maximal site of the continuous murmur is lower down the left sternal edge and not in the second left interspace. It is demonstrated by aortography.

Aneurysm of sinus Valsalva

If an aneurysm of the sinus of Valsalva ruptures into one of the cardiac chambers there is sudden congestive heart failure associated with a collapsing pulse and a continuous or to-and-fro murmur, but again the murmur is maximal in the third and fourth left intercostal spaces. Occasionally, a fistula is present between the sinus and one of the cardiac chambers from birth. The lesion is confirmed by aortography.

Ventricular septal defect and aortic regurgitation

Ventricular septal defect and aortic regurgitation gives rise to a murmur which has a to-and-fro rather than continuous rhythm, and is best heard in the third and fourth left interspaces. Cardiac catheterization and retrograde aortography differentiate it from patent ductus arteriosus.

The other causes of continuous murmurs are not easily confused with patent ductus arteriosus but worth mentioning.

Peripheral pulmonary stenosis

Multiple stenoses of the peripheral pulmonary arteries produce continuous murmurs all over the chest. The electrocardiogram usually shows evidence of right ventricular hypertrophy.

Murmurs of collateral vessels

Murmurs of collateral vessels may be heard in pulmonary atresia. They are well heard at the back and the patients usually show some degree of cyanosis (*see* p. 171).

Pulmonary arteriovenous fistula

The continuous murmur of pulmonary arteriovenous fistula is best heard usually over one lung and is associated with cyanosis and finger clubbing.

Continuous murmur associated with obstructed anomalous pulmonary veins

The murmur is usually heard in the pulmonary area and is due to blood flowing through the stenosed anomalous vein.

Sequestrated segment of lung

The systemic blood supply to a sequestrated segment of the lung may result in a continuous murmur which is confined to the area of the lung so supplied.

Systemic ateriovenous fistula

When such a fistula occurs in the thorax a continuous murmur may be heard over the chest or thoracic inlet. This however is less common than an arteriovenous malformation within the skull which gives rise to a continuous murmur heard over the temporal region or in babies over the anterior fontanelle. In addition if the fistula is large the pulses will be collapsing and the heart enlarged.

VENTRICULAR SEPTAL DEFECT

Incidence

Ventricular septal defect is by far the commonest congenital heart lesion, accounting for 30 per cent of all cases.

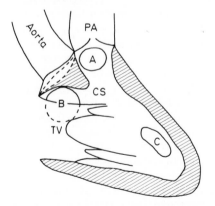

Figure 6.4. Types of ventricular septal defect. A: supracristal; B: infracristal (note that both of these are close to the aortic valve); C: muscular; PA: pulmonary artery; TV: tricuspid valve; CS: crista supraventricularis

Definition

The defect usually occurs in the membranous part of the ventricular septum below the aortic valve. Viewed from the right ventricle it lies below the crista supraventricularis. Less commonly it is situated in the lower, muscular septum or, occasionally, immediately below both pulmonary and aortic rings (*Figure 6.4*). Usually the defect is single, but occasionally multiple small defects may occur.

Natural history

The natural history of this lesion has proved to be a fascinating one and has only been fully appreciated over the last few years, as a result of serial clinical and laboratory studies. A retrospective study by Bloomfield (1964) has helped to clarify the natural history, but there is still a need for further careful follow-up studies in this lesion, particularly in infants. The prognosis is mainly related to the size of the defect, the changes which may occur with growth and the alterations which may occur in the pulmonary circulation. Unless a careful study is made of *infants* with this defect, the evolution of the condition will not be fully appreciated. This lesion more than any other illustrates that congenital heart lesions are not static conditions but that changes gradually occur throughout life, the most dramatic ones in the first year of life.

In series where infants have been studied, those investigated have usually had symptoms due to a defect of moderate or large size and patients with smaller lesions have not been subjected to cardiac catheterization. Kidd and co-workers (1965) studied the haemodynamics in infancy and early childhood and showed that progressive pulmonary vascular obstruction developed in those patients who, during infancy, had a high pulmonary blood flow with a low pulmonary vascular resistance. They found that during infancy the pulmonary vascular resistance was raised above normal in only 25 per cent of patients. Although in patients with large defects the pulmonary vascular resistance gradually rises over the first few years of life, it is unusual for it to reach systemic levels in infancy; however, this has been reported (Anderson *et al.*, 1967).

After infancy, death is rare until after 25 years of age, but in large defects the patient's improvement may be due to the onset of pulmonary vascular disease; although this is initially beneficial in reducing the left-to-right shunt, it may become progressive and irreversible and make surgical closure impossible. In patients with large defects who survive the first few years, heart failure is likely to occur sometime between the ages of 25 and 40 years. Patients who develop the Eisenmenger complex usually die before the end of the fourth decade.

The following changes may occur in ventricular septal defect (*Figure 6.5*).

1. About 50 per cent of them will close spontaneously. Many of those that close are small and symptomless but closure can also occur in moderate and large defects. The commonest time for closure is during the first year of life but later closure does occur.

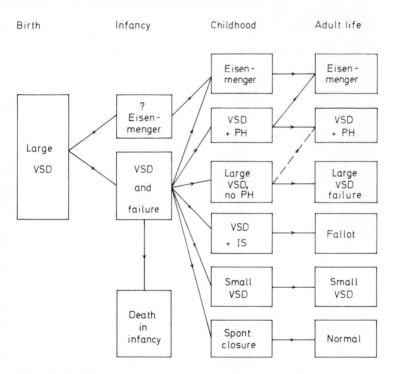

Birth   Infancy   Childhood   Adult life

Figure 6.5. Possible outcome in patients born with large ventricular septal defects (VSD). PH: pulmonary hypertension; IS: infundibular stenosis

2. The defect becomes relatively smaller. As growth of the heart takes place the defect remains the same size and becomes relatively smaller. This relative change is most obvious in the first year of life. Both closure and reduction in size is commonly associated with the development of a thin, mobile part of the

membranous septum which projects into the right ventricle during systole – the 'aneurysm of the interventricular septum' (Freedom *et al.*, 1974). Over 50 per cent of patients with small or closing defects have such an aneurysm, but it causes no haemodynamic problems and presumably eventually shrinks, since it is very seldom found at autopsy in adults. These defects have been demonstrated by angiography (although this is seldom justified on clinical grounds) and by echocardiography (*Figure 6.6*).

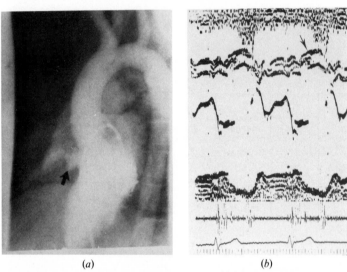

(*a*)   (*b*)

Figure 6.6. Aneurysm of interventricular septum. (a) left ventricular angiogram. The aneurysm is arrowed and there is a small jet of contrast entering the right ventricle. (b) Echocardiogram. The aneurysm (arrowed) is shown as an echo moving anteriorly in systole

3. Infundibular stenosis develops. Serial catheter studies (Gasul and co-workers, 1957) have shown that infundibular stenosis may develop in patients who previously had none. In some of these the degree of stenosis remains mild and a left-to-right shunt through the defect continues, but the pulmonary arteries are protected from a high pressure. In others, the infundibular narrowing is progressive and a right-to-left shunt through the ventricular septal defect develops and the lesion becomes the tetralogy of Fallot. Infundibular stenosis occurs particularly in those who have a right-sided aorta (Varghese *et al.*, 1970). Development of infundibular stenosis and closure of the defect may occur in the

same patient, resulting in what appears to be isolated infundibular stenosis.
4. Progressive pulmonary vascular obstruction develops. This occurs most commonly in patients who, during infancy, have had a high flow, low resistance, pulmonary circulation. Closure of the defect in patients in whom the pulmonary vascular resistance is increasing does not always halt its progress and the pulmonary vascular resistance may continue to rise after satisfactory surgical closure. There does seem to be a group of cases, inadequately studied, in whom the pulmonary vascular resistance does not fall sufficiently in the weeks after birth to allow a large shunt ever to occur, even though the defect is a large one. Such patients have few symptoms but do go on to develop increasing pulmonary vascular obstruction. When the pulmonary vascular resistance rises above the systemic resistance, a right-to-left shunt occurs through the defect and the Eisenmenger complex results.

Clinical presentation

Clinical presentation varies so much with the size of the defect and pulmonary vascular changes, that it is better, for clarity, to divide the cases into four groups.

GROUP 1: SMALL VENTRICULAR SEPTAL DEFECTS

Patients with small ventricular septal defects will have no symptoms and will grow and develop normally. The heart disease is discovered during routine examination. The heart is not enlarged, or only slightly so, there is a pansystolic murmur and thrill maximal in the third and fourth interspaces at the left sternal edge. The second sound is normal. In very small defects there may be no thrill and the murmur does not continue throughout systole. These defects are particularly associated with the development of an aneurysm of the membranous septum (Freedom *et al.*, 1974). When the defect becomes very small the murmur becomes soft and short and may be preceded by an early systolic click.

Alpert *et al.* (1979) reported that of 50 patients with small ventricular septal defects followed from soon after birth for 10 years, 75 per cent closed spontaneously, mainly by the age of 2 years.

Radiology

Radiology shows slight or no cardiac enlargement and there may be slightly increased or normal pulmonary vascularity.

Electrocardiography

The electrocardiogram may be normal or show slight increase in left ventricular activity.

Investigation

Cardiac catheterization is seldom performed in this group and indeed is not necessary, but it shows a small left-to-right shunt at ventricular level and normal right vetricular and pulmonary artery pressures.

Treatment

No treatment is required in this group other than prophylaxis against bacterial endocarditis. The lifetime risk of this complication is 30 per cent and the risk of death is 5 per cent. Apart from this hazard the life expectancy with this lesion is more than 60 years, so that the operative mortality would have to be well below 1 per cent for surgery to be recommended.

GROUP 2: MEDIUM-SIZED VENTRICULAR SEPTAL DEFECTS

Medium-sized ventricular septal defects will often cause symptoms in infancy; the child is breathless on feeding, takes longer to feed and often does not finish his feeds. His weight gain is slower than normal. He is prone to chest infections, which take longer to resolve than in a normal child. Heart failure may develop in the first three months of life, often precipitated by a chest infection, but responds readily to treatment. Slow but steady progress is made and when spoon-feeding is introduced the infant feeds better, is less exhausted than by sucking a bottle and his weight gain improves. As he gains more weight the defect often becomes relatively smaller; he becomes less breathless and his general condition improves. Thereafter he makes reasonable progress although lagging behind normal. He may rest more than a normal child after activity and becomes more easily tired than his friends. He is more disturbed by chest infections than a normal child but these distress him less as he becomes older and by the time school age is reached he is symptomatically little different from normal.

On examination, in infancy, there may be slight breathlessness at rest. There is some cardiac enlargement with prominent activity of the left ventricle and some increase in the right ventricular activity. A well marked thrill is felt in the third and fourth left interspaces close to the sternum and there is a loud, harsh, impressive pansystolic murmur maximal in the same area and conducted all over the chest.

A mid-diastolic murmur can be heard in the mitral area where it is fairly localized and gives a to-and-fro rhythm. The presence of this murmur indicates that there must be a moderate or large left-to-right shunt through the defect, for, when a large amount of blood flows to the lungs, there is a large amount of blood returning to the left atrium and flowing through the normal mitral valve. This excessive flow through a normal valve causes the mitral diastolic murmur. It usually occurs when the amount of blood flowing to the lungs is more than twice that flowing in the systemic circulation.

The second sound may be normally split, but in cases where the pulmonary artery pressure is increased the splitting may be closer than normal and the second element increased in intensity.

Some patients with medium-sized defects have normal pulmonary artery pressures, but with others it is raised although not as high as systemic level.

Radiology

Radiology shows moderate cardiac enlargement, a prominent pulmonary artery, moderately increased hilar vessels and an increased vascularity of the lungs (*Figure 6.7*).

Electrocardiography

The electrocardiogram shows an increase in right and left ventricular activity, the left greater than the right. Frequently the right ventricular hypertrophy appears as a right bundle branch block type pattern (*Figure 6.8*).

Investigation

Cardiac catheterization may be undertaken in infancy if there is doubt about the diagnosis or if some other lesion (for example, patent ductus) is thought to be present. If the diagnosis seems certain on clinical grounds and the infant is making satisfactory progress, catheterization is unnecessary at this stage. Catheterization should subsequently be performed in the fourth or fifth years, unless it is clear on clinical grounds that the defect has become small, and shows that there is a rise in oxygen saturation of the blood in the right ventricle such that the pulmonary blood flow is about two to three times that in the systemic circulation. The right ventricular pressure and pulmonary artery systolic pressure may be normal or slightly or moderately raised (*Figure 6.9*).

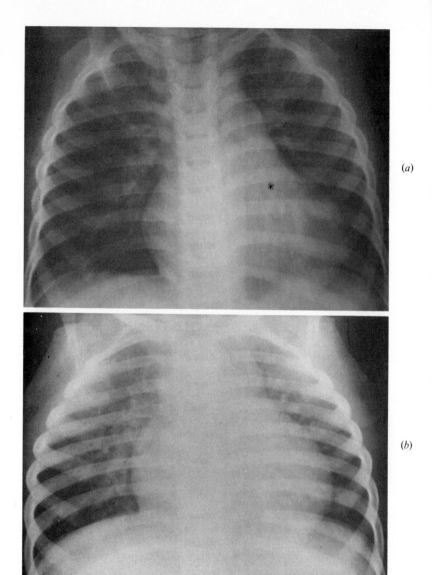

(a)

(b)

Figure 6.7. Radiology of ventricular septal defects. (*a*) Fairly small
defect (pulmonary to systemic flow ratio 2 : 1 with normal pulmonary
artery pressure). The left ventricle is enlarged and there is minimal
plethora. (*b*) Moderate-sized defect (P : S about 4 : 1 and slight elevation
in pulmonary artery pressure). The heart is enlarged and there is
pulmonary plethora. (*c*) Large defect with equal pulmonary artery and
aortic pressures and P : S flow ratio 4 : 1. (*d*) Large defect and high
pulmonary vascular resistance (P : S flow ratio 1.5 : 1). The heart is not
enlarged overall, the main pulmonary artery is prominent but the
peripheral vessels are pruned

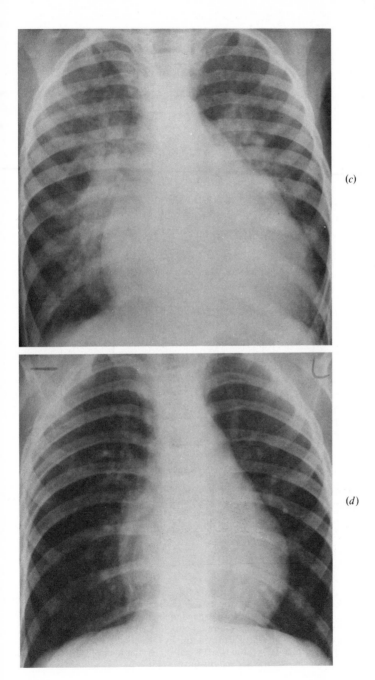

(c)

(d)

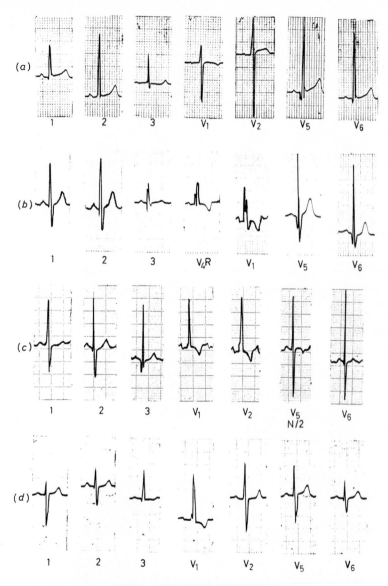

Figure 6.8. Electrocardiograms of patients with ventricular septal defects whose haemodynamic states correspond to those of *Figure 6.7.* (*a*) Mild left ventricular hypertrophy (10-year-old). (*b*) Left ventricular hypertrophy and mild right ventricular hypertrophy (3-year-old). (*c*) Biventricular hypertrophy (3-year-old). (*d*) Right ventricular hypertrophy with normal left ventricular activity (3-year-old)

Treatment

If there is evidence of heart failure, digoxin will be required. Diuretics are rarely necessary. Medical help should be summoned when there is any respiratory infection so that if this infection reaches the lungs, antibiotics can be given promptly. Early introduction of spoon-feeding will often result in an improved weight gain. Prophylaxis against bacterial endocarditis is very important.

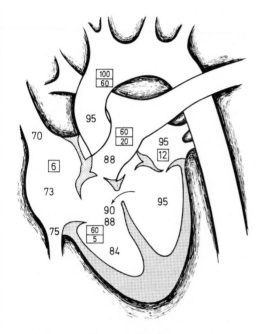

Figure 6.9. Ventricular septal defect of moderate size. Pressures in mmHg, within squares; percentage oxygen saturations, unsquared

Children should be observed frequently throughout the first few years of life. Often the defect becomes relatively smaller, but if by the third or fourth year the child still has symptoms and there is cardiac enlargement and plethora, closure of the defect is advised before the child starts school. Closure of any ventricular septal defect requires some form of cardiopulmonary bypass (*see* p. 54). Most of the commonest defects, in the membranous septum, are approached through an incision in the right atrium and visualized through the tricuspid valve. Supracristal and large complex defects are best dealt with through an incision in the right ventricular wall. Multiple defects in the muscular septum are difficult to locate when viewed from the right ventricular aspect as they are hidden by the trabeculae and may require an incision into the apex of the left ventricle.

The mortality from closing a single defect in the membranous septum in a child over the age of 1 year is low, about 1 per cent, but the overall mortality for all defects at this age is about 5 per cent as many of the larger defects are multiple or complex. Apart from the usual postoperative complications the main morbidity is from damage to the conducting system, but this can usually be avoided by careful placement of sutures in the part of the defect near the conducting tissue.

GROUP 3: LARGE VENTRICULAR SEPTAL DEFECTS

Children with large defects are often very ill early in life. Some of these have multiple defects in the septum. Symptoms usually begin after the second or third weeks of life and heart failure usually occurs at around 6 weeks, often precipitated by a chest infection. It is unusual for even large defects to cause symptoms in the first week or two of life, probably because the pulmonary arteries take that long to dilate to a size sufficient to take a high flow. Feeding is usually poor after the first 2 weeks of life and becomes increasingly difficult. Dyspnoea is also progressive as the left-to-right shunt increases in the first few weeks of life. These infants fail to thrive satisfactorily at first despite treatment of the heart failure. They may need tube-feeding, but slowly, after maximal medical treatment, the majority of them begin to improve and start to gain weight. Prolonged hospitalization is often required, however, and when the infant is discharged home, repeated admission to hospital because of chest infection may be necessary. Nevertheless, many of these infants do make satisfactory progress after 6 months of age; in some of them the defect lessens in size and the left-to-right shunt diminishes. It is in patients with large defects, however, that there is the greatest danger of improvement taking place at the expense of change in the vasculature of the lungs, which increases the pulmonary vascular resistance and reduces the left-to-right shunt.

Infants show marked dyspnoea at rest (*Figure 6.10*); they may be slightly cyanosed out of oxygen, due to their respiratory difficulty. The heart is markedly enlarged with increased activity of both ventricles. Where the systolic murmur is maximal a systolic thrill is palpable in the third and fourth left interspaces. The thrill and murmur, however, do not occupy the whole of systole and may fade away before the end of systole. This is because there is increased pressure in the right ventricle due to some increase in pulmonary vascular resistance and the systolic pressures in the two ventricles equalize before the end of systole. When the defect is very large there may be no systolic murmur from the defect; instead a

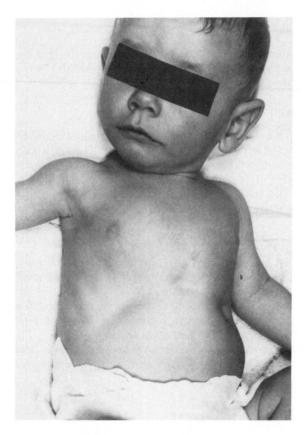

Figure 6.10. Infant aged 4 months with large ventricular septal defect. Note the incession of the lower chest. At the age of 5 years the patient was symptom-free and had only a very small defect, which does not require closure

pulmonary systolic ejection murmur is heard. A short, quite loud, mid-diastolic murmur is audible at the apex which is often displaced well out into the anterior axillary line. The second sound is loud owing to hyperdynamic pulmonary hypertension.

Radiology

Radiology shows marked cardiac enlargement with a very large pulmonary artery, large hilar vessels and increased peripheral vascularity (*see Figure 6.7*).

Electrocardiography

The electrocardiogram shows a marked increase in both right and left ventricular activity and sometimes there are inverted T waves over the left ventricular leads (*see Figure 6.8*).

Echocardiography

The echocardiogram is useful, if non-specific. All cardiac chambers are enlarged, as is the left ventricular stroke volume. The aorta is not enlarged and the ratio of the size of the left atrium to aorta (normally between 1.0 and 1.3) is a guide to the size of the shunt. The investigation is also useful in excluding more complex anomalies such as single ventricle and truncus arteriosus.

Investigation

Investigation is usually required in this group in infancy to confirm the diagnosis and exclude additional lesions. The right ventricular and pulmonary artery systolic pressures are at systemic level and angiography is required to exclude such lesions as double outflow right ventricle (in which both great vessels arise from the right ventricle), common ventricle and persistent truncus arteriosus. The pulmonary blood flow is at least three times the systemic blood flow. The pulmonary vascular resistance may be normal in infancy but increases with age.

Treatment

It is the group with large defects in which surgery will be required in all but a few, and ideally the defects should be closed as early in life as possible. The age at which closure can be carried out safely continues to fall and in the future direct closure will become the treatment of choice. The problem is, however, that among the patients subjected to surgery would be some whose progress would be favourable if they were left alone. There is no way of differentiating between those patients whose defects will become smaller or will develop infundibular stenosis to protect their pulmonary vasculature and those who will develop irreversible pulmonary hypertension by 2 years of age, making surgery impossible. The mortality of closing a single, large ventricular septal defect in an infant in heart failure is about 2–5 per cent, but unfortunately about a third of defects are multiple, in which case the mortality is higher—10 to 20 per cent. If heart failure can be controlled and growth continues, albeit slowly, it is best to wait until after the age of 1 year before attempting closure.

In the past it has been customary to 'band' the pulmonary artery, in infants with large ventricular septal defects, that is to constrict it with tape to reduce the pulmonary blood flow. The risks of surgical closure of large but uncomplicated defects in infancy are now sufficiently low to make this generally unnecessary, although the procedure still has a place when there are multiple septal defects, or a large defect occurring in association with some other major lesion such as coarctation of the aorta. Subsequently the banded area has to be repaired and the defect itself closed.

GROUP 4: LARGE VENTRICULAR SEPTAL DEFECTS WITH HIGH PULMONARY VASCULAR RESISTANCE

Patients with large defects and high pulmonary vascular resistance will rarely be seen before 2 years of age and are becoming uncommon as large defects can now be closed safely within the first year of life. The development of a marked increase in pulmonary vascular resistance reduces the left-to-right shunt so that the pulmonary blood flow is only slightly increased when the pulmonary artery pressure is the same as the systemic pressure. The pulmonary artery pressure is high because of the resistance to blood flow by the narrowed muscular arteries in the lungs. As this resistance increases, the left-to-right shunt through the defect further diminishes and when the pulmonary vascular resistance equals the systemic resistance there is no net flow through the defect in either direction. The pulmonary vascular resistance continues to rise gradually and, when it is greater than the systemic resistance, a right-to-left shunt through the defect occurs, producing the so-called Eisenmenger complex (*see* p. 274).

At first, patients are not cyanosed and have few if any symptoms; the heart is not enlarged or only slightly so. The left ventricle is not overworking because of the small shunt, and the right ventricle, although working at systemic pressure, is not working with a volume overload as in the two previous groups. There is no systolic thrill and there is only a short systolic murmur and no apical diastolic murmur. The second heart sound is very loud, usually single, and may be palpable. As the left-to-right shunt lessens, the systolic murmur becomes shorter and then disappears when the shunt ceases. The heaving of the right ventricle increases and the second sound is very loud. When a right-to-left shunt occurs the patient becomes cyanosed and presents the picture of the Eisenmenger complex (*see* p. 274).

Radiology

Radiology shows only a slight increase in heart size or a normal size. The pulmonary artery is prominent, the hilar vessels are large but there is poor vascularity in the periphery of the lungs, an appearance often described as 'pruning' (from its resemblance to a pruned tree with spindly new growth (*see Figure 6.7*).

Electrocardiography

The electrocardiogram shows right ventricular hypertrophy and there is often a qR pattern in V_4R and V_1. The left ventricular activity is normal (*see Figure 6.8*).

Investigation

Cardiac catheterization is carried out in this group to measure the pulmonary vascular resistance to ascertain whether operation is possible. At catheterization there is a small rise in oxygen saturation in samples high up in the ventricle, and as the pulmonary vascular resistance increases a sample of blood from the aorta shows that there may be a small right-to-left shunt which may often be insufficient to cause cyanosis clinically. The amount of right-to-left shunt increases when the pulmonary vascular resistance rises above the systemic resistance.

Treatment

When the pulmonary vascular resistance is more than half the systemic resistance, closure of the defect carries a high mortality and many surgeons do not advise it. Treatment is symptomatic only. The risks of operation must be balanced against the relatively good prognosis for 20 years if nothing is done. There is also the risk that closing the defect may accelerate the development of hypertensive pulmonary vascular disease and so shorten, rather than lengthen, the patient's life.

It must be emphasized that although the lesion has been divided into groups for the purpose of description, many patients overlap between one group and another, and individual patients may move from one group to another as they grow up. Some will move from group 2 to group 1 if the defect becomes smaller; others will move from group 3 to 4 if the defect is not closed and the pulmonary vascular resistance rises. Others will develop infundibular stenosis and some of these cases will become indistinguishable from those with tetralogy of Fallot.

THE EISENMENGER SYNDROME

Patients with ventricular septal defects in whom the resistance in the pulmonary vascular bed rises higher than that in the systemic vascular bed and who have a right-to-left shunt through the defect are described as having the Eisenmenger complex. It was in ventricular septal defect that the presence of cyanosis was first described by Eisenmenger. There are many other heart lesions, however, in which the presence of severe pulmonary vascular disease is associated with a right-to-left shunt and cyanosis. If these patients are seen for the first time when they are already cyanosed, it is very difficult to differentiate one from another. The Eisenmenger syndrome is dealt with in more detail in Chapter 15 since, from the clinician's viewpoint, it presents as a problem of diagnosis of pulmonary hypertension.

General factors affecting operability of ventricular septal defect

In the previous few pages the general principle used to select patients with ventricular septal defects for operation have been discussed. Much weight is placed upon the size of the shunt, the pulmonary artery pressure and the pulmonary vascular resistance as measured at cardiac catheterization. It should be stressed, however, that the haemodynamic figures are not the only factors guiding the cardiologist, and that these figures are always studied in conjunction with the physical signs and radiological appearances. It should also be realized that, although figures for pulmonary vascular resistance can be calculated from the haemodynamic data, the actual value may vary from day to day and from hour to hour, according to the condition of the patient. It will be clear that the information obtained at cardiac catheterization is only a guide to treatment.

VENTRICULAR SEPTAL DEFECT WITH AORTIC REGURGITATION

In ventricular septal defect with aortic regurgitation the defect is high up and there is no tissue between it and the aortic valve. In infancy there is evidence only of a ventricular septal defect but later in life, usually after 3 years of age, a blowing diastolic murmur develops down the left sternal edge. One of the cusps of the aortic valve, usually the right anterior cusp, prolapses into the ventricular septal defect and aortic regurgitation results. The pansystolic murmur and early diastolic murmur may mimic a continuous murmur and the lesion be mistaken for a patent ductus arteriosus. The degree of regurgitation may increase as the child becomes older and result in progressive cardiac enlargement and left ventricular hypertrophy on the electrocardiogram. In other patients the degree of regurgitation is slight and remains unchanged for several years.

The condition is confirmed at cardiac catheterization, there being a left-to-right shunt at ventricular level, and a retrograde aortogram shows the prolapsing cusp. Sometimes the bulging cusp causes narrowing of the outflow tract of the right ventricle.

Treatment

The decision about operation depends upon the severity of the aortic regurgitation. If there is congestive heart failure or considerable cardiomegaly, operation is necessary since medical treatment will fail. If, however, symptoms are few or absent, surgery can be delayed until the child is big enough for valve replacement when it is indicated. Repair of the aortic valve, when possible, may halt the progress of the aortic regurgitation but it seems likely that most patients will require valve replacement at some time. Some workers (Somerville, Brandao and Ross, 1970) believe that closure of the ventricular septal defect will halt the progress of the aortic regurgitation.

LEFT VENTRICLE TO RIGHT ATRIAL COMMUNICATION (GERBODE DEFECT)

In the Gerbode defect there is a fault in the part of the septum between the left ventricle and the right atrium, at the base of the tricuspid valve, which is frequently cleft. The precise anatomical abnormality is variable but in every case as the left ventricle contracts, a jet of blood streams into the right atrium.

Clinically a patient presents as with a ventricular septal defect but the electrocardiogram frequently shows an rSr' complex in V_4R and

V_1 and peaked P waves indicate right atrial hypertrophy. The radiograph shows a prominent right atrium with left ventricular enlargement.

The diagnosis is confirmed at cardiac catheterization when there is a rise of oxygen saturation in the blood at atrial level but the catheter cannot be passed into the left atrium. A left ventricular angiogram shows dye streaming from the left ventricle into the right atrium.

Treatment

Closure is usually simpler than in a ventricular septal defect and can be carried out through the right atrium. Operation is recommended because there is a high incidence of bacterial endocarditis associated with the jet lesion and spontaneous closure does not occur.

ATRIAL SEPTAL DEFECTS

Atrial defects may be divided into two groups.

1. The simplest form of atrial septal defect is the *ostium secundum defect* in which there is an opening in the atrial septum in the region of the fossa ovalis.
2. The more complex form is made up of the *endocardial cushion defects*. These include the ostium primum defect and the common, or persistent, atrioventricular canal.

Ostium secundum defects

Incidence

Atrial septal defects of all types constitute about 10 per cent of all congenital heart defects; 80 per cent of these are of the ostium secundum type.

Definition

There is an opening between the two atria in the region of the fossa ovalis (*Figure 6.11a*). There may be more than one opening. The amount of blood shunting through the defect depends more on the filling resistances of the two ventricles than on the size of the defect.

In the early months of life, the right and left ventricles have walls of equal thickness and, since the filling characteristics of the two ventricles are similar, very little blood flows through the defect. As the pulmonary vascular resistance falls, so does the right ventricular pressure, and the right ventricular muscle becomes thinner. The right ventricle becomes more distensible and offers less resistance to filling than the left ventricle and so blood flows from the left to the right atrium to enter the right ventricle.

Atrial septal defects are often associated with partial anomalous drainage of pulmonary veins which enter the superior vena cava or the right atrium directly. The haemodynamic effect of this anomalous drainage is the same as that of atrial septal defect and it is not possible to determine clinically whether there is anomalous drainage as well as an atrial septal defect. Occasionally, partial anomalous pulmonary venous drainage occurs without an atrial septal defect.

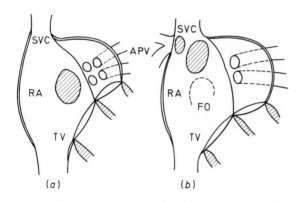

Figure 6.11. Atrial septal defects (*a*) Ostium secundum defect. (*b*) Sinus venosus defect associated with anomalous pulmonary veins (APV). SVC: superior vena cava; RA: right atrium; TV: tricuspid valve; FO: fossa ovalis. The large shaded circle is the atrial defect in each case

A special type of atrial septal defect occurs near the entrance of the superior vena cava and is associated with one or more pulmonary veins from the right lung draining into the superior vena cava. This is called a sinus venosus defect (*Figure 6.11b*).

Natural history

It is very uncommon for an atrial septal defect alone ever to give rise to symptoms in infancy, when the resistance to filling in the two ventricles is the same. Only in very large shunts are symptoms present in childhood and more usually a heart murmur is found during a routine examination. Most patients do well in childhood and rarely develop symptoms before the third decade. They may then develop pulmonary hypertension, heart failure or atrial arrhythmias. Pregnancy often aggravates the condition and causes heart failure.

Pulmonary hypertension is rare before the third decade, but when it becomes severe the right ventricle hypertrophies and is less compliant, the flow through the defect becomes from right to left and cyanosis occurs. The reason why pulmonary hypertension does not occur in childhood is probably related to the fact that the left atrial pressure never rises significantly and so the pulmonary venous pressure is normal (unlike with ventricular septal defects and patent ductus arteriosus). The pulmonary hypertension in atrial septal defects is secondary to increased pulmonary flow.

Clinical presentation

Only when there is a very large flow of blood through the atrial septal defect do the patients have symptoms. They are excessively tired and breathless on exertion and may suffer from frequent chest infections. Most children are free of symptoms.

The patients are usually normal in size but some are tall and thin with long fingers and toes. When the shunt is large they may be below average weight. The patient is pink, the pulses are normal or of small volume and usually do not show any respiratory variation in rate. The heart is only slightly enlarged or normal in size but there is palpable pulsation of the right ventricle. There is no thrill but an ejection systolic murmur is heard which is loudest in the second left interspace. This murmur is due to excessive flow through the normal pulmonary valve. When the amount of blood flowing to the lungs is more than twice that flowing to the systemic circulation, an additional, diastolic murmur can be heard in the tricuspid area due to increased flow of blood through the tricuspid valve. This murmur increases with inspiration and fades with expiration. Flow through the defect causes no murmur as the defect is large and there is no pressure gradient and therefore no turbulence. The two components of the second sound are more widely split than normally and the splitting no longer varies with respiration and is described as being 'fixed'.

Occasionally the patient may have a tinge of cyanosis due to some inferior vena-caval blood being deflected to the left atrium by a large

96

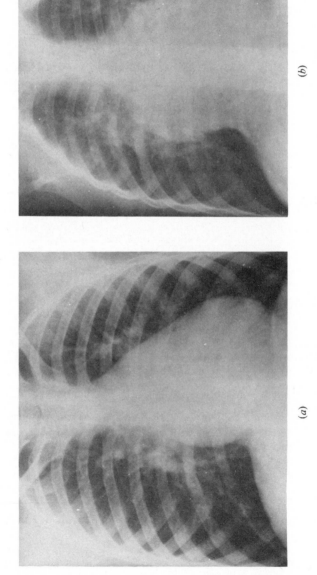

(a)

(b)

Figure 6.12. Chest radiographs of patients with atrial septal defects. (*a*) Ostium secundum defect, pulmonary flow four times systemic. The right ventricle is enlarged, the main pulmonary artery is prominent and there is moderate pulmonary plethora. (*b*) Ostium primum (endocardial cushion defect). The heart is larger and the pulmonary vessels are more prominent.

Eustachian valve on the inferior vena cava, so that desaturated blood enters the systemic circulation.

Radiology

The degree of cardiac enlargement varies with the size of the shunt, the right atrium is prominent and the pulmonary artery and its branches are enlarged and there is increased vascularity in the periphery of the lungs (*Figure 6.12*). In the lateral view the right ventricle bulges forward under the sternum. The aorta is small and the superior vena cava shadow is not usually visible.

Electrocardiography

The electrocardiogram shows right axis deviation and right ventricular hypertrophy. Leads V_4R and V_1 show an rsR' complex and this is present in 95 per cent of all ostium secundum atrial septal defects (*Figure 6.13*) – its *absence* makes the diagnosis of ostium secundum suspect. It must be stressed, however, that this rsR' complex occurs in other lesions and its *presence* does not mean that the lesion is an atrial septal defect. The P–R interval may be prolonged but the P waves are usually normal. The rhythm is usually regular; atrial fibrillation is rare in childhood but occurs in adults.

Echocardiography

The echocardiogram reflects the high flow through the right side of the heart. The right ventricle is enlarged and the movement of the interventricular septum paradoxical in large defects. The hole can be seen on 2-D echocardiography (*Figure 6.14a*). The turbulence caused by the increased blood flow produces fluttering of the tricuspid valve in diastole and of the pulmonary valve in systole. These features are sufficiently characteristic to allow differentiation between large defects requiring surgery and small defects or patients with functional murmurs.

Investigation

The diagnosis can be made with certainty clinically in most cases and cardiac catheterization is only carried out if there is suspicion of an additional lesion. A right heart catheterization shows a rise in oxygen saturation in the right atrial samples (*Figure 6.15*) and the defect is usually crossed by the catheter. Occasionally, because of

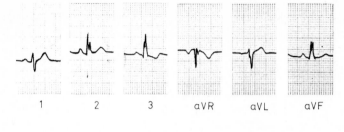

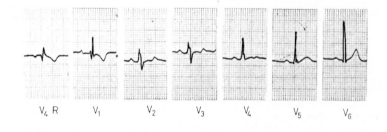

(a)

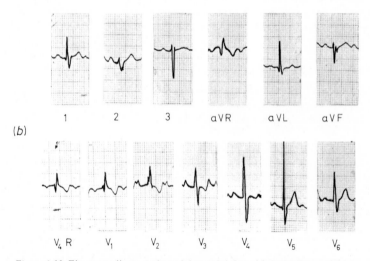

(b)

Figure 6.13. Electrocardiograms in atrial septal defect. (*a*) Ostium secundum defect. Right bundle branch block pattern and right axis deviation (+110 degrees). (*b*) Ostium primum. Right bundle branch block pattern and left axis deviation (−60 degrees) with P–R interval of 0.20 seconds which is above the normal limit for the age (3 years) of the patient

streaming, a significant rise in oxygen saturation is not evident until a ventricular sample is taken. The right ventricular and pulmonary artery pressures are normal or only slightly raised. In large shunts there may be a gradient of up to 20 mmHg across the pulmonary valve. It is thought to be due to 'functional' pulmonary stenosis associated with excessive blood flow. If the gradient is more than 20 mm, organic pulmonary valve stenosis should be suspected.

Diagnosis

Difficulty is sometimes experienced in distinguishing the systolic murmur of a small atrial septal defect from a functional murmur. The second heart sound is the best guide, for if it shows clear variation with respiration a defect large enough to warrant surgical closure can definitely be excluded.

With large defects the main problem is to exclude a more complicated lesion. Total anomalous pulmonary venous connection produces similar signs, and the degree of cyanosis may be mild enough to escape detection clinically. It is also important to exclude obstruction to the left side of the heart, or left ventricular disease, both of which increase the amount of left-to-right shunting. Certainly, if cardiac failure occurs in childhood a more complex lesion should be suspected.

Treatment

Ostium secundum defects are closed using cardiopulmonary bypass. The hole may be sutured directly or a patch used to cover it. Most cardiologists advise operation when the pulmonary to systemic flow ratio is more than 2:1. When the ratio is less they are usually left alone. The mortality rate is of the order of 1 per cent and surgery is usually recommended some time between 5 and 14 years depending on the size of the shunt and the presence of symptoms. Occasionally, the defects are closed earlier if there are severe symptoms due to a very large shunt.

Operation is not advised when there is severe pulmonary vascular disease resulting in a right-to-left or very small left-to-right shunt, but this is virtually never seen in childhood.

Complications

Paroxysmal atrial tachycardia is a recognized complication of ostium secundum atrial septal defects, but only occurs in about 5 per cent of patients. It is more common in infancy and adolescence than in the middle years of childhood.

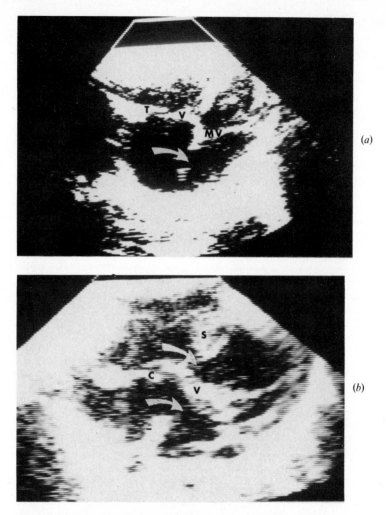

Figure 6.14(a). Ostium secundum atrial septal defect. Two-dimensional echocardiogram—subxiphoid 4-chamber view. The arrow shows the defect between the right atrium (on left of picture) and left atrium (on right of picture). The tricuspid valve (TV) is seen between the right atrium and right ventricle. The mitral valve (MV) is seen between left atrium and left ventricle. There is septal tissue forming the margin of the defect between the defect and the tricuspid and mitral valves. *(b)*. Complete atrioventricular defect. Two-dimensional echocardiogram—subxiphoid 4-chamber view. The atrial defect (lower arrow) is seen and there is no septum between the defect and the common atrioventricular valve (CV). The upper arrow points to the defect in the ventricular septum (S)

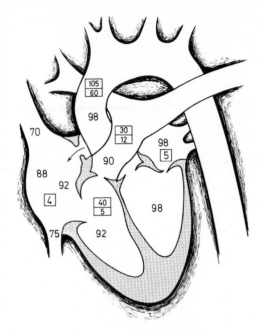

Figure 6.15. Ostium secundum defect. Pressures in
mmHg, within squares; percentage oxygen saturations,
unsquared

Atrioventricular defects

Definition

The term 'endocardial cushion defect' includes all the abnormalities
which occur due to abnormal development of the endocardial
cushions.

In the most severe form (persistent or common atrioventricular
canal) there is a large defect in the lower part of the atrial septum, a
defect in the upper part of the ventricular septum and both
atrioventricular valves are deformed (*Figure 6.16*). In the mildest
form (the ostium primum defect) there is a low atrial septal defect
above the atrioventricular valves and there is a cleft in the anterior
leaflet of the mitral valve, the tricuspid valve is normal and the
ventricular septum is intact. There are intermediate types between
these two.

Ostium primum defect

In ostium primum defect the fault is in the lower part of the atrial septum just above the atrioventricular valves. There is usually a cleft in the aortic leaflet of the mitral valve, the cusp is thickened and the cleft may be very small or extend up to the valve ring. It causes incompetence of the mitral valve. Less commonly there is cleft in the tricuspid valve as well. The ventricular septum is functionally intact, although its crest is depressed downwards (*Figure 6.16*).

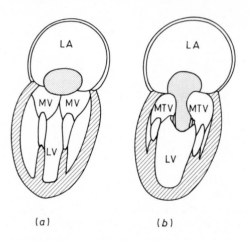

(a)   (b)

Figure 6.16. Atrioventricular canal defects. (*a*) Ostium primum. (*b*) Common atrioventricular canal. Both viewed from the left side. LA: left atrium; LV: left ventricle; MV: cleft mitral valve; MTV: common leaflets of mitral and tricuspid valves; the defect is stippled

The haemodynamic changes are similar to those of ostium secundum defects but there is mitral incompetence in addition. The degree of mitral incompetence is determined by the size of the cleft in the mitral valve; it may range from a trivial to a severe degree. The presence of mitral regurgitation increases the left-to-right shunt through the defect. If there is a cleft in the tricuspid valve there is also tricuspid regurgitation.

Natural history

The overall prognosis in patients with ostium primum defects is much worse than in those with ostium secundum defects. Patients fail to thrive and require treatment at an earlier age than those with ostium secundum defects. This is due to the effect of the associated mitral regurgitation.

Clinical presentation

If there is no significant mitral incompetence the situation is the same as with an ostium secundum defect and there are no symptoms. There is more disability, however, when mitral regurgitation is significant and half the patients have excessive dyspnoea, are easily tired and have frequent chest infections.

The patient presents as with an atrial septal defect with mitral incompetence. There is no cyanosis and the pulse is small or normal in volume. Children are often below normal size and may show a sulcus around the chest and a bulged praecordium. The heart is usually enlarged and there is increased left, as well as right, ventricular activity. The murmurs are as described in the secundum defects with the additional apical pansystolic murmur of mitral incompetence. The apical murmur is not always very obvious, however, even when there is significant mitral regurgitation.

Radiology

As in secundum defects, the right ventricle is enlarged and the pulmonary artery is prominent. There is an increased vascularity of the hilar and peripheral pulmonary vessels. The left atrium and left ventricle are also enlarged when there is a significant degree of mitral incompetence (*see Figure 6.12*). Overall, cardiomegaly is much commoner than in ostium secundum defects.

Electrocardiography

The electrocardiogram is very characteristic and helpful in making the diagnosis (*see Figure 6.13*). There is left axis deviation and evidence of hypertrophy of both ventricles. The rsR' pattern in leads V_4R and V_1 found in secundum defects, is often present, but there is usually a greater degree of right ventricular hypertrophy. The P waves may be tall due to right atrial hypertrophy but when there is considerable mitral regurgitation they are bifid due to left atrial enlargement. Splintered S waves are common in leads 2, 3 and aVF. The P–R interval is frequently prolonged.

Echocardiography

The same evidence of volume overload is shown as in secundum defects, but in addition there is usually some abnormality of the mitral valve. The anterior cusp in diastole reaches to or in front of the line of the interventricular septum and anterior aorta, and often shows a double echo due to the two portions on either side of the cleft moving differently. The 2-D echo from the subxiphoid position shows the defect most clearly (*Figure 6.17*).

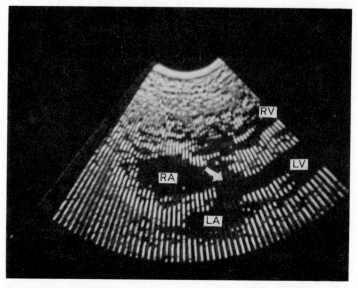

Figure 6.17. Echocardiogram of ostium primum defect (arrowed) in the septum between right atrium (RA) and left atrium (LA), in a 4 month old infant. (Subxiphoid view.)

Investigation

Cardiac catheterization shows evidence of a left-to-right shunt at atrial level; the defect is easily traversed at a low level and the left ventricle is easily entered. The pulmonary artery pressure is usually normal or only moderately raised. A left ventricular angiogram helps to assess the degree of mitral regurgitation and shows the distortion of the left ventricular outflow tract. This appearance is diagnostic of endocardial cushion defects. It is due to two factors (Macartney *et al.*, 1979). Firstly the attachment of the mitral valve is displaced towards the apex of the left ventricle and secondly the crest of the interventricular septum is depressed and the anterior cusp of the mitral valve is largely attached to it producing a scalloped edge in which the cleft is usually visible.

Treatment

Operation is required in patients with obvious symptoms or with progressive cardiac enlargement on radiography. Since these patients deteriorate more rapidly than those with ostium secundum defects, surgery is usually advised at an earlier age, at 2–3 years. The results of operation are good and the mitral valve can usually be repaired satisfactorily, leaving trivial or no incompetence. Occasionally, however, the shortness of chordae tendineae and a wide cleft makes repair impossible and mitral valve replacement is necessary. The proximity of the atrioventricular bundle to the defect resulted in a high incidence of postoperative heart block in early series, but this has not proved as common in recent years.

The overall risks of operation are higher than in patients with ostium secundum defects, partly because of the greater complexity of the operation and partly because of the risks of heart block. For this reason, surgery is not advised in patients with no symptoms and nearly normal-sized hearts.

Common atrium or single atrium

Common atrium as an isolated lesion is rare and its natural history and presentation resemble that of ostium primum defects since it is often associated with a cleft mitral valve. Mitral regurgitation is present and symptoms usually occur in infancy. Mild cyanosis is usual. Pulmonary hypertension develops early in childhood. The two atria can be separated at operation using a patch and the mitral valve repaired as in ostium primum defects. In association with abnormalities of cardiac position it is rather more common and there are then additional abnormalities of systemic and pulmonary venous drainage.

Complete atrioventricular defect

Definition

There has been much disagreement about the classification of these defects formerly referred to as endocardial cushion defects. Piccoli *et al.* (1979) have classified them into partial and complete forms. The partial form has separate mitral and tricuspid orifices. The complete form has a common atrioventricular orifice. Both the partial and complete forms may or may not be associated with an ostium primum atrial septal defect, clefts in the mitral or tricuspid valves or perimembranous inlet ventricular septal defect. The latter always occurs in the complete form. (The defect is therefore a 3-dimensional one extending in both directions within the plane of the interventricular and interatrial septa and at right-angles across the mitral and tricuspid valve rings).

Natural history

The prognosis is poor. Infants usually have repeated episodes of chest infection and cardiac failure and there is a high death rate. Of those who survive infancy, improvement may occur because of the development of pulmonary vascular disease. About one-third of patients with atrioventricular defects are mongols and atrioventricular defect is one of the commonest lesions in the 40 per cent of mongols who have congenital heart disease.

Clinical presentation

Symptoms occur in the first few weeks of life. The infants feed poorly, are slow to gain weight and are excessively breathless. Cyanosis usually occurs, but may be slight. Congestive heart failure commonly occurs in the first few months. Examination reveals a breathless, slightly cyanosed infant with a markedly enlarged heart. The pulses are normal or of small volume. There is usually evidence of pulmonary hypertension with a loud single second sound and a heaving right ventricle. There is an ejection systolic murmur over the pulmonary area and very often a tricuspid diastolic murmur due to excessive flow of blood through the tricuspid valve. There may be a pansystolic murmur at the apex due to mitral incompetence.

Radiology

There is marked cardiac enlargement with pulmonary plethora and often interstitial oedema. The left atrium is usually enlarged but may be difficult to identify in the presence of generalized cardiac enlargement.

Electrocardiography

The electrocardiogram shows left axis deviation with combined right and left ventricular hypertrophy. Deep and splintered S waves are seen in leads 2, 3 and aVF. The P–R interval is usually prolonged.

Echocardiography

The most important point is that the mitral and tricuspid echoes are superimposed in the region of the atrioventricular ring, but a septum

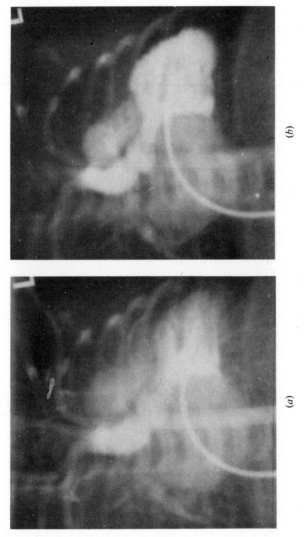

(a)
        (b)

Figure 6.18. Left ventricular angiogram of a 3-week infant with an atrioventricular canal defect. (*a*) Systole. The medial wall of the left ventricle is irregular due to the abnormal mitral valve. (*b*) Diastole. The mitral valve balloons abnormally far into the outflow region of the ventricle producing a 'goose-neck' deformity

can be demonstrated nearer the apex. This is best demonstrated by a two-dimensional technique with the transducer in the subxiphoid position (*Figure 6.14b*) (Hunter *et al.*, 1979).

Investigation

Cardiac catheterization confirms the lesions. The catheter readily flicks from one chamber to another and it is difficult to maintain it in a stable position. Blood oxygen saturations show a left-to-right shunt at atrial and ventricular levels and there is usually slight desaturation of the arterial blood due to a small right-to-left shunt. Angiography from the left ventricle shows the classic 'goose-neck' appearance of the outflow tract of the left ventricle, caused by the abnormal anterior leaflet of the mitral valve (*Figure 6.18*).

The complete nature of the defect is best shown with cineangiography in the left anterior oblique or '4-chambered view' when it is possible to demonstrate dye passing direct from left ventricle to right ventricle (Macartney *et al.*, 1979).

Treatment

Medical treatment is required first to control heart failure. This is often unsuccessful, especially when there is severe mitral regurgitation.

Total correction is now practicable in older children and possible in infants though with a high mortality. It must be carried out before pulmonary vascular disease develops. Both ventricular and atrial components of the defect need to be patched and the mitral and tricuspid valves repaired or, occasionally, replaced.

BIBLIOGRAPHY AND REFERENCES

Patent ductus arteriosus
Campbell, M (1955). Patent ductus arteriosus. Some notes on prognosis and on pulmonary hypertension. *Br. Heart J.* **17**, 511
Campbell, M (1968). Natural history of persistent ductus arteriosus. *Br. Heart J.* **30**, 4
Cosh, J. A. (1957). Patent ductus arteriosus: a follow-up study of 73 cases. *Br. Heart J.* **19**, 13
Gibson, G. A. (1900). Clinical lectures in circulatory affections. 1. Persistence of the arterial duct and its diagnosis. *Edinb. med. J.* **N.S. 8**, 1
Gittenberger-de-Groot, A. C. (1977). Persistent ductus arteriosus: most probably a primary congenital malformation. *Br. Heart J.* **40**, 610
Gittenberger-de-Groot, A. C. (1979). Patent ductus arteriosus in the newborn: histological observations. In *Paediatric Cardiology* Vol. 2. Eds M. J. Godman and R. M. Marquis. London: Churchill Livingstone
Keys, A. and Shapiro, M. J. (1943). Patency of the ductus arteriosus in adults. *Am. Heart J.* **25**, 158

Mark, H. and Young, D. (1965). Congenital heart disease in the adult. *Am. J. Cardiol.* **15**, 293

Olley, P. M. and Coceani, F. (1979). Mechanism of closure of the ductus arteriosus. pp. 15–31. In *Paediatric Cardiology* Vol. 2. Eds M. J. Godman and R. M. Marquis. London, Edinburgh and New York: Churchill Livingstone

Olley, P. M., Rowe, R. D., Freedom, R. M., Swyer, P. R. and Coceani, F. (1979). Pharmacological manipulation of the ductus arteriosus. pp. 32–44. In *Paediatric Cardiology* Vol. 2. Eds. M. J. Godman and R. M. Marquis. London, Edinburgh and New York: Churchill Livingstone

Rudolph, A. M., Mayer, F. E., Nadas, A. S. and Gross, R. E. (1958). Patent ductus arteriosus. A clinical and hemodynamic study of 23 patients in the first year of life. *Pediatrics, Springfield* **33**, 892

Wood, P. H. (1958). The Eisenmenger syndrome. *Br. med. J.* **2**, 701, 755

Ventricular septal defect

Alpert, B. S., Cook, D. H., Varghese, P. J. and Rowe, R. D. (1979). Spontaneous closure of small ventricular septal defects: ten year follow-up. *Pediatrics* **63**, 204

Anderson, R. A., Levy, A. M., Naeye, R. L. and Tabakin, B. S. (1967). Rapidly progressing pulmonary vascular obstructive disease: association with ventricular septal defects during early childhood. *Am. J. Cardiol.* **19**, 854

Blackstone, E. H., Kirklin, J. W., Bradley, E. L., Dushane, J. W. and Applebaum, A. (1976). Optimal age and results in repair of large ventricular septal defects. *J. thorac. cardiovasc. Surg.* **72**, 661

Bloomfield, D. K. (1964). The natural history of ventricular septal defect in patients surviving infancy. *Circulation* **29**, 914

Campbell, M. (1971). Natural history of ventricular septal defect. *Br. Heart J.* **33**, 246

Clarkson, P. M., Frye, R. L., Dushane, J. W., Burchell, H. B., Wood, E. H. and Weidman, W. H. (1968). Prognosis for patients with ventricular septal defect and severe pulmonary vascular obstructive disease. *Circulation* **38**, 129

Freedom, R. M., White, R. D., Pieroni, D. R., Varghese, P. J., Krovetz, L. J. and Rowe, R. D. (1974). The natural history of the so-called aneurysm of the membranous ventricular septum in childhood. *Circulation* **49**, 375

Gasul, B. M., Dillon, R. F., Vrla, V. and Hait, G. (1957). Ventricular septal defects; their natural transformation into those with infundibular stenosis or into cyanotic or noncyanotic type of tetralogy of Fallot. *J. Am. med. Ass.* **164**, 847

Glancy, D. L. and Roberts, W. C. (1967). Complete spontaneous closure of ventricular septal defect. *Am. J. Med.* **43**, 846

Hallidie-Smith, K. A., Holman, A., Cleland, W. P., Beltall, H. H. and Goodwin, J. (1969). Effects of surgical closure of ventricular septal defects upon pulmonary vascular disease. *Br. Heart J.* **31**, 246

Hallidie-Smith, K. A., Wilson, R. S. E., Hart, A. and Zeidfard, E. (1977). Functional studies of patients with large ventricular septal defects and pulmonary vascular disease 6 to 16 years after surgical closure of their defect in childhood. *Br. Heart J.* **40**, 1093

Henry, J. G., Kaplan, J., Helmsworth, J. A. and Schrieber, J. T. (1970). Management of infants with large ventricular septal defects. *Am. J. Cardiol.* **26**, 637

Hoffman, J. I. E. and Rudolf, A. M. (1965). The natural history of ventricular septal defects in infancy. *Am. J. Cardiol.* **16**, 634

Horiuchi, T. Koyamada, K., Matano, I., Mohri and co-workers (1963). Radical operation for ventricular septal defect in infancy. *J. thorac. cardiovasc. Surg.* **46**, 180.

Kidd, L., Rose, V., Collins G. and Keith, J. (1965). Ventricular septal defect in infancy. *Am. Heart J.* **69**, 4

Kidd, L., Rose, V., Collins, G. and Keith, J. (1965). The haemodynamics in ventricular septal defect in childhood. *Am. Heart J.* **70**, 732

Lambert, M. E., Widlansky, E., Franken, E. A., Hurwitz, R., Nielson, R. and Nasser, W. K. (1974). Natural history of ventricular septal defects associated with ventricular septal aneurysm. *Am. Heart J.* **88**, 566

McNicholas, K., de Leval, M., Stark, J., Taylor, J. F. N. and Macartney, F. J. (1979). Surgical treatment of ventricular septal defect in infancy. Primary repair versus banding of pulmonary artery and later repair. *Br. Heart J.* **41**, 133

Moss, A. J. (1970). The conquest of ventricular septal defect – a period of uncertainty. *Am. J. Cardiol.* **25**, 457

Sapire, D. W. and Black, I. F. S. (1975). Echocardiographic detection of aneurysm of the interventricular septum associated with ventricular septal defect. A method of non-invasive diagnosis and follow-up. *Am. J. Cardiol.* **36**, 797

Varghese, P. J., Allen, J. R., Rosenquist, G. C. and Rowe, R. D. (1970). Natural history of ventricular septal defect with right sided aortic arch. *Br. Heart J.* **32**, 537

Vogen, J. H. K., McNamara, D. G. and Blount, S. G. Jr. (1967). The role of hypoxia in determining pulmonary vascular resistance in infants with ventricular septal defects. *Am. J. Cardiol.* **20**, 346

Ventricular septal defect with aortic regurgitation

Somerville, J., Brandao, A. and Ross, D. N. (1970). Aortic regurgitation and ventricular septal defect. Surgical management and clinical features. *Circulation* **41**, 311

Atrial septal defects

Baron, M. G., Wolf, B. S., Steinfeld, L. and Van Mierop, L. H. S. (1964). Endocardial cushion defects – specific diagnosis by angiocardiography. *Am. J. Cardiol.* **13**, 162

Craig, R. J. and Selzer, A. (1968). Natural history and prognosis of atrial septal defect. *Circulation* **37**, 805

Griffiths, S. P., Ellis, K., Burris, J. O., Bumenthal, S., Bowman, F. O. and Malm, J. R. (1969). Postoperative evaluation of mitral valve function in ostium primum defect with cleft mitral valve (partial form of atrioventricular canal). *Circulation* **40**, 21

Mueller, T. M., Kerber, R. E. and Marcus, M. L. (1978). Comparison of interventricular septal motion studied by ventriculography and echocardiographically in patients with atrial septal defect. *Br. Heart J.* **40**, 984.

Rahimtoola, S. H., Kirklin, J. W. and Burchell, H. B. (1968). Atrial septal defect. *Circulation* **37**, Suppl. 5, 2

Atrioventricular defects

Macartney, F. J., Ress, P. G., Daly, K., Piccoli, G. P., Taylor, J. F. N., de Laval, M. R., Stark, J. and Anderson, R. H. (1979). Angiographic appearances of atrioventricular defects with particular reference to distinction of ostium primum atrial septal defect from common atrioventricular orifice. *Br. Heart J.* **42**, 640

Piccoli, G. P., Gerlis, L. M., Wilkinson, J. L., Lozsadi, K., Macartney, F. J. and Anderson, R. H. (1979). Morphology and classification of atrioventricular defects. *Br. Heart J.* **42**, 621

Piccoli, G. P., Wilkinson J. L., Macartney, F. J., Gerlis, L. M. and Anderson, R. H. (1979). Morphology and classification of complete atrioventricular defects. *Br. Heart J.* **42**, 633

Pieroni, D. R., Homcy, E. and Freedom, R. M. (1975). Echocardiography in atrioventricular canal defect. A clinical spectrum. *Am. J. Cardiol.* **35**, 54

Somerville, J. and Jefferson, K. (1968). Left ventricular angiography in atrioventricular defects. *Br. Heart J.* **30**, 446

CHAPTER 7

Acyanotic Lesions with Left Heart Abnormalities

AORTIC VALVE STENOSIS

Incidence

Isolated aortic stenosis accounts for 5 per cent of all congenital heart disease. Congenital bicuspid valves probably account for a rather larger number of cases, although they are not diagnosed in childhood since they may function normally early in life with only a soft systolic murmur, and become stenotic in adult life and may then be difficult to differentiate from acquired aortic stenosis. Aortic stenosis may occur with coarctation of the aorta and patent ductus arteriosus.

Definition

There is obstruction to flow of blood from the left ventricle. The deformity of the aortic valve is variable (*Figure 7.1*); at times all three cusps may be fused and at other times two cusps are fused. The opening in the valve is often eccentric. Some degree of aortic regurgitation often exists with the stenosis.

Natural history

Campbell's study (1968) shows that there is a mortality of 1.2 per cent per annum during the first two decades. This rises to 3.0, 3.5, 6.0 and 8.5 per cent per annum in the third, fourth, fifth and sixth

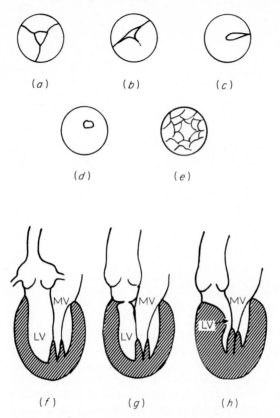

Figure 7.1. Types of aortic obstruction. (*a*) to (*e*) are types of valvar stenosis: (*a*) tricuspid; (*b*) bicuspid; (*c*) unicuspid; (*d*) non-cusped; and (*e*) myxomatous. (*f*) Supravalvar stenosis. (*g*) Discrete subaortic stenosis. (*h*) Hypertrophic obstructive cardiomyopathy. LV: left ventricle; MV: mitral valve

decades respectively; 60 per cent of patients are dead by the age of 40 years. Campbell's study, however, did not include infants, in whom heart failure may occur in the first few weeks of life. If the lesion is not recognized and treated in these severe cases, the patients will die. The mortality of untreated aortic stenosis in infants with symptoms is probably about 50 per cent. The risk of sudden death is at least 0.4 per cent per annum in the first three decades; that is, 12 per cent of patients will die before they are 30 years old. Glew and co-workers (1969), however, had only 8 cases of sudden death (1 per cent of their patients, seen over 20 years) and all had either symptoms or electrocardiographic changes. Bacterial endocarditis occurs in about 1 per cent per annum. Although this can be cured, it may cause progressive aortic regurgitation. Hossack *et al.* (1980) followed 218 patients under the age of 25 for periods up to 25 years. They found good correlation between clinical and ECG signs of severity and the presence of a gradient of 80 mmHg or more at catheterization. Six developed significant regurgitation, four as a result of infective endocarditis.

Children who present with mild aortic stenosis early in life may deteriorate as the stenosis becomes more critical with growth, or when calcification occurs on the valve in later life.

Clinical presentation

Severe aortic stenosis may be seen in infancy, when it causes heart failure or sudden death (Scott and Feldman, 1964). In older children the heart murmur is discovered at a routine examination and few have any symptoms. When symptoms do occur they are breathlessness, substernal pain on effort and syncope or dizziness on effort.

The patient is acyanotic and the pulse is usually normal in character except in severe stenosis when the characteristic small volume pulse is felt. Severe stenosis can, however, exist with a normal pulse. There is forceful pulsation of the left ventricle and in moderate and severe stenosis there may be a presystolic impulse at the cardiac apex, due to forceful atrial contraction filling the ventricle. In children, a systolic thrill may not be felt at the base of the heart but is obvious in the suprasternal notch and over the carotid vessels. If a thrill is not palpable the obstruction is usually mild. The systolic murmur is ejection in type and is best heard in the aortic area, but is also loud at the cardiac apex. It is well conducted up into the neck over the carotid arteries. When the aortic valve is mobile the murmur is preceded by an ejection click, usually best heard at the apex during expiration. The more severe the stenosis, the closer the ejection click becomes to the first sound, because the rapid rise of pressure in the left ventricle opens the aortic valve soon after the mitral valve has closed. The second heart sound is normal in mild stenosis but in severe stenosis it may be single due to prolonged left ventricular systole and the aortic element occurring late. In very severe stenosis the aortic closure sound may occur after the pulmonary closure and this results in paradoxical splitting with respiration.

Radiology

The overall heart size is usually normal but there may be rounding of the apex due to thickening of the left ventricle. The ascending aorta commonly shows poststenotic dilation. In very severe obstruction the left ventricle may enlarge and there may be a prominent left atrium.

Electrocardiography

When the electrocardiogram shows evidence of left ventricular hypertrophy and strain the aortic stenosis is severe. On the other hand, severe aortic stenosis may exist in the presence of a normal electrocardiogram. The presence of symptoms or clinical evidence of severe aortic stenosis are more reliable than the electrocardiogram.

In severe stenosis the P waves in lead 2 are broad and bifid. In moderate stenosis the QRS axis in the standard leads is normal but there is increased voltage of the R wave in all standard leads and the precordial leads V_5 and V_6 which are over the left ventricle. In severe stenosis the electrical axis is directed more posteriorly and there are deep S waves in the anterior chest leads V_2 and V_3. As the disease increases in severity the T waves in V_5 and V_6 become flattened and then inverted, and the QRS duration may be increased (*Figure 4.8*).

Echocardiography

When the valve is thick and rigid this is reflected in the echo which shows multiple echoes in diastole and poor systolic opening (*Figure 7.2*). However a mobile, but severely stenotic valve may show an apparently normal opening movement if the echo beam is directed across the cusps near the aortic root. Bicuspid valves usually show eccentric closure in diastole (*Figure 7.2*). The degree of left ventricular hypertrophy can be accurately assessed (*Figure 7.2*) and this is useful in longitudinal studies pre- and postoperatively. Two-dimensional studies are usually more accurate in predicting the nature of the valve stenosis as it is possible to scan up and down the valve.

Investigation

The gradient across the aortic valve should always be measured if the patient has symptoms, if the electrocardiogram shows severe left ventricular hypertrophy or shows progressive changes, or if clinically

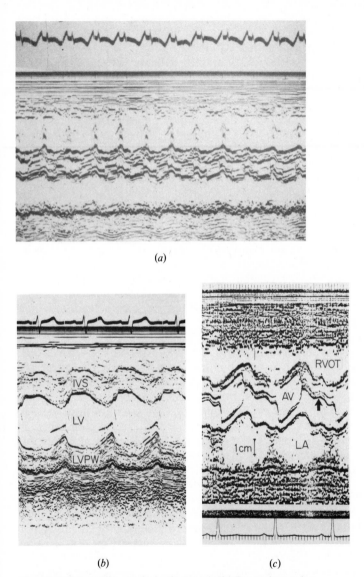

Figure 7.2. Echocardiogram in aortic stenosis. (*a*) Eccentric opening and multiple echoes in diastole. (*b*) Left ventricular hypertrophy involving septum (IVS) and posterior wall (LVPW). (*c*) Eccentric closure but normal opening in bicuspid aortic valve

the lesion seems severe. The gradient is usually measured in children by passing a catheter in a retrograde manner through an artery and into the left ventricle, or by puncturing the atrial septum from the right side to enter the left atrium and left ventricle. The gradient may vary from 60 to 120 mmHg in patients with severe stenosis (*Figure 7.3*). The gradient depends on the stroke volume of the heart as well as the severity of the stenosis. The gradient is related to the square of the stroke output of the left ventricle, which means that if the output is doubled the gradient is quadrupled. Ideally the cardiac output should be measured as well as the gradient. In severe stenosis the left atrial pressure wave produced by atrial systole is increased.

Radio-opaque dye injected into the left ventricle shows the size of its cavity and the thickness of the wall. It provides information about the thickness of the valve and the mobility of the valve leaflets.

Treatment

Patients who, on clinical or electrocardiographic grounds, have more than trivial aortic stenosis should not be allowed to take part in *competitive* athletics, swimming or football. If there is doubt, it is wise to suspend these activities until echocardiography or cardiac catheterization has been performed. Severe exertion leads to severe left ventricular hypertrophy and a 'muscle-bound' ventricle, and carries a definite risk of sudden death.

Infants who present with heart failure should be regarded as emergencies and investigated immediately with a view to operation. Satisfactory results can be obtained now that cardiopulmonary bypass is possible in small infants. The operative mortality in this group is in the region of 10–20 per cent, but in some of these there is associated endocardial fibroelastosis.

Operation is advised when the peak systolic gradient across the aortic valve exceeds 70 mmHg in the presence of a normal cardiac output. The gradient may increase as the patient grows and it may need to be measured again when the patient is older. Operation is performed using cardiopulmonary bypass and the aorta is opened just above the valve. The valve is often thickened and irregular and it is difficult to relieve the stenosis completely without producing some degree of regurgitation. The surgeon therefore incises the valve just sufficiently to convert the severe stenosis to a mild or moderate one. Shackleton and co-workers (1972) found that, following surgery, both residual obstruction and excessive regurgitation were responsible for deterioration. Parents must be warned that a further operation, with valve replacement, may be necessary later in life. The mortality of operation at present is of the order of 1–2 per cent.

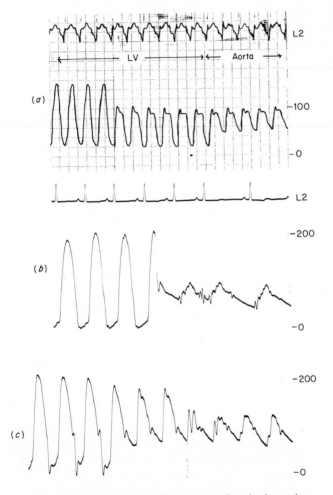

Figure 7.3. Pressure gradients in different types of aortic obstruction demonstrated by withdrawing a catheter from the left ventricle into the aorta. (*a*) Hypertrophic obstructive cardiomyopathy in a 3-month-old infant. The gradient is within the ventricle and the aortic pressure shows a rapid upstroke. (*b*) Aortic valve stenosis in a 10-year-old boy. (*c*) Supra-aortic stenosis in a 4-year-old girl who had facies of infantile hypercalcaemia and also multiple pulmonary artery stenosis

Aortic valve replacement

Aortic valve replacement is usually impracticable under the age of five years, due simply to the limited size of the aorta. In older children there are two fundamental problems: firstly that any implanted valve, tissue or prosthetic, will fail to grow with the patient; secondly that all valves available commercially have an effective orifice less than their overall diameter and are therefore to various degrees stenotic. The surrounding flange is the same size for all sizes of valve and there is therefore a critical diameter below which there is effectively no room for a central orifice. Homograft or heterograft valves without a stent (or frame) are free of this disadvantage, but tend to become rigid and calcify, particularly in small children. Additionally the valve ring in severe congenital aortic stenosis is often hypoplastic, and to overcome this problem Somerville and Ross (1977) have advocated excising the valve and valve ring and inserting a gusset between the mitral valve and interventricular septum, enlarging the whole left ventricular outflow. A homograft valve of suitable size is then inserted.

Prosthetic valves of the Starr–Edwards and Björk–Shiley types, which work well in adults, have the additional disadvantage of requiring permanent anticoagulants, and are rarely used in children.

A simple valve replacement in a child of 10 years upwards is a relatively safe operation with a mortality of about 1–2 per cent. However, the poor function of small valves and doubts as to the longterm life of tissue valves (currently estimated at 10–12 years) still mean that a palliative procedure is often preferable to valve replacement.

Bacterial endocarditis

Bacterial endocarditis is a particularly important complication of aortic valve disease, for it can convert trivial aortic stenosis into gross aortic reflux. Strict dental hygiene needs to be advised and full antibiotic cover is required for dental extractions or other operations. This applies equally after any surgery on the valve.

AORTIC REGURGITATION

Incidence

Aortic regurgitation occurs both as a congenital lesion and as a result of acute rheumatic fever. Occasionally it is produced by acute bacterial endocarditis on a previously normal valve, and subacute bacterial endocarditis can convert a slightly stenotic bicuspid aortic valve into a freely regurgitant one. At present congenital aortic regurgitation is rather more common than the acquired forms in childhood. Several of our patients have had a family history of a similar abnormality. In the congenital form the lesion is only about one-tenth as common as aortic stenosis.

Definition

Severe regurgitation occurs as a result of rolling up and rigidity of the cusps or from weakness and prolapse of one or more cusps. It also occurs in association with aneurysms of the sinuses of Valsalva, and with high ventricular septal defects which extend into the fibrous ring of the aortic valve and weaken it. Marfan's syndrome is associated with dilatation of the aorta and aortic regurgitation due to prolapse of valve cusps.

Clinical presentation

Severe aortic regurgitation may present with heart failure in infancy or with breathlessness in older children. Most patients, however, are asymptomatic and are referred because a murmur has been heard on routine examination. The pulses are of large volume or collapsing if the regurgitation is severe, capillary pulsation is visible in the fingers and the muscle of arms and legs are felt to pulsate. The blood pressure shows a high systolic and a low diastolic pressure. The left ventricle is palpably enlarged and hyperdynamic. As well as the characteristic early diastolic murmur heard at the aortic area and left sternal border, there is usually also a systolic murmur due to the high stroke output. Occasionally a short, mid-diastolic (Austin Flint) murmur is heard at the apex. This has been shown by echocardiography to be due to fluttering of the anterior cusp of the mitral valve due to the combined effects of the regurgitant jet on one side and the normal flow through the mitral valve on the other. In addition the rapid rise in pressure in the left ventricle in diastole may close the mitral valve prematurely so that flow is restricted to the early part of diastole, and has therefore to be more rapid than normal.

In mild aortic regurgitation the only abnormality is the soft, early diastolic murmur normally best heard in the 3rd left intercostal space.

Radiology

In moderate or severe regurgitation the left ventricle is enlarged. Owing to the large stroke volume there is a considerable difference in the size of the heart in different parts of the cardiac cycle. Single films are therefore unreliable, but screening the heart gives a better idea of its size.

Electrocardiography

The electrocardiogram shows left ventricular hypertrophy of a degree commensurate with the degree of regurgitation.

Echocardiography

The fluttering of the anterior mitral valve cusp and, in severe regurgitation, its early closure, can be demonstrated. The LV cavity is enlarged and calculation of the stroke volume gives a good indication of the severity of the regurgitation. Contractility is usually normal. Sometimes the prolapse of aortic cusps can be shown, particularly with two-dimensional scans.

Investigation

The diagnosis can be made clinically with a fair degree of accuracy. Cardiac catheterization is indicated in infants with symptoms to distinguish it from other lesions which may be more readily amenable to surgery. In older children catheterization should be reserved for those with severe or progressive symptoms in whom operation is contemplated. The important investigation is an aortogram, which reveals the extent of the reflux and something of the pathology of the valve.

Treatment

In infancy, if there are symptoms, digoxin and diuretics are indicated, but it is doubtful whether surgical exploration is indicated since the chances of the valve being repairable are remote. In older children attempts to repair the valve by various techniques may prove moderately successful, but in general the results have been disappointing, and replacement by a homograft or prosthesis is now favoured (*see* p. 118). In view of the uncertain life of both homografts and prosthetic valves, operation is clearly reserved for patients with severe or progressive symptoms.

SUPRAVALVULAR STENOSIS

There is a diffuse or localized narrowing of the aorta above the valve in supravalvular stenosis. Although this lesion may occur sporadically, it is usually either familial or associated with some of the features of the hypercalcaemic syndrome (*see* p. 350). The clinical presentation is similar to that of aortic valve stenosis, but there is no ejection click and no poststenotic dilatation on the chest radiograph. The electrocardiogram shows left ventricular hypertrophy.

The site of the pressure gradient is shown by retrograde aortic catheterization (*see Figure 7.3*) and aortography demonstrates the narrowing which may be just above the coronary arteries (which are often dilated) or extend up to the arch of the aorta (*see Figure 7.1.*). Operation is advised when the patient has symptoms or the narrowing is localized and there is a gradient of 70 mmHg or more across it. The narrowed area is enlarged by placing a gusset of Dacron across it using cardiopulmonary bypass. Peripheral pulmonary artery stenosis may occur in association with supravalvular stenosis.

SUBAORTIC STENOSIS

Incidence

Discrete subaortic stenosis is much less common than aortic valve stenosis. Its incidence is about 0.3 per cent of all congenital heart disease.

Definition

The obstruction is fibrous and takes the form of a diaphragm. It is usually attached to the anterior cusp of the mitral valve and to the membranous portion of the interventricular septum. It is in close proximity to the main atrioventricular bundle and its left branch (*see Figure 7.1*).

Clinical presentation

As in aortic valve stenosis, the murmur is often discovered at a routine examination. The signs are the same as those of aortic valve stenosis except that an ejection click is not heard. As well as the systolic ejection murmur a faint and early diastolic murmur is often heard. This is probably due to regurgitation from the aortic valve. The aortic valve cusps become thickened as a result of the jet effect of blood coming through the subvalvular obstruction and there is a high risk of bacterial endocarditis in this lesion.

Electrocardiography

The electrocardiogram is the same as in aortic valve stenosis.

Radiology

The chest X-ray shows evidence of left ventricular hypertrophy, but there is no poststenotic dilatation of the ascending aorta.

Echocardiography

The distinction between valvar and subvalvar aortic stenosis can usually be made by echocardiography. Sometimes the obstruction can be seen on the M-mode echo as an additional echo between the anterior mitral valve leaflet and the septum (*Figure 7.4a*). This is seen better with a two-dimensional scan. The particular diagnostic feature however is in the tracing from the aortic valve. One or both cusps show that, immediately after the initial opening movement, the cusp closes again (*Figure 7.4b*). This is due to the fact that the subvalvar stenosis directs a jet towards one cusp and therefore allows the other ones to close. The degree of left ventricular hypertrophy can also be assessed.

Cardiac catheterization

The presence of a gradient within the left ventricle is clearly shown as the catheter is withdrawn to the aorta from the left ventricle (*see Figure 7.3*). The stenosis is also shown by angiography.

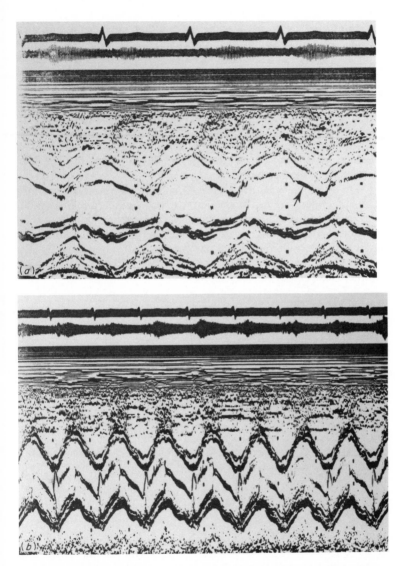

Figure 7.4. Echocardiogram from a patient with discrete subaortic stenosis. (*a*) Echo (arrowed) between mitral valve and septum due to the diaphragm. (*b*) Early systolic closure of aortic valve

Treatment

Since the diaphragm can be excised without interfering with the normal aortic valve a cure can be effected. However, the relationship of the diaphragm to the interventricular septum indicates that care is required to avoid producing an interventricular or left-ventricle-to-right-atrial tear.

The stenosis is also intimately related to the mitral valve, which may also be damaged. Sometimes the mitral valve itself may be abnormal, stenotic or regurgitant, and the only way to treat the condition satisfactorily is then to excise the mitral valve and replace it with a heterograft or prosthesis. The development of complete heart block is another hazard.

Even if the patient avoids these complications, the longterm results of surgery are not always satisfactory. Somerville, Stone and Ross (1980) found evidence of functional obstruction similar to that in hypertrophic obstructive cardiomyopathy, or poor left ventricular function in almost two-thirds of patients studied postoperatively. To some extent this may be preventable by earlier operation and complete excision of the stenosis.

MUSCULAR SUBAORTIC STENOSIS

(*See* Hypertrophic obstructive cardiomyopathy, p. 327.)

COARCTATION OF THE AORTA

Incidence

Coarctation accounts for about 7 per cent of all cases of congenital heart disease.

Definition

There have been many attempts to classify coarctation and describe its pathogenesis. These have been reviewed by Ho and Anderson (1979). The term coarctation is used to describe a localized constriction of the aorta, almost always in the region where the ductus joins it — juxtaductal coarctation. This would have been described as postductal coarctation in the past. A diffuse narrowing of the isthmus proximal to the ductus is described as tubular isthmal hypoplasia. It frequently coexists with juxtaductal coarctation and may be found with a large ductus arteriosus filling the descending aorta. This would correspond to the older term of 'preductal coarctation'. It is the type frequently found with other intracardiac abnormalities, such as large VSD or primitive ventricle. The rare condition in which there is an extreme narrowing of the aortic arch proximal to the left subclavian artery is described as coarctation of the aortic arch.

Developmental anatomy and physiology

It is now well established that juxtaductal coarctation is caused by spread of the specialized ductal tissue into the adjacent aorta, forming a sling around the aorta (Ho and Anderson, 1979). It is probable that this results from displacement of the junction of the isthmus proximally (*Figure 7.5*). After birth, the ductus closes and the aorta is constricted. Since the closure initially involves only the centre of the ductus, there is a short period during which blood can still flow relatively easily from the isthmus into the descending aorta,

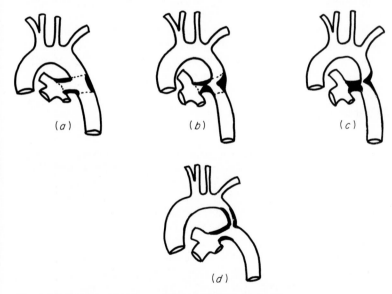

Figure 7.5. Development of coarctation. (*a*) Prior to birth. (*b*) Immediately following closure of ductus. (*c*) Obliteration of the aortic end of the ductus leads to further obstruction. (*d*) Tubular hypoplasia of the isthmus. The contractile tissue, normally confined to the ductus, is shown in solid black

but as this closes (*Figure 7.5*), the constriction becomes almost complete. This process may take up to a few weeks and this allows the left ventricle to adapt gradually to the increasing load and also for the development of collaterals, so that symptoms may not occur. If, however, the narrowing develops rapidly, severe consequences—cardiac failure and oliguria—result.

Associated conditions

About two-thirds of patients with coarctation have other lesions of which aortic stenosis and ventricular septal defect are the commonest. Mitral valve abnormalities also occur. Additionally many babies with coarctation seen in the neonatal period, have a patent ductus arteriosus.

Natural history

About half of patients with isolated coarctation and most of those with ventricular septal defect, aortic stenosis and more complex lesions present with severe symptoms in the first week or two of life. Few will survive without appropriate treatment. The other half survive infancy without symptoms, but Campbell (1970) estimated that 50 per cent of those would be dead by the age of 32 years and 75 per cent by 46 years.

Clinical presentation

IN THE NEWBORN INFANT

When symptoms occur in the neonatal period, they are frequently dramatic. An infant who has been well for the first few days of life, is suddenly found to be breathless with poor peripheral circulation and a large liver. Oliguria or anuria often ensues. Usually it is possible to determine that the brachial pulses are palpable and the femoral pulses not, but sometimes the overall cardiac output is so poor that even the brachial pulses cannot be easily felt. Sometimes the strength of the femoral pulses varies from hour to hour, either because the ductus is opening and closing or, when the ductus is widely patent, reflecting the varying pressures in the pulmonary artery. In other cases the infant becomes breathless on feeding, starts to cough (due to pulmonary oedema) and the liver becomes enlarged. The classic finding of strong brachial pulses with absent or much diminished femoral pulses, is then easily demonstrated. The blood pressure should be taken in both arms to avoid missing the rare coarctation above the left subclavian artery. It must be stressed that in a normal newborn, using the Doppler technique, the systolic pressure in the arms is often 20 mm higher than in the legs, presumably due to some isthmal narrowing. There are usually no heart murmurs audible or a soft systolic murmur may be heard in the pulmonary area.

Radiography

Chest X-ray shows moderate cardiomegaly and pulmonary venous congestion.

Electrocardiography

In the newborn, right ventricular hypertrophy is commonly seen on the cardiography.

Echocardiography

It is difficult to demonstrate the coarctation by conventional techniques, but two-dimensional scanning from the suprasternal notch has been used. The main use has been in demonstrating abnormalities of mitral and aortic valves and the hypoplastic or poorly functioning left ventricle which may be associated.

Investigation

This is a matter of urgency. Catheterization with angiocardiography is necessary to show the coarctation and the size of the aorta. Critically ill infants require resuscitation first. Prostaglandins may be given (p. 173) to keep the ductus open, if possible, to perfuse the lower half of the body. Acidosis must be corrected and hypothermia avoided. Hypoglycaemia and hypocalcaemia are also treated. Dopamine (as used in persistent fetal circulations, p. 257) will improve perfusion of the kidneys and the baby will begin to pass urine. Diuretics can then be given to reduce the fluid overload.

Treatment

There was a tendency in the past to treat these babies medically but the results of surgery have improved considerably and most of them are referred for operation. The babies are resuscitated as above and if necessary ventilated and they are then in a much better condition before operation begins. Where the aorta above the coarctation is narrow, as is usual when operation is required in infancy, a better longterm result can be obtained by a modified operation (Hamilton *et al.*, 1978). The aorta is incised longitudinally across the coarctation and the incision extended up into the left subclavian artery which is then ligated and divided (*Figure 7.6*). The coarctation is excised within the aortic lumen and the subclavian flap brought down as a gusset. This not only enlarges the size of the aortic lumen but also leaves an elongated, rather than circumferential scar, so that there is less tendency for a stricture to redevelop with the growth of the child.

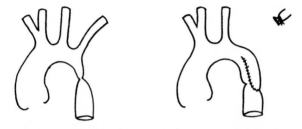

Figure 7.6. Subclavian flap operation for coarctation (*see* text)

The management of any associated ventricular septal defect is the same as that of a simple ventricular septal defect. If the defect is large enough to give equal pressure in pulmonary artery and aorta and a large left-to-right shunt, it may be wise to band the pulmonary artery at the same time as operating on the coarctation. Smaller defects take a favourable course in the postoperative period and if they do not, direct closure may be carried out later.

IN OLDER CHILDREN

In patients who do not have symptoms in infancy, the diagnosis is usually made at a routine medical examination. Headaches, pain in the legs and frequent nosebleeds are described by some authors in children with coarctation, but we have not been convinced that they occur any more frequently than in normal children.

The classic sign, which establishes the diagnosis of coarctation is that the femoral pulses are absent or very weak in the presence of normal or increased brachial pulses. Delayed, but easily palpable femoral pulses are seen only when there are extensive collateral vessels allowing filling of the lower segment and are rarely seen in childhood. The blood pressure in the right arm will usually be raised. It is however important to compare the two brachial pulses and pressures. An absent or diminished left brachial pulse indicates that there may be a coarctation at the site of origin of this vessel or proximally in the aortic arch, and such patients definitely require angiography before surgery. From the age of about four years, it is usually possible to feel collateral vessels around the lower edge of the scapulae and in the adjacent intercostal spaces, but, since most patients have been operated on by this age, this sign has become something of a rarity. Similarly, palpable left ventricular hypertrophy is seen mainly in older children where the diagnosis has been missed. If the coarctation is not associated with other lesions, there are no significant murmurs over the praecordium but a soft interscapular murmur. Failure to hear such a murmur in a patient with otherwise classic signs of coarctation, suggests there may be a large atretic segment and indicates the need for preoperative angiography.

Examination should also include a search for signs of associated abnormalities.

The murmur of ventricular septal defect is usually obvious, but the ejection click and soft systolic murmur of a biscuspid aortic valve less so. Mitral regurgitation or stenosis are also associated lesions.

Radiology

The heart may appear normal, but left ventricular enlargement is frequently seen. In severe cases the left atrium is prominent. In an overpenetrated posteroanterior film the aorta assumes a figure 3 shape, the first bulge being the aorta above the coarctation and the second bulge the poststenotic dilatation. The barium-filled oesophagus is similarly indented to give a reverse-3 pattern. In older children and adults notching of the ribs by the collateral vessels is evident. This is rarely seen before 6 years of age (*Figure 7.7*).

Electrocardiography

The electrocardiogram may be normal or show left ventricular hypertrophy, depending on the severity of the lesion. Severe left

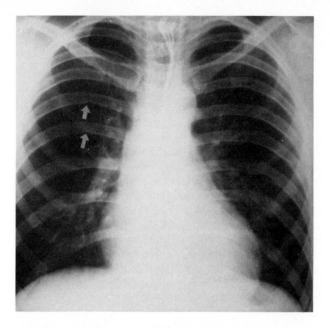

Figure 7.7. Chest radiograph of a patient with coarctation of the aorta, showing left ventricular enlargement and notching of the ribs (arrowed)

ventricular hypertrophy with inverted T waves over V_5 and V_6 is rare in childhood and its presence usually means that there is an additional lesion such as aortic stenosis. A right bundle branch block pattern is sometimes seen.

Investigation

Investigation is required to exclude additional lesions if these are suspected, but where a simple coarctation alone is diagnosed surgery may be recommended without further investigation. The aorta is best shown by retrograde aortography, but if there is no other lesion a pulmonary artery angiogram shows the coarctation well when the dye reaches the systemic circulation. If the interatrial septum is patent a left ventricular angiogram demonstrates the lesion (*Figure 7.8*).

Treatment

In children who are symptom-free and in whom the coarctation is discovered as an incidental finding, no medical treatment is required

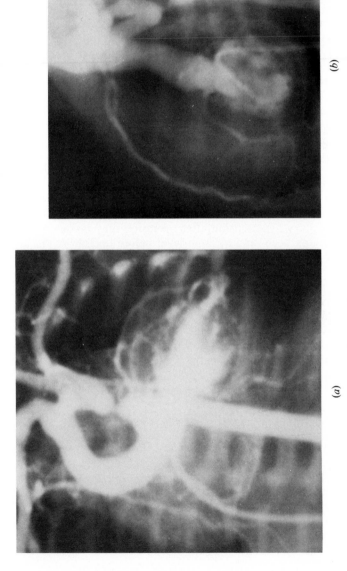

Figure 7.8. Angiogram of coarctation. The catheter has been passed across the foramen ovale and into the left ventricle. Although this is from a 4-week-old infant the coarctation is of the 'adult' type since there is a localized narrowing and the ductus arteriosus is not patent. (*a*) Anteroposterior and (*b*) left lateral views

and the child should be allowed to live a normal life. Advice should be given regarding prophylaxis against bacterial endarteritis.

The tendency nowadays is to operate on coarctation when it is diagnosed. Follow-up studies have shown that if a patient is left with systemic hypertension for some years, then it will not return to normal in some patients even after successful surgery (Nauton and Olley, 1976). Now that the subclavian flap operation is available or a Gor-Tex tube may be used across the coarctation if it is long, then there is no reason to delay surgery. Some patients may require a repeat operation but it is better to accept that than leave the patient to develop irreversible hypertension.

The mortality of operation if performed at 3 or 4 years is about 1 per cent. Reactive hypertension may occur within 36 hours of surgery in a few patients and this usually responds well to treatment with antihypertensive drugs for a few days. In some patients, however, the hypertension comes on three or four days after operation and is then accompanied by abdominal pain, nausea and vomiting. Abdominal distension occurs and symptoms may persist for one to three weeks. It is often difficult to control the hypertension with drugs but it gradually subsides. Laparotomy is best avoided unless perforation of a viscus is suspected.

The temporary hypertension after operation may be due to the pressure having been set at a high level before operation and an attempt by the body to maintain that high level after operation. The risks of surgery are increased by aneurysm of the aorta below the coarctation and by bacterial endarteritis. Surgery will not prevent bacterial endocarditis when a bicuspid aortic valve occurs as an associated lesion. Since minimal aortic valve disease may be difficult to diagnose clinically it is advisable to continue to observe precautions against bacterial endocarditis in all patients following resection of the coarctation.

AORTIC RING

In the course of development of the great arteries, the only primitive aortic arch which remains complete is the fourth left arch, which forms the definitive aortic arch. Occasionally, only the right fourth arch remains, this occurring particularly in association with Fallot's tetralogy. Functionally it is of no significance. Very rarely, both left and right fourth arches persist and a vascular ring then encircles the trachea and oesophagus, leading to stridor and difficulty in swallowing in early infancy. There are no abnormal signs in the cardiovascular system, but good radiographs of the chest show compression of the trachea and a barium swallow shows compression of oesophagus. These findings can be confirmed by oesophagoscopy and laryngoscopy. Angiography is required to show which of the arches is the larger (*Figure 7.9*), and the opposite arch is divided at thoracotomy.

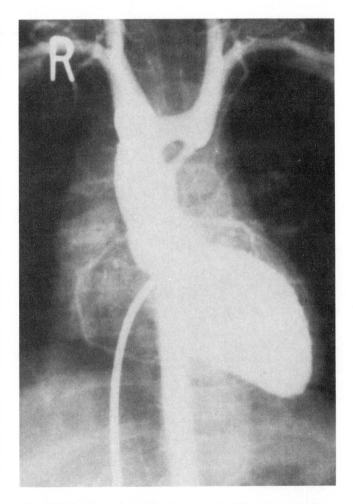

Figure 7.9. Double aortic arch. In this patient the left arch is, unusually, much smaller then the right

ANOMALOUS RIGHT SUBCLAVIAN OR INNOMINATE ARTERIES

Atrophy of the proximal rather than the distal portion of the right fourth aortic arch results in a right subclavian artery (less commonly an innominate artery) which arises from the descending aorta and passes behind the oesophagus or between the oesophagus and trachea. Stridor may occur during childhood, and in later life mild dysphagia may occur. Occasionally, a continuous murmur is produced. Otherwise there are no abnormal signs. A barium swallow shows an oblique impression across the oesophagus.

AORTIC ATRESIA

Complete atresia of the aortic valve is dealt with in the chapter on heart disease in the newborn (p. 245).

MITRAL STENOSIS

Isolated congenital mitral stenosis is a very rare lesion although it occurs occasionally in association with aortic atresia and coarctation. The valve cusps are poorly formed and often myxomatous. Breathlessness or pulmonary oedema occurs at any time from the neonatal period onwards. Occasionally, the presentation is that of pulmonary hypertension. The murmur so characteristic in adolescents and adults is frequently not heard in the neonatal period, but in older children it enables the condition to be diagnosed clinically. Otherwise, radiological evidence of pulmonary oedema, and left atrial enlargement, is a helpful guide to the diagnosis which can be confirmed at cardiac catheterization by demonstrating a gradient during diastole between the left atrial (or pulmonary wedge) and left ventricular pressures. Owing to the poor cusp development valvotomy is seldom satisfactory but may, in a young child, produce relief until the child is large enough for prosthetic valve replacement.

MITRAL ATRESIA

Complete obstruction of the mitral valve is one cause of the 'hypoplastic left heart syndrome' and is dealt with in the chapter on heart disease in the newborn (p. 245).

MITRAL REGURGITATION

Formerly mitral regurgitation was regarded as being invariably due to rheumatic fever, but the diminution in the disease together with the early investigation of infants with heart disease has shown up a small number of patients with isolated congenital mitral regurgitation. In addition, mitral regurgitation is well recognized in endocardial cushion defects, L-(corrected)transposition, endocardial fibroelastosis, hypertrophic obstructive cardiomyopathy and in association with coronary artery or myocardial disease causing left ventricular dilatation. In reviewing isolated mitral regurgitation, Berghius and co-workers (1964) found cleft anterior mitral valve cusps, shortened or absent chordae tendineae, accessory orifices, redundant posterior cusps and deficient posterior cusps.

Natural history

Severe lesions can cause death in infancy. Minor defects are compatible with a normal life-span.

Clinical presentation

Apart from those patients who have heart failure in infancy the lesion is usually discovered at routine examination. Left ventricular enlargement is palpable in moderate or severe disease. In all but the most trivial lesions (when the murmur may be late systolic) there is a loud apical pansystolic murmur. With a large regurgitant flow there is also a short diastolic murmur due to rapid filling of the left ventricle. Signs of pulmonary arterial hypertension may be present.

Radiology

The left atrium and left ventricle are enlarged in moderate and severe regurgitation and the pulmonary veins are congested. If the left atrial pressure is very high, signs of pulmonary oedema (either a diffuse hilar haze or Kerley lines) may be seen. When the lesion is complicated by reactive pulmonary hypertension the main pulmonary artery is prominent.

Electrocardiography

The electrocardiogram shows left atrial and left ventricular hypertrophy.

Cardiac catheterization

Cardiac catheterization is not required in mild lesions nor, in the absence of symptoms, when the diagnosis is made clinically. Even in fairly severe regurgitation the left atrial (or 'wedge') pressure may be normal, or nearly normal at rest. The lesion is best demonstrated by left ventricular cineangiography, which demonstrates the nature of the mitral valve abnormality.

Treatment

Treatment is usually medical. In the severe lesions causing death in infancy it is impracticable to attempt operation. In older children repair of the valve or annuloplasty (reducing the size of the mitral valve ring) may be possible, but replacement may be the only solution. Under the age of 1 year the mitral valve orifice is too small to accept either a prosthesis or a biological valve, but over that age, and particularly where the left heart is enlarged due to severe regurgitation it is usually possible to insert a small adult-size valve. Both from the point of view of valve performance and avoiding anticoagulants, the newer tissue valves, made up of porcine aortic valves, or homologous or heterogenous dura mater or pericardium are preferred to prosthetic valves although they have a tendency to thicken and calcify in young children. However, if the left ventricular cavity is small the 'low profile' Björk–Shiley type of prosthesis is preferred as it has no frame or stent to project into the left ventricle. It does however require permanent anticoagulants. Either type of valve will need subsequent operation, either because of growth of the patient or gradual deterioration of the valve, although the time span is uncertain.

MITRAL VALVE PROLAPSE

In children as well as adults mitral valve prolapse has been increasingly reported over the past decade, although it appears to be uncommon under the age of 10 years, except in association with

Marfan's syndrome. Becker and de Wit (1979) have drawn attention to the variable length of cordae tendiniae and cusps and it is probable that those diagnosed as 'floppy valves' are one end of a spectrum.

The classic signs are a loud midsystolic click (or series of clicks) and a late systolic murmur. Occasionally the murmur is pansystolic. The signs in mild cases may vary from day to day and according to posture—often being loudest when the child is standing. Occasionally the murmur is very loud when the child stands up and a loud honk is heard. The condition is usually diagnosed without difficulty clinically, but can be elegantly shown by either M-mode or 2-dimensional echocardiography (*Figure 7.10*) Apart from the risk of bacterial endocarditis the condition is benign and requires no treatment or restriction other than penicillin cover for dental extractions.

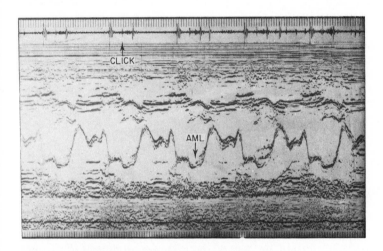

Figure 7.10. Echocardiogram and phonocardiogram of patient with midsystolic click due to mitral valve prolapse. There is an abrupt backward movement of the anterior mitral leaflet (arrowed) in mid-systole, corresponding to the click recorded on the phonocardiogram

MITRAL REGURGITATION DUE TO PAPILLARY MUSCLE DYSFUNCTION

A syndrome of abnormal function of the papillary muscles or of the ventricular wall close to them has recently been reported (Ehlers and co-workers, 1970). Excessively rapid contraction of the muscle prevents the mitral valve closing. In the early stages the only sign is a loud, midsystolic click at the apex but later a late, and finally a pansystolic, murmur can be heard. The reported cases have been mainly adolescent girls and there appears to be a familial tendency. The electrocardiogram frequently shows T wave inversion in leads 3 and aVF and sometimes V_6, and angiography shows an indentation during systole in the inferior wall of the left ventricle. The condition seems to be benign, although both supraventricular and ventricular arrhythmias are seen in older patients.

SUPRAVALVE AND SUBVALVE MITRAL OBSTRUCTION

Obstruction may occur from a fibrous ring in the region of the mitral valve ring and the signs and natural history are identical with those in congenital mitral stenosis. Another rare cause of mitral valve obstruction is the parachute mitral valve in which there is a single, large papillary muscle, to which the free margin of the mitral cusps are attached by short, and often thickened cordae, so that the valve cannot open fully. These anomalies can be demonstrated by angiography (Macartney *et al.*, 1974) or by echocardiography. Supravalve rings can be excised but parachute mitral valves are difficult to treat—although incision of the mitral valve cusps and papillary muscle may increase the size of the orifice, regurgitation usually results and it may be necessary to replace the mitral valve.

COR TRIATRIATUM

An unusual defect, cor triatriatum consists of a septum, usually with a small hole in it, across the left atrium, separating the pulmonary veins from the mitral valve orifice. The condition is thought to arise either from failure of incorporation of the common pulmonary vein into the left atrium, or from an incorrect positioning of the septum primum. Physiologically the condition simulates mitral stenosis.

Patients usually present in the first two years of life either with cough and breathlessness due to pulmonary oedema or with signs of pulmonary hypertension. There are no murmurs. Radiology shows right ventricular enlargement and pulmonary venous congestion or oedema. Unlike the picture in mitral stenosis the left atrial appendage is not prominent. The electrocardiogram shows right ventricular hypertrophy and, a helpful pointer, left atrial hypertrophy. Cardiac catheterization reveals pulmonary artery hypertension with raised pulmonary artery and pulmonary wedge pressures. Contrast medium injected into the pulmonary artery outlines the left atrium and shows the septum after circulation through the lungs.

The septum can be excised using cardiopulmonary bypass and the heart is then anatomically and physiologically normal. The pulmonary hypertension regresses.

BIBLIOGRAPHY AND REFERENCES

Aortic valve stenosis
Campbell, M. (1968). The natural history of congenital aortic stenosis. *Br. Heart J.* **30**, 514
Blackwood, R. A., Bloom, K. R. and Williams, C. M. (1978). Aortic stenosis in children. Experience with echocardiographic prediction of severity. *Circulation* **57**, 263
Glew, R. H., Varghese, P. J., Krovetz, J., Dorst, J. P. and Rowe, R. D. (1969). Sudden death in congenital aortic stenosis. A review of eight cases with an evaluation of premonitory clinical features. *Am. Heart J.* **78**, 615
Hossack, K. F., Neutze, J. M., Lowe, J. B. and Barratt-Boyes, B. G. (1980). Congenital valvar aortic stenosis. Natural history and assessment for operation. *Br. Heart J.* **43**, 561
Johnson, A. M. (1971). Aortic stenosis, sudden death and the left ventricular baroceptors. *Br. Heart J.* **33**, 1
Mulder, D. G., Katz, R. D., Moss, A. J. and Hurwitz, R. A. (1968). The surgical treatment of congenital aortic stenosis. *J. thorac. cardiovasc. Surg.* **55**, 786
Roberts, W. C. (1970). The congenitally bicuspid aortic valve. *Am. J. Cardiol.* **26**, 72
Scott, L. P. and Feldman, B. H. (1964). Aortic stenosis in infancy. *Pediatrics, Springfield* **33**, 931
Shackleton, J., Edwards, F. R., Bickford, B. J. and Jones, R. S. (1972). Long term follow up of congenital aortic stenosis after surgery. *Br. Heart J.* **34**, 47
Somerville, J. and Ross, D. N. (1977). Atypical aortic valve stenosis—a diffuse congenital cardiovascular disease—recognition and surgical treatment. *Br. Heart J.* **39**, 930

Subaortic stenosis
Krueger, S. K., French, J. W., Forker, A. D., Caudill, C. C. and Popp, R. L. (1979). Echocardiography in discrete subaortic stenosis. *Circulation* **59**, 506
Somerville, J., Stone, S. and Ross, D. (1980). Fate of patients with fixed subaortic stenosis after surgical removal. *Br. Heart J.* **43**, 629

Coarctation of the aorta
Becker, A. E., Becker, M. J. and Edwards, J. E. (1970). Anomalies associated with coarctation of the aorta. Particular reference to infancy. *Circulation* **41**, 1067
Campbell, M. (1970). Natural history of coarctation of the aorta. *Br. Heart J.* **32**, 637
Hamilton, D. L., Di Eusanio, G., Sandrasagra, F. A. and Donnelly, R. J. (1978). Early and late results of aortoplasty with a left subclavian flap for coarctation of the aorta in infancy. *J. thorac. cardiovasc. Surg.* **75**, 699
Hartmann, A. F., Goldring, D., Hernandez, A., Behrer, M. R., Schad, N., Ferguson, T., Burford, T. and Crawford, C. C. (1970). Recurrent coarctation of the aorta after successful repair in infancy. *Am. J. Cardiol.* **25**, 405
Ho, S. Y. and Anderson, R. H. (1979). Coarctation, tubular hypoplasia and the ductus arteriosus—a histological study of 35 specimens. *Br. Heart J.* **41**, 268
Ho, S. Y. and Anderson, R. H. (1979). Coarctation of the aorta. In: *Paediatric Cardiology*. Vol. 2 (*Heart Disease in the Newborn*). Eds M. J. Godman and R. M. Marquis. p. 173. London: Churchill Livingstone

Mays, E. and Sergeant, C. K. (1965). Post-coarctectomy syndrome. *Archs Surg.* **91**, 58

Nauton M. A. and Olley, P. M. (1976). Hypertension after coarctectomy in children. In *The Child with Congenital Heart Disease After Surgery*, p. 143. Eds Langford Kidd and Richard Rowe. London: Futura Press

Parsons, C. G. and Astley, D. M. R. (1966). Recurrence of aortic coarctation after operation in childhood. *Br. Med. J.* **1**, 573

Pelletier, C., Daugnon, A., Ethier, M. F. and Stanley, P. (1969). Coarctation of the aorta in infancy. Post-operative follow-up. *J. thorac. cardiovasc. Surg.* **57**, 171

Shinebourne, E. A., Tam, A. S. Y., Elseed, A. M., Paneth, M., Lennox, S. C., Cleland, W. P., Lincoln, C., Joseph, M. C., Anderson, R. H. (1976). Coarctation of the aorta in infancy and childhood. *Br. Heart J.* **38**, 375–380

Sinha, S. N., Kardatzke, M. L., Cole, R. B., Muster, A. J., Wessel, H. V. and Paul, M. H. (1969). Coarctation of the aorta in infancy. *Circulation* **40**, 385

Verska, J. J., DeQuattro, V. and Woolley, M. M. (1969). Coarctation of the aorta. The abdominal pain syndrome and paradoxical hypertension. *J. thorac. cardiovasc. Surg.* **58**, 746

Weidman, P., Baumann, K., Gysling, E., Wirz, P. and Siegenthaler, W. (1969). Plasma renin activity in patients with coarctation of the aorta; a comment on the pathogenesis of prestenotic hypertension. *Circulation* **40**, 731

Mitral regurgitation

Berghuis, K. H., Kirklin, J. W., Edward, J. E. and Titmus, J. L. (1964). The surgical anatomy of congenital mitral insufficiency. *J. thorac. cardiovasc. Surg*, **47**, 799

Ehlers, K. H., Engle, M. A., Levin, A. R., Grossman, H. and Fleming, R. J. (1970). Left ventricular abnormality with late mitral insufficiency and abnormal electro-cardiogram. *Am. J. Cardiol.* **26**, 353

Cor triatriatum

Ahn, C., Hosier, D. M. and Sirak, H. D. (1968). Cor triatriatum. A case report and review of other operative cases.' *J. thorac. cardiovasc. Surg.* **56**, 177

CHAPTER 8

Acyanotic Lesions with Right Heart Abnormalities

PULMONARY VALVE STENOSIS

Incidence

Isolated pulmonary valve stenosis accounts for 10 per cent of all cases of congenital heart disease.

Definition

The pulmonary valve cannot open normally. The valve cusps are not well formed and the valve is dome-shaped with a central or near central orifice (*Figure 8.1*). It is thickened and at times almost cartilaginous in consistency. The size of the orifice varies in diameter from 1 mm to two-thirds of that of the valve ring. The right ventricle thickens in relation to the severity of the stenosis and in severe stenosis the cavity of the right ventricle is reduced by the hypertrophied muscle which can cause secondary obstruction to blood flow. The pressure gradient between the right ventricle and pulmonary artery varies from 10–20 mmHg in very mild stenosis, to 100 or even 200 mmHg in severe stenosis. The gradient increases with activity when the cardiac output increases.

Natural history

Severe stenosis may cause death in infancy from right heart failure. Otherwise, severe symptoms or death are unusual in childhood, but

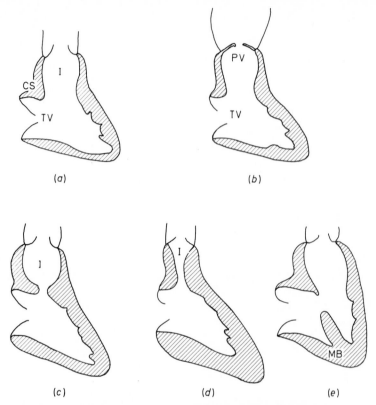

Figure 8.1. Types of right ventricular obstruction. (*a*) Normal anatomy
of right ventricle. (*b*) Pulmonary valve stenosis. (*c*) Localized infundibular stenosis. (*d*) Generalized muscular thickening of infundibulum.
(*e*) Double right ventricle (obstruction by anomalous muscle bundle).
CS: crista supraventricularis; I: infundibulum; TV: tricuspid valve;
PV: pulmonary valve; MB: muscle bundle

most patients with severe stenosis are disabled by 20 years of age. As
the right ventricle hypertrophies to try to overcome the obstruction,
the infundibulum of the right ventricle becomes narrowed and itself
then forms an obstruction to the flow of blood from the right
ventricle. Moderate stenosis causes progressive muscular hypertrophy and ultimately fibrosis of the right ventricular muscle, leading to
limitation of cardiac output and, not infrequently, to attacks of
ventricular tachycardia or fibrillation. Mild stenosis is compatible
with normal activities and normal life expectation. We are uncertain
whether some of the moderate cases develop a rise in pressure over
the years or remain the same.

Clinical presentation

The heart murmur is usually an incidental finding and the child has no symptoms even though the stenosis is severe. When the cardiac output becomes low, however, breathlessness, fatigue, ischaemic chest pain and syncope follow and relief of the stenosis becomes urgent or sudden death may occur, probably due to arrhythmia. Palpitations due to extrasystoles may occur.

The physical appearance is often helpful in making the diagnosis. The child is well nourished, chubby and healthy looking with a moon face and rather a high colour. The lips and tongue however are quite pink. The extremities are often cold with peripheral vasoconstriction. The peripheral pulses are normal in mild to moderate stenosis but are reduced when there is severe obstruction. In moderate stenosis the A wave in the jugular pulse is accentuated but in severe stenosis it may be 5 cm or more in height and may be palpable. Presystolic pulsation of the liver may also then be felt. There is increased heaving over the right ventricle and this increases with the severity of the stenosis. The left ventricle at the apex may be difficult to feel or is 'tapping' in quality. A systolic thrill in the second left interspace is palpable except in the mildest and most severe forms.

Auscultation is valuable in assessing the severity of the stenosis. The first heart sound is normal and is followed by an ejection click which occurs when the dome-shaped stenotic valve is fully open. The valve must be mobile for an ejection click to occur so it is not heard when the valve is dysplastic and immobile. The click is best heard in the second left interspace and is loudest in expiration. As the stenosis becomes more severe the right ventricular pressure rises more rapidly and the valve opens earlier so that the click occurs earlier. In very severe stenosis the click may disappear completely. The systolic murmur is a rough, loud ejection murmur and is well conducted to the lung apex and particularly over the left lung because the jet through the stenotic valve is carried into the left pulmonary artery which originates as a continuation of the main pulmonary artery. In infants with pinpoint pulmonary stenosis, the stenotic murmur may be very soft. In mild stenosis, right ventricular systole is only slightly prolonged so the murmur is symmetrical and ends before the aortic component of the second sound. In moderate stenosis the murmur ends after the aortic component and in severe stenosis the aortic component may be obliterated by the murmur which is longer because of the prolongation of the emptying of the right ventricle. (*Figure 8.2.*)

The second sound also gives clues to the severity of the stenosis.

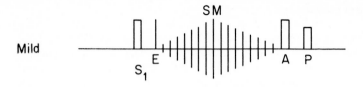

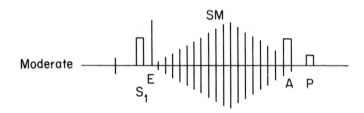

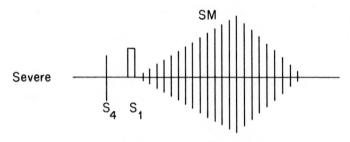

Figure 8.2. The systolic murmur in pulmonary valve stenosis

S₁ = first heart sound   A₂ = aortic component of second sound
E = ejection click   P₂ = pulmonary component of second sound
SM = systolic murmur   S₄ = fourth heart sound
Note: The ejection click is heard nearer to the first heart sound as the
severity of the stenosis increases; in very severe stenosis it disappears

The more severe the stenosis, the longer the duration of the right
ventricular ejection; pulmonary valve closure is therefore delayed
and the split between the aortic and pulmonary components of the
second sound widens. In severe stenosis the split is fixed and in the
most severe stenosis the pulmonary component may be inaudible.

Noonan's syndrome

Children with this syndrome have the phenotype of a Turner's
syndrome but the chromosomes are normal. One often sees children
who have a characteristic facies with widely separated and

downward sloping eyes, often with a flattened nasal bridge, and have none of the other features of Noonan's syndrome, but who, like those with Noonan's syndrome, have pulmonary stenosis in which the valve is thick and dysplastic and associated with a small valve ring. Such cases are much more difficult to operate on than the classic thin dome-shaped valves and it is being increasingly recognized that many of these children have cardiomyopathy as well.

RADIOLOGY

The most striking finding is dilatation of the pulmonary artery with a heart of normal size and no increase in the vascularity of the lungs (*Figure 8.3*). There is no direct correlation between the size of the pulmonary artery and the degree of pulmonary stenosis—it is sometimes obvious in mild stenosis and small in severe stenosis. It is due to the jet of blood coming through the narrowed pulmonary valve and impinging on the wall of the pulmonary artery. There is prominence of the right atrium in moderate and severe cases and in this group the peripheral vascularity in the lungs is diminished. The small size of these vessels is thought to be due to lack of pulsatile flow in them because all the output from the right ventricle must in fact enter the lungs and there is no diminution in the amount of blood reaching them. Enlargement of the heart usually occurs only when the patient is developing symptoms and the heart is beginning to fail (*Figure 8.3*).

Electrocardiography

The degree of right ventricular hypertrophy is a good guide to the severity of the stenosis. Typical tracings of mild, moderate and severe stenosis are shown in *Figure 4.9* (p. 36). In moderate and severe stenosis there is evidence of right atrial hypertrophy (peaked P waves in lead 2).

Investigation

When the clinical findings, electrocardiogram and radiograph all suggest that the stenosis is mild, no further investigation is necessary. If the narrowing is thought to be moderate or severe, cardiac catheterization is carried out and the pressure gradient across the pulmonary valve measured. Contrast medium is injected into the

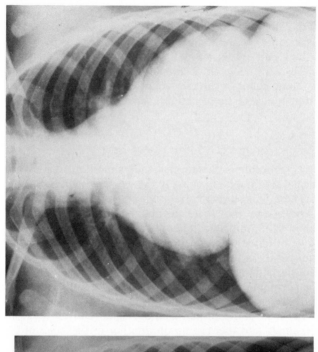

(a)

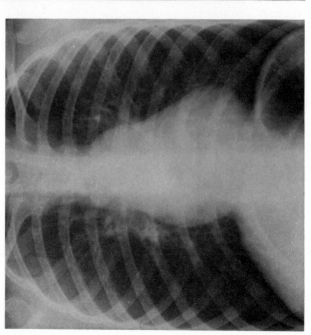

(b)

Figure 8.3. Pulmonary stenosis: chest radiographs. (*a*) Usual picture in moderate or severe stenosis. The main pulmonary artery is prominent (poststenotic dilatation) but there is no generalized cardiac enlargement. (*b*) Uncommon picture in a 7-year-old girl with severe pulmonary stenosis who presented with effort syncope and a right ventricular pressure over 200 mmHg at rest. The right atrium and right ventricle are dilated and the lungs are oligaemic

right ventricle so that the stenosis is visualized (*Figure 8.4*) and any secondary infundibular narrowing noted. Angiography also confirms that the ventricular septum is intact.

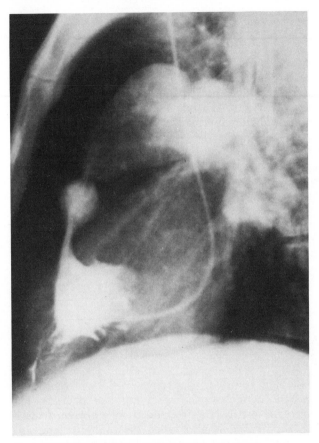

Figure 8.4. Right ventricular angiogram of a patient with pulmonary valvar stenosis (left lateral view). The right ventricle is hypertrophied, especially in the infundibular part, the pulmonary valve is thickened and domed and there is a jet of contrast medium through the centre. The main pulmonary artery shows poststenotic dilatation

Differential diagnosis

Mild pulmonary stenosis may be confused with a *small* atrial septal defect, but the differentiation of these lesions is not important since neither of them requires treatment. In significant pulmonary stenosis there is a thrill palpable and in an atrial septal defect of significant size a tricuspid diastolic flow murmur is heard.

Treatment

Pulmonary valvotomy is indicated if the resting right ventricular pressure is greater than 70 mmHg. It is a safe and simple operation. Any pulmonary incompetence which may occasionally follow division of the valve is of no clinical significance. The operation should be performed before severe secondary infundibular hypertrophy has occurred; otherwise the risks of operation are increased because the right ventricular pressure remains high after valvotomy and the cardiac output is poor in the postoperative period. Operation is performed using cardiopulmonary bypass; the valve is approached through the pulmonary artery and cut in three places to make a valve with three cusps. Some surgeons operate without bypass, using inflow occlusion of the superior and inferior venae cavae and again approaching the valve from above. Just two minutes of such circulatory arrest can be allowed and only a few expert surgeons find this method as safe as the first.

PULMONARY INFUNDIBULAR STENOSIS

Definition

The cavity of the right ventricle is separated into inflow and outflow portions by a band of muscle, the crista supraventricularis. The outflow portion of the ventricle, between the crista supraventricularis and the pulmonary valve, is also called the infundibulum, and stenosis of any portion of this chamber is known as infundibular stenosis.

Although in Fallot's tetralogy infundibular obstruction is common, when the interventricular septum is intact, infundibular stenosis is rare, occurring only about one-tenth as commonly as pulmonary valvar stenosis. The stenosis may be fibrous, muscular or a combination of both. Two types are described, according to the size of the chamber between the stenosis and the pulmonary valve. A large infundibular chamber is usually associated with a fibrous stricture and a small chamber with muscular narrowing (*see Figure 8.1*)

Presentation

When there is no interatrial communication there are usually no symptoms. When an atrial septal defect or patent foramen ovale is present, cyanosis may occur due to the right-to-left interatrial shunt.

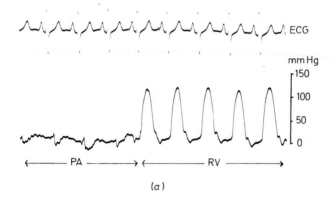

(a)

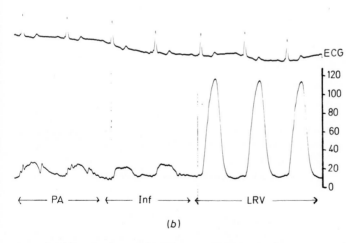

(b)

Figure 8.5. Pressure traces as the catheter is withdrawn from the pulmonary artery to the body of the right ventricle. (*a*) Pulmonary valvar stenosis. PA: pulmonary artery; RV: right ventricle. (*b*) Infundibular stenosis. Inf: infundibulum; LRV: low right ventricle. The systolic pressure in the infundibulum is the same as in the pulmonary artery, the diastolic pressure the same as in the body of the right ventricle

In severe obstruction there may be an accentuated 'a' wave in the venous pulse. The cardiac impulse is usually normal but a loud systolic murmur is heard, maximal in the third or fourth left intercostal space, usually with a thrill. There is no ejection click and the pulmonary element of the second heart sound is usually faint or inaudible.

Investigation

Radiographs of the chest in the frontal view are usually unremarkable unless there is a right-to-left shunt, in which case the lung fields are oligaemic. In the lateral view the right ventricle may be seen to be prominent. The electrocardiogram usually shows right ventricular hypertrophy.

Diagnosis

Although the lower site of the murmur and the absence of an ejection click are useful in distinguishing the condition from pulmonary valvar stenosis, cardiac catheterization is usually required to establish the diagnosis. On withdrawal of the catheter from the pulmonary artery, the pulmonary artery and infundibular systolic pressures are normal but a gradient is shown on further withdrawal into the body of the right ventricle (*Figure 8.5*). The angiogram demonstrates the obstruction.

Treatment

Operation is usually advised if the pressure in the right ventricle proximal to the obstruction is 80 mmHg or more at rest. Cardiopulmonary bypass or profound hypothermia is required and the obstruction is excised through a right ventriculotomy.

DOUBLE CHAMBERED RIGHT VENTRICLE

Occasionally, obstruction due to muscle bands is found below the level of the infundibulum. The effect is to divide the right ventricle into two roughly equal chambers (*see Figure 8.1*). The physical signs are the same as for infundibular stenosis, but the electrocardiogram frequently does not show right ventricular hypertrophy, owing to the relatively small size of the proximal, high pressure chamber.

RIGHT VENTRICULAR INVOLVEMENT IN
HYPERTROPHIC OBSTRUCTIVE CARDIOMYOPATHY

In patients with hypertrophic obstructive cardiomyopathy the interventricular septum may bulge into the right ventricle, producing obstruction. A gradient of up to 50 mmHg may be found at cardiac catheterization.

PULMONARY REGURGITATION

Isolated pulmonary regurgitation is extremely rare. A few of the patients are shown to have complete absence of the pulmonary valve. The condition may complicate diseases of connective tissue, such as Marfan's syndrome. (Functional pulmonary regurgitation occurs in severe pulmonary hypertension and a mild degree is common after repair of Fallot's tetralogy.)

Presentation

The condition is asymptomatic in children although tiredness and right heart failure have been reported in patients in late middle-age. A murmur is heard on routine examination or a routine chest radiograph draws attention to the condition. Usually the only sign is a soft diastolic murmur or systolic and diastolic murmurs heard in the pulmonary area, but absence of the pulmonary component of the second sound may be noted. The electrocardiogram in children is normal but in adults may show a right bundle branch block pattern. The chest radiograph in older children shows dilatation of the main pulmonary artery, which becomes more marked with increasing age.

Treatment

The condition is benign and no restrictions are required except for prophylaxis against bacterial endocarditis.

ABSENCE OF THE PULMONARY VALVE

This very rare abnormality is invariably associated with a ventricular septal defect. The pulmonary valve annulus is constricted and there is massive dilatation of the pulmonary arteries. The infundibulum is often long, narrow and tortuous. The valve is represented by nodular tissue like primitive valve tissue.

Symptoms occur immediately after birth. There is respiratory distress and dilatation of the heart which may lead to heart failure. Initially the baby may be cyanosed due to right-to-left shunting but as the pulmonary vascular resistance falls, blood flows from left to right and the baby becomes pink. There is a systolic thrill in the second and third left interspaces immediately after birth which is pathognomonic of an absent pulmonary valve. There are impressive systolic and early diastolic murmurs giving a to-and-fro rhythm down the left sternal edge. There may be respiratory infection secondary to tracheobronchial obstruction by the dilated pulmonary arteries. Such infections may be troublesome during the first year of life but after that are less common.

Radiography

There is marked enlargement of the heart with large dilated pulmonary arteries.

Electrocardiography

There is right ventricular hypertrophy and if there is a large left-to-right shunt, there is increased left ventricular activity also.

Treatment

Conservative treatment is best in infancy and definitive correction with pulmonary valve replacement can be done later in life.

PULMONARY ARTERY STENOSIS

Obstruction to the flow of blood on the right side of the heart may occur from stenosis of the main pulmonary artery above the valve or from multiple stenoses of peripheral branches. Peripheral pulmonary artery stenosis is one of the lesions caused by maternal rubella and also occurs with the tetralogy of Fallot and in association with infantile hypercalcaemia. Further details are given in the section on infantile hypercalcaemia in Chapter 20.

TRICUSPID STENOSIS

As a congenital lesion, tricuspid stenosis probably does not occur. It may result from rheumatic fever, but in childhood it occurs so rarely that it can be ignored.

TRICUSPID REGURGITATION

Tricuspid regurgitation occurs in association with tricuspid stenosis when the valve is affected by rheumatic endocarditis. As a congenital lesion it occurs in association with Ebstein's anomaly and may also occur as a result of right ventricular outflow tract obstruction due to severe pulmonary stenosis or pulmonary atresia.

EBSTEIN'S ANOMALY

Incidence

Ebstein's anomaly is rare, less than 1 per cent of children with congenital heart disease being affected.

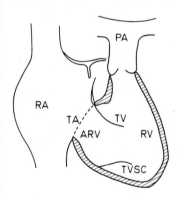

Figure 8.6. Ebstein's anomaly of the tricuspid valve. The septal leaflet of the tricuspid valve (TVSC) originates within the ventricular cavity, so that there is a portion of the right ventricular cavity (ARV) which is 'atrialized' as far as pressure is concerned. RA: right atrium; TA: tricuspid annulus; TV: tricuspid valve; RV: main cavity of the right ventricle; PA: pulmonary artery

Definition

The posterior and septal leaflets of the tricuspid valve are not attached to the annulus fibrosus but to the endocardium of the right ventricle below the annulus (*Figure 8.6*). The anterior leaflet usually arises normally. The leaflets are often thickened and inserted into chordae tendineae which are attached directly to the wall rather than to the papillary muscles, and the valve assumes a conical shape.

It is narrowed and incompetent. The part of the heart above the valve has atrial and ventricular portions, although both are functionally atrium, and it is divided into these two parts by the annulus fibrosus. The ventricle distal to the valve is small and the atrial and ventricular muscle is unusually thin. The infundibulum is thick and muscular. There is usually a patent foramen ovale or atrial septal defect. The right ventricle is unable to eject the normal blood volume and the flow of blood to the lungs is reduced. The right atrium and ventricle proximal to the valve are dilated and a right-to-left shunt may occur between the two atria.

The degree of the abnormality varies and there is a whole spectrum of these malformations ranging from mild to severe forms.

Natural history

The effects of the condition are manifest most strikingly soon after birth, when the high pulmonary vascular resistance produces an obstruction to forward flow which the right ventricle is unable to overcome with an incompetent tricuspid valve. If the first few days of life are survived the prognosis in childhood is good except for the few who have severe cyanosis or attacks of paroxysmal tachycardia.

Symptoms

Breathlessness, mild cyanosis and congestive heart failure occur in infancy in the more severe forms, but in the milder forms symptoms develop later with mild cyanosis and excessive dyspnoea becoming apparent after exercise.

Signs

Although a few patients are acyanotic, the majority show mild cyanosis associated with mild clubbing. The pulse has a small volume and the venous pulse may show prominent 'a' or 'v' waves, but is often normal. The heart action is quiet and the apex beat diffuse and difficult to locate. A systolic murmur at the left sternal edge occurs when there is significant tricuspid regurgitation. Three or four heart sounds can be heard, giving rise to a triple or quadruple rhythm. A characteristic scratchy diastolic murmur is usually present, best heard at the lower left sternal edge.

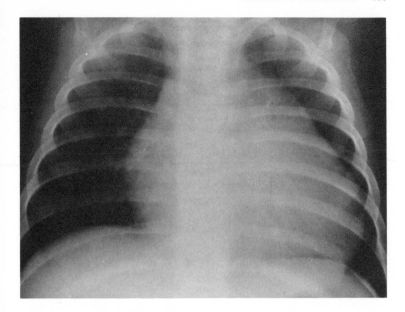

Figure 8.7. Ebstein's anomaly. Chest radiograph showing right atrial and right ventricular enlargement and pulmonary oligaemia in a 9-month-old infant with a right-to-left shunt through an atrial septal defect

Radiology

Radiology is characteristic in the overt case, there being marked cardiac enlargement with a large right atrium and oligaemia of the lung fields (*Figure 8.7*). In milder forms, prominence of the right atrium may be the only abnormal finding.

Electrocardiography

The electrocardiogram is pathognomonic in the majority of patients. The P waves in lead 2 are tall and peaked, often being higher than the QRS complexes. The P–R interval may be prolonged. Right bundle branch block, complete or incomplete, is seen (*Figure 8.8*). Pre-excitation, as in the Wolff–Parkinson–White syndrome, occurs frequently and arrhythmias, particularly paroxysmal atrial tachycardia and atrial flutter, are common. In mild cases a right bundle branch block may be the only finding.

156

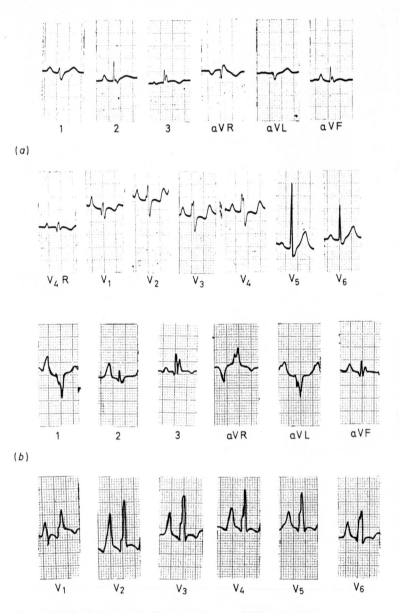

Figure 8.8. Ebstein's anomaly. Electrocardiograms. (*a*) Showing right atrial hypertrophy, slightly prolonged P–R interval and right bundle branch block pattern with small voltage QRS complexes. (*b*) Another patient, showing giant P waves

Echocardiography

The diagnosis can usually be confirmed by M-mode or two-dimensional studies. The most characteristic finding on the M-mode is greatly prolonged opening time of the tricuspid valve, extending 60 to 140 milliseconds after mitral valve closure. Valve movement is usually increased and septal movement paradoxical (Daniel *et al.*, 1980). Two-dimensional studies show the right atrial enlargement and displacement of the valve into the right ventricular cavity.

Investigation

Investigation carries a greater risk than in other lesions because of the danger of arrhythmias. It is not carried out when the clinical diagnosis is certain unless operation is being contemplated. Occasionally, there is difficulty in differentiating Ebstein's anomaly from severe pulmonary stenosis with a reversed interatrial shunt and then investigation is mandatory because the latter lesion can and must be corrected by surgery. Intracardiac electrocardiograms help to establish the diagnosis when they show an intraventricular pattern in the electrocardiogram in the presence of an atrial pressure wave. Similarly ventricular ectopics may be elicited in the 'atrialized' right ventricle.

Treatment

When symptoms occur in the first few days of life, oxygen (to reduce the pulmonary vascular resistance) and digoxin are required. Asymptomatic children require no treatment, but competitive sports are best avoided in view of the risks of arrhythmias. Attacks of paroxysmal atrial tachycardia can be suppressed by propranolol. Surgical repair of the valve has proved disappointing but valve replacement is now established in adolescents and adults. Another form of treatment is to close the tricuspid annulus and place a conduit between the right atrium and the pulmonary artery (Fontan operation, *see* p. 182).

BIBLIOGRAPHY AND REFERENCES

Pulmonary stenosis
Benton, J. W. Jr., Elliott, L. P., Adams, P. Jr., Anderson, R. C., Hong, C. T. and Lester, R. G. (1962). Pulmonary atresia and stenosis with intact ventricular septum. *Am. J. Dis. Child.* **104**, 161

Boyle, D. M., Morton, P. and Pantridge, J. F. (1964). The electrocardiogram in pulmonary valve stenosis with intact ventricular septum. *Br. Heart J.* **26**, 477

Engle, M. A., Ito, T. and Goldberg, H. P. (1964). The fate of the patient with pulmonic stenosis. *Circulation* **30**, 554

Gersony, W. M., Bernhard, W. F., Nadas, A. S. and Gross, R. E. (1967). Diagnosis and surgical treatment of infants with critical pulmonary outflow obstruction. *Circulation* **35**, 767

Hartmann, A. F., Tsifutis, A. A., Arvidsson, H. and Goldring, D. (1962). The two-chambered right ventricle. *Circulation* 26, 279

Lucker, R. D., Vogel, J. H. K. and Blount, S. G. Jr. (1970). Regression of valvular pulmonary stenosis. *Br. Heart J.* **32**, 779

Mustard, W. T., Jain, S. C. and Trusler, G. A. (1968). Pulmonary stenosis in the first year of life. *Br. Heart J.* **30**, 255

Tandon, R., Nadas, A. S. and Gross, R. E. (1965). Results of open heart surgery in patients with pulmonic stenosis and intact interventricular septum. *Circulation* **31**, 190

Tinkler, J., Howitt, G., Markman, P. and Wade, E. G. (1965). The natural history of isolated pulmonary stenosis. *Br. Heart J.* **27**, 151

Ebstein's anomaly

Daniel, W., Rathsack, P., Walpurger, G., Kahill, A., Gizbertz, R., Schmitz, J. and Lichtlen, P. R. (1980). Value of M-mode echocardiography for non-invasive diagnosis of Ebstein's anomaly. *Br. Heart J.* **43**, 38

Kumar, A. E., Fyler, D. C., Miettinen, O. S. and Nadas, A. S. (1971). Ebstein's anomaly. Clinical profile and natural history. *Am. J. Cardiol.* **28**, 84

Lillehei, C. W., Kalke, B. R. and Carlson, R. G. (1967). Evolution of corrective surgery for Ebstein's anomaly. *Circulation* **36**, Suppl. 11, 111

Newfeld, E. A., Cole, R. B. and Paul, M. H. (1967). Ebstein's malformation of the tricuspid valve in the neonate. Functional and anatomic pulmonary outflow tract obstruction. *Am. J. Cardiol.* **19**, 727

Pocock, W. A., Tucker, R. B. K. and Barlow, J. B. (1969). Mild Ebstein's anomaly. *Br. Heart J.* **31**, 327

Simcha, A. and Bonham Carter, R. E. (1971). Ebstein's anomaly. Clinical studies of 32 patients in childhood. *Br. Heart J.* **33**, 46

Watson, H. (1974). Natural history of Ebstein's anomaly of tricuspid valve in childhood and adolescence. An international co-operative study of 505 cases. *Br. Heart J.* **36**, 417

CHAPTER 9

Cyanotic Lesions with Diminished Pulmonary Blood Flow

TETRALOGY OF FALLOT

Incidence

Fallot's tetralogy accounts for about 7 per cent of all congenital cardiac deformities and *after the first year of life* it is the commonest cyanotic lesion.

Definition

The two important primary specific defects which constitute the so-called 'tetralogy' of Fallot are ventricular septal defect and pulmonary stenosis (*Figure 9.1*). The ventricular defect is large, about the size of the aortic orifice, and it lies beneath the aortic valve more anteriorly than the usual ventricular septal defect. Stenosis is always present in the infundibulum of the right ventricle and in about one-third of cases there is stenosis of the pulmonary valve as well. The stenosis is of sufficient severity for the peak systolic pressures in the right and left ventricles to be the same.

Patients with tetralogy of Fallot cover a wide spectrum. At one extreme the patient is almost pink at rest and cyanosis is noticed only after exercise; at the other end of the scale is the patient who is deeply cyanosed at rest. The factor which determines the severity of the condition is the degree of pulmonary or infundibular stenosis. When the narrowing of the outflow tract is severe, more of the desaturated blood in the right ventricle flows into the aorta. When the stenosis is not so severe, most of the right ventricular blood passes to the lungs and it is only during exercise that a significant amount of right ventricular blood enters the aorta.

After birth, the degree of stenosis in the outflow tract from the right ventricle may be mild and such patients may have a left-to-right shunt through the ventricular septal defect. As growth occurs, the narrowing in the infundibular region of the right ventricle

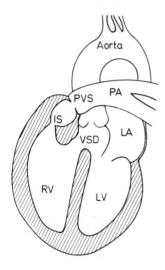

Figure 9.1. Anatomy of Fallot's tetralogy. View from left side to show the ventricular septal defect (VSD) and the overriding aorta. In this diagram both valvar (PVS) and infundibular (IS) stenoses are shown. PA: pulmonary artery; LA: left atrium; LV left ventricle; RV: right ventricle

increases and by 2, 3 or 4 years of age the left-to-right shunt ceases, and the lesion is then called tetralogy of Fallot.

The right ventricular hypertrophy and overriding aorta which are the other two findings in the 'tetralogy' are not important in the understanding of the haemodynamics of the lesion. The aorta tends to be displaced anteriorly but there is considerable variation in its relationship to the left and right ventricles. When looked at from above, because of the presence of the high ventricular septal defect, the right ventricular cavity may be seen and this appearance gave rise to the term 'overriding of the aorta'. The size of the right-to-left shunt is determined by the degree of pulmonary valve or infundibular stenosis and not by the amount of override. The right ventricular hypertrophy is secondary to the raised pressure within the right ventricle.

Natural history

The natural history was not documented before surgical help became possible and will never now be accurately known. In Abbott's series (1936) the average age at death was 12 years. There is a high death rate in severe cases in the first year of life and this falls after 2 years of age. The study of Bertranon (1978) shows that only half of the children born with this lesion survive their third birthday. There is then a progressive deterioration around puberty, and death usually occurs in the second decade.

The prognosis depends almost entirely on the degree of pulmonary valvar or infundibular obstruction and, therefore, the degree of right-to-left shunt. Patients who have little or no right-to-left shunt at rest may remain virtually asymptomatic, well into middle age. Even in these patients, however, there is a tendency for polycythaemia to develop and for thromboembolism to occur. There is also a tendency, particularly in the first three or four years of life for the infundibular muscular obstruction to become worse.

Clinical presentation

Infants are usually pink or only slightly cyanosed at birth and become more cyanosed as they grow. Some infants may present with signs of a ventricular septal defect with a left-to-right shunt and minimal pulmonary stenosis; then after two or three years the pulmonary stenosis increases and cyanosis follows.

In infants who appear pink at rest, the first indication that anything is wrong may be the occurrence of a 'cyanotic attack'. This comes on suddenly, often after waking up after a good sleep, or after crying, defaecation or feeding. The infant becomes increasingly blue, breathes rapidly and finally loses consciousness. There is usually spontaneous recovery but occasionally infants may die during an attack. It is emphasized that such an infant may seem very well between attacks, but examination reveals a heart murmur.

Some children may survive without 'attacks'. It is interesting that apparently mild cases may have severe attacks whereas more deeply cyanosed children may not have them. The attacks are thought to be due to spasm of the muscle of the infundibulum.

If there are no attacks, the disability usually becomes more evident when the child begins to walk, cyanosis develops or increases with exertion, and after bouts of exercise the child may be observed to 'squat'. He sits with his knees up to his chest and, as he does so, becomes gradually less cyanosed and less breathless, and then resumes activity again (*Figure 9.2*). *Squatting* is a very important finding because its occurrence makes tetralogy of Fallot the most likely diagnosis. Squatting in any other lesion is exceptionally rare.

The way in which squatting benefits the patient has been imperfectly understood. It is best first to consider what happens when a patient with tetralogy of Fallot exercises. During the period of exercise a large oxygen debt is built up, the muscle vascular beds are dilated and there is an increase in the extraction of oxygen locally so that the amount of oxygen in the systemic venous blood is reduced more than usual. In tetralogy of Fallot such a reduction of

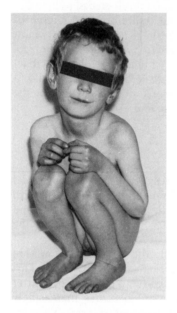

Figure 9.2. Squatting demonstrated by a patient with Fallot's tetralogy

oxygen in the venous blood causes a further fall of oxygen content in the arterial blood, because some of the venous return to the right heart is shunted directly into the aorta. Furthermore, the vasodilatation in the muscles lowers the systemic vascular resistance, and thus lowers the systemic blood pressure which favours an increase in the amount of blood flowing from the right ventricle into the aorta. The patient therefore becomes intensely blue.

Squatting helps to counteract the effects of exercise in two ways.

1. The arterial blood flow to the legs is reduced during squatting and this helps to maintain the systemic resistance so that more blood enters the lungs.
2. The venous return from the legs is slowed and therefore the oxygen debt after exercise can be paid off over a longer period and this corrects the sudden fall in arterial oxygen saturation.

Guntheroth and co-workers (1968) have shown that there is a diminished flow of blood in the inferior vena cava in the squatting position and this is accompanied by a rise in systemic arterial pressure and a rise in arterial oxygen saturation.

In some children the progress of the disease is slow and they continue to live reasonable, though slightly restricted, lives until they reach puberty. It is worth mentioning that heart failure in tetralogy of Fallot is extremely rare in childhood. Its presence makes the diagnosis doubtful or raises the possibility of bacterial endocarditis complicating the disease.

The degree of cyanosis and clubbing of fingers and toes varies with the severity of the disease. The conjunctivae are often injected. A prominent A wave may be seen in the neck. There is usually a systolic thrill in the second, third and fourth left interspaces close to the left of the sternum and a systolic murmur of the ejection type is heard in the same area. The murmur is caused by infundibular stenosis and not by blood flowing through the ventricular septal defect—it must be remembered that the peak systolic pressure is the same in both ventricles.

Blood count

The red cell count and haematocrit level are elevated. This usually correlates well with the severity of the arterial desaturation and the severity of the pulmonary stenosis. An exception occurs when the infant is iron deficient. The haemoglobin may then be normal or low although there is nearly always some polycythaemia and a normal or raised packed cell volume.

Radiology

The heart is not enlarged. The aortic arch can usually be identified lying on either the left or the right side of the trachea (*Figure 9.3*). It is on the right side in 25 per cent of patients. The size of the ascending aorta can often be assessed. The small apex of the heart suggests right ventricular enlargement. Marked concavity in the upper left cardiac border suggests a small pulmonary artery; a convex shadow in that region suggests that the pulmonary artery is of good size. The vascularity of the lungs is reduced to a degree depending on the severity of the pulmonary stenosis.

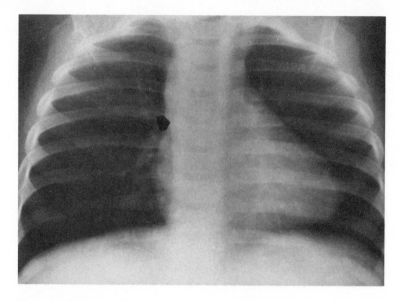

Figure 9.3. Chest radiograph in Fallot's tetralogy. The arrow points to
the right-sided aorta

Electrocardiography

In the newborn infant, the electrocardiogram may differ little from
normal, although the T wave may be positive in V_1 in infants with
tetralogy of Fallot. As the infant with the severe form of the disease
becomes older, severe right ventricular hypertrophy is seen. The R
wave in V_4R and V_1 is tall and there is an S wave in V_5 and V_6. The
P wave in lead 2 is often peaked in appearance, indicating right
atrial hypertrophy. A Q wave in V_4R or V_1 is unusual in tetralogy of
Fallot and suggests the possibility of corrected transposition of the
great vessels with pulmonary stenosis, or severe pulmonary stenosis
and atrial septal defect.

Echocardiography

The most characteristic feature is the overriding of the septum by
the aorta (*See Figure 9.4*). Usually the drop-out of septal echoes in
the region of the ventricular septal defect can be shown. In severe
cases, with a narrow outflow to the right ventricle, it is not possible
to demonstrate the pulmonary valve. The relative size of the aorta

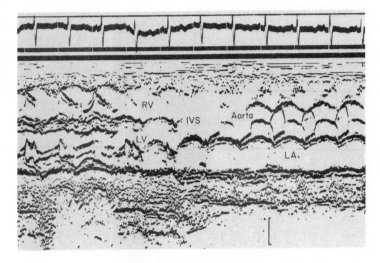

Figure 9.4. Tetralogy of Fallot. Echocardiogram showing 'drop-out' of echoes from the interventricular or septum (IVS) and the overriding aorta with its anterior wall in front of the line of the septum. Compare with normal UCG on p. 41)

and right ventricular outflow (infundibulum) has been used as a guide to surgical treatment, as a very large aorta and diminutive outflow will necessitate reconstruction with some form of patch.

Cardiac catheterization and angiography

Although a reliable diagnosis of tetralogy of Fallot can be made after a careful history, clinical examination, radiography and electrocardiography, further investigation by cardiac catheterization and angiography is indicated to define the precise anatomy inside the heart before considering complete correction of the defects (*Figure 9.5*). It is also useful to show the size of the pulmonary arteries and on which side the aorta lies before recommending palliative operations.

Complications

Cerebral thrombosis

Cerebral thrombosis is most common in severely cyanosed infants and young children and may cause hemiplegia. Such children may

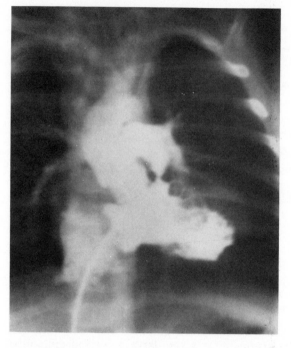

Figure 9.5. Right ventricular angiogram of a 6-month-old infant
with Fallot's tetralogy. The infundibular stenosis is well shown,
the pulmonary arteries are small and most of the contrast has
passed backwards through the ventricular septal defect and
entered the aorta

have high haematocrit values and should always be kept well
hydrated so that the viscosity of their blood is not further increased
by dehydration. Martelle and Linde (1961), however, have found a
closer relationship between the presence of relative anaemia and
hemiplegia, than between high haematocrit levels and hemiplegia.

Cerebral abscess

A diagnosis of cerebral abscess should always be considered in a
child with tetralogy of Fallot who presents with headaches, fever
and a change of personality followed by vomiting, convulsions and
localizing cerebral signs. A hemiplegia may occur insidiously.
Cerebral abscess is hardly ever associated with bacterial endocarditis. It is possible that there is some localized cerebral damage
following thrombosis and that infection subsequently occurs when

there is a systemic bacteraemia. Early diagnosis with prompt treatment nowadays carries a good prognosis in this condition. It must be stressed that a shunt operation does not alter the incidence of cerebral abscess and is another reason why complete correction is a preferable operation if the child's size permits it. Taussig (1971), in her long follow-up study of patients who had shunt operations, found an incidence of 5.5 per cent.

Bacterial endocarditis

Bacterial endocarditis should be suspected in patients with unexplained fever. The associated anaemia in bacterial endocarditis may not be appreciated in tetralogy of Fallot because the haematocrit value is usually very much higher than normal, so a normal blood count in a patient with tetralogy of Fallot indicates some degree of anaemia. Taussig's (1971) follow-up showed an incidence of bacterial endocarditis of 14.3 per cent and a mortality rate of 21.4 per cent.

Haemorrhagic tendency

Any operation in patients with tetralogy of Fallot may be associated with excessive bleeding. This is probably associated with the lowered platelet count and is best controlled by transfusing with fresh whole blood. Sudden blood loss in a child with tetralogy of Fallot may aggravate the hypoxia to a dangerous degree.

Treatment

Restriction of exercise is unnecessary since such patients restrict themselves. It should be ensured that infants and young children have adequate supplies of iron so that they do not become relatively anaemic. If a child with tetralogy of Fallot is found to have a *relatively* low haemoglobin the response to iron therapy may be dramatic and cause marked improvement in symptoms. There should be scrupulous care of the teeth and prophylactic penicillin should be given to cover dental extraction. Dehydration should be prevented during intercurrent illnesses. Loss of blood from any cause may require transfusion to prevent hypotension occurring.

Cyanotic attacks are thought to be associated with narrowing of the outflow tract from the right ventricle due to infundibular spasm. Infants are helped by being placed in the knee/elbow position and morphine (0.2 mg/kg) may terminate an attack; 100 per cent oxygen should be given by mask, and acidosis which develops should be corrected by intravenous sodium bicarbonate. More recently, propranolol (0.1 mg/kg) i.v. as a bolus has been found to be of value in terminating attacks (Cumming, 1970). An alternative method of terminating attacks is to give a drug which increases the peripheral vascular resistance, such as metaraminol (0.2 mg/kg i.m. or i.v.) or methoxamine, 0.2 mg/kg. The occurrence of cyanotic attacks is an indication for surgery. *Digoxin should not be used in patients with cyanotic attacks.* It may be dangerous because it increases the contraction of the heart muscle and may further narrow the outflow tract from the right ventricle.

If surgery has to be delayed for any reason or if a shunt operation has not been successful, propranolol may be used to prevent or reduce the frequency of the attacks (Eriksson, 1969). It has been more effective in infants than in older children and should be given orally 6 hourly in a dose of 1.0 mg/kg. The longterm results of propranolol, however, are not as good as a successful shunt operation.

Surgical treatment

All patients require surgery at some time but the choice of operation and the time it is carried out varies with the clinical severity of the lesion, the size of child and the anatomy demonstrated at angiography.

Some surgeons recommend total correction at all times (Radley-Smith *et al.*, 1980; Norwood *et al.*, 1980; Starr *et al.*, 1973) but the mortality in most centres would then be unacceptably high. At present most workers are agreed that in the first year of life palliative surgery is safest and after that (unless the pulmonary arteries are very small and the outflow tract from the right ventricle grossly underdeveloped), total repair is advised sometime before school age (Levy *et al.*, 1980).

The two usual procedures are Blalock–Taussig shunt and Waterston anastomosis (*see* p. 52). Lincoln *et al.* (1980) found that when the pulmonary artery diameter before the bifurcation was less than 5 mm, the best operation was enlargement of the right ventricular outflow tract with a patch, valved conduit or infundibulectomy. A subsequent operation to relieve the remaining obstruction and close the ventricular septal defect is then carried out in a few years' time when the increased blood flow has enabled the pulmonary arteries to grow.

Patients with a mild form of tetralogy of Fallot do not need palliative surgery in infancy and can wait for total repair sometime before school age. The definitive operation consists of closure of the ventricular septal defect and relief of the right ventricular outflow obstruction, either by resecting the obstruction or combining this with an onlay patch to enlarge the outflow tract. Depending on the exact anatomy the patch may be confined to the infundibulum or extend across the valve ring into the pulmonary artery. The operation is carried out with cardiopulmonary bypass on profound hypothermia.

It is often impossible for the surgeon to relieve the obstruction fully, but the aim is to reduce the right ventricular pressure to one-third or less of the left ventricular pressure. Following the operation almost all patients have a residual systolic murmur and most have a diastolic murmur due to pulmonary regurgitation—particularly those in whom a patch has been inserted across the pulmonary valve. Nevertheless there is usually a dramatic improvement in exercise tolerance following operation and postoperative studies (Finnegan *et al.*, 1976) have shown near normal exercise tolerance.

As in most operations nowadays, the aim is to make the heart as normal as possible as soon as possible so that the heart muscle is not overloaded for a long time and can return to normal function after surgery as the child grows.

PULMONARY ATRESIA WITH VENTRICULAR SEPTAL DEFECT

Incidence

About one-fifth of patients who present with symptoms similar to those of tetralogy of Fallot have pulmonary atresia, although it is more common than Fallot's tetralogy as a cause of cyanosis in the newborn infant.

Definition

This deformity is distinct from tetralogy of Fallot, although the ventricular septal defect lies in the same position or even more anteriorly. There is no way through to the pulmonary artery from the right ventricle and all the right ventricular blood enters the aorta. The site of atresia varies. There may be atresia of the valve alone, the pulmonary artery and its branches being well formed, or there may be complete obstruction of the infundibulum of the right ventricle. Blood may enter the pulmonary arteries by a patent ductus or by aortopulmonary collateral vessels. Recognizable pulmonary arteries are absent in some cases of pulmonary atresia and the lungs are supplied by large tortuous vessels arising from the aortic arch or the upper portion of the descending thoracic aorta.

170

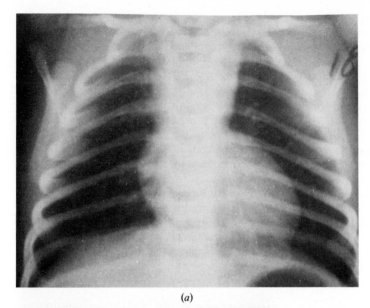

(a)

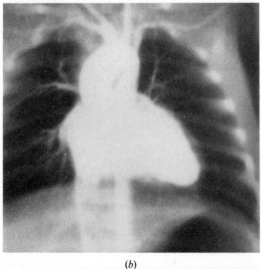

(b)

Figure 9.6. Pulmonary atresia with ventricular septal defect. (*a*) Three-day-old infant. A plain chest radiograph showing oligaemic lungs. (*b*) Right ventricular angiogram showing AP and (*c*) showing lateral absence of filling of the outflow portion of the right ventricle, filling of the left ventricle and aorta and opacification of the pulmonary artery through a small ductus arteriosus.

Usually in cases of pulmonary atresia with ventricular septal defect, the pulmonary blood flow is decreased, but occasionally the patent ductus arteriosus is very large or there are large aortopulmonary collateral vessels and the blood flow to the lungs is increased.

Natural history

Patients tend to become increasingly blue and breathless and many would die in the first few years of life without surgery. A few who have a good pulmonary blood flow from collateral vessels, lead restricted lives into the third decade.

Clinical presentation

The patient usually presents with cyanosis earlier than tetralogy of Fallot, frequently in the first few weeks of life. Subsequently there is no history of sudden cyanotic attacks and no squatting. There is no systolic murmur over the outflow tract of the right ventricle. Continuous murmurs may be heard anteriorly or posteriorly, due to blood flowing through collateral vessels to the lungs. There are a few patients in whom there is a high pulmonary blood flow (more than

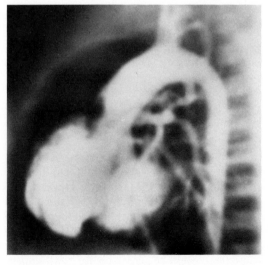

(c)

Figure 9.6

twice the systemic flow) due to large collateral vessels. Such patients are only mildly cyanosed, the heart is large and hyperactive and heart failure may be present early in life. Such patients may initially be diagnosed as having patent ductus arteriosus, but the widespread continuous murmurs, usually heard posteriorly as well as anteriorly, the slight cyanosis and the right ventricular hypertrophy on the electrocardiogram contradict this.

Radiology

Radiological appearances are similar to tetralogy of Fallot but there is marked pulmonary oligaemia and a longer left cardiac border (*Figure 9.6*).

Electrocardiography

The electrocardiogram resembles that seen in tetralogy of Fallot, with right axis deviation and right atrial and right ventricular hypertrophy.

Echocardiography

The overriding aorta with drop-out of septal echoes just below can usually be demonstrated (*Figure 9.4*). The aorta is large and no pulmonary valve can be shown.

Investigation

Investigation is necessary to try to show whether central pulmonary arteries are present and if so how big they are. In older children the collateral vessels have been catheterized (Macartney, Deverall and Scott, 1973) and are at systemic pressure. Many of them have stenoses on them as they enter the hilum of the lung and there is a fall in pressure across the stenoses. Many such vessels enter the lung directly without entering a pulmonary artery proper and the pressure in them (at a point where they would be accessible for anastomosis) is too high to permit an anastomotic operation. It is often difficult to demonstrate central pulmonary arteries at angiography because they fill late by retrograde flow from the collateral vessels. Injection into pulmonary veins however will fill these low pressure central pulmonary arteries retrogradely and demonstrate their size (Singh *et al.*, 1980).

Treatment

In newborn infants sometimes the only way in which blood reaches the lungs is through a patent ductus arteriosus. Closure of this tends to occur and death results. Nowadays prostaglandins can be used to encourage the ductus to stay open until some palliative surgery—either a Blalock or Waterston shunt—can be performed. The prostaglandins E1 or E2 are given intravenously in a dose of 0.1 μg/kg per min. This is a temporary procedure but results in better oxygenation of the child and ensures that he goes for surgery in a much better condition. Oral preparations of prostaglandin E2 have been found to be effective and can be used for several weeks in a dose of 62.5 μcg to 250 μcg hourly to 3 hourly (Silove *et al.*, 1979). Toxic effects of prostaglandins are uncommon but they do cause vasodilatation and hypotension and the blood pressure must be watched. High temperatures have also been observed. When central pulmonary arteries are demonstrated, they are usually small. Howarth and Macartney (1980) have shown that the branches of these central pulmonary arteries supply fewer than half of the bronchopulmonary segments, so that demonstration of central pulmonary arteries does not mean that they can be used to carry adequate blood flow to the lungs. Also, when the peripheral pulmonary arteries were studied, they found that the intra-acinar arteries could be hypoplastic or show hypertensive obliterative change and there was a variation in pulmonary vascular resistance from one segment of lung to another.

In infancy a palliative procedure such as a Blalock or Waterston's operation may be performed if there is a central pulmonary artery present which is suitable for anastomosis. Surgical repair of the lesion is only possible if there are well defined pulmonary arteries to both lungs but as Howarth *et al.* (1980) have shown, satisfactory total repair is not possible in a large number of patients because there are stenoses between the central pulmonary arteries and the lobar pulmonary arteries, and the peripheral vessels continue to be abnormally small. In these cases only rarely will a conduit from the right ventricle to central pulmonary arteries, closure of the ventricular septal defect and ligation of collateral vessels, give satisfactory results.

PULMONARY VALVE STENOSIS WITH RIGHT-TO-LEFT SHUNT AT ATRIAL LEVEL

Incidence

The incidence of pulmonary valve stenosis is 10 per cent of all congenital heart lesions, and about one-quarter of patients have a right-to-left shunt at atrial level. The most severe form presents in infancy.

Definition

The degree of stenosis at the pulmonary valve is severe and there is a very high right ventricular pressure. This results in a high right atrial pressure and the foramen ovale is forced open so that there is a right-to-left shunt at atrial level. Occasionally, an atrial septal defect is present. It is of interest that some infants and children can withstand very high pressures in the right ventricle without developing tricuspid incompetence and without having any right-to-left shunt.

Natural history

The stenosis is usually so severe in these children that, if it is not relieved, right heart failure and death will follow in infancy or early childhood. Occasionally, patients survive into adult life.

Clinical presentation

Symptoms usually begin in infancy but the patients usually gain weight satisfactorily initially and are often moon-faced healthy-looking babies. Cyanosis is usually slight initially and the infants are thought to have a healthy colour until they gradually or suddenly become more cyanosed and dyspnoeic or develop heart failure. There is an ejection systolic murmur in the second left interspace but a thrill is often absent because the stenosis is so severe. The murmur becomes softer when there is a large right-to-left shunt, because there is a reduced blood flow through the stenotic valve. In a small number of cases a loud pansystolic murmur is audible in the tricuspid area due to tricuspid incompetence.

Radiology

In contrast to tetralogy of Fallot the heart is enlarged and there is conspicuous enlargement of the right atrium. The lung fields are oligaemic.

Electrocardiography

The electrocardiogram shows right atrial hypertrophy with peaked P waves in lead 2 and right ventricular hypertrophy with deeply inverted T waves in the right ventricular leads. When there is a large right-to-left shunt there is evidence of increased activity over the left ventricle also.

Investigation

Investigation demonstrates the high right ventricular pressure, but in small infants it may be impossible to pass the catheter across the pulmonary valve. The pulmonary stenosis is then best demonstrated by right ventricular angiography. If, as is usually the case, the interatrial communication is only a foramen ovale, the right atrial pressure is higher than the left and shows a prominent 'a' wave.

Treatment

When there is cardiac enlargement and right-to-left shunt at atrial level, surgery is indicated. Operation becomes a matter of emergency if dyspnoea or heart failure occurs. Medical treatment will not help the heart failure for any length of time in the presence of severe mechanical obstruction. Now that cardiopulmonary bypass can be safely used in infants and young children the risks of surgery are diminishing and the benefits of surgery are dramatic in these patients. Mustard, Jain and Trusler (1968) achieved excellent results in infancy (mortality of 4 per cent) using transarterial valvotomy with inflow occlusion of the venae cavae.

PULMONARY ATRESIA WITH INTACT VENTRICULAR SEPTUM

Incidence

Pulmonary atresia with intact ventricular septum comprises less than 1 per cent of all cardiac malformations.

Definition

There is no way out for the blood from the right ventricle and no ventricular septal defect so that the blood from the right atrium has to pass through a foramen ovale (or an atrial septal defect) to the left heart. The only way blood can reach the lungs is through a patent ductus arteriosus or the bronchial circulation (*Figure 9.7*).

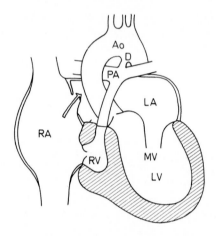

Figure 9.7. Pulmonary atresia with intact ventricular septum and hypoplastic right ventricle. D: ductus arteriosus; PA: pulmonary artery; RA: right atrium; RV: hypoplastic right ventricle; LA: left atrium; MV: mitral valve; LV: left ventricle

Zuberbuhler *et al.* (1979) carried out careful measurements of the right ventricle in this lesion and found that it was usually smaller than normal and only a few specimens had large right ventricles. In most cases the infundibulum was stenotic or atretic and the outflow tract obstruction was rarely at the valve only. There is often tricuspid regurgitation and Ebstein's anomaly of the tricuspid valve sometimes occurs.

Natural history

Death usually occurs in the first few months of life if no treatment is available (Moller and co-workers, 1970).

Clinical presentation

Cyanosis is present at birth and shortly becomes intense; dyspnoea and heart failure develop rapidly. There may be no heart murmurs but sometimes there is a systolic murmur due to tricuspid regurgitation or to flow through the patent ductus arteriosus.

Radiology

The chest radiograph shows some cardiomegaly after the first day or two of life. The right atrium is prominent. The pulmonary vascular markings are usually diminished unless the ductus is widely patent.

Electrocardiography

The electrocardiogram shows peaked, tall P waves indicating right atrial enlargement. There is a normal QRS axis. In the cases with hypoplastic right ventricle the anterior precordial leads (V_1 and V_2) show less right ventricular activity than is usually seen in infancy (or there may be left ventricular hypertrophy) and this pattern, in a severely cyanosed infant with oligaemic lung fields, is highly suggestive of pulmonary atresia with intact ventricular septum.

Echocardiography

It is usually possible to demonstrate the slit-like right ventricular cavity surrounded by thick muscle and a relatively large left ventricle and aorta. (*Figure 9.8*)

Cardiac catheterization

Cardiac catheterization shows elevation of the right atrial pressure; the right ventricular pressure usually exceeds systemic pressure. The blood in the right side of the heart is markedly desaturated. The pulmonary artery cannot be entered but the catheter will pass through the foramen ovale or atrial septal defect to the left atrium and left ventricle where there is also desaturation of the blood because of the large right-to-left shunt. The degree of desaturation in the left ventricle depends on the amount of blood flowing to the lungs through a patent ductus. If there is a small pulmonary blood

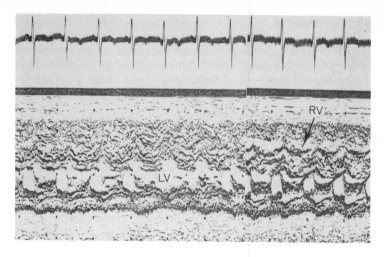

Figure 9.8. Pulmonary atresia with intact interventricular septum. The ultrasound cardiogram shows a muscular right ventricle with a small cavity (shown only in the portion on the right)

flow, only a small amount of oxygenated blood will return to the left atrium; if there is an unusually large pulmonary blood flow to the lungs through a patent ductus, then there will be a large amount of oxygenated blood returning to the left heart and the oxygen saturation is only a little less than normal.

Angiography

Angiography shows pulmonary obstruction and the dye refluxes back through the tricuspid valve to the right atrium and then enters the left side of the heart. The size of the right ventricle is shown and the ductus arteriosus demonstrated.

Treatment

Kachener (1979) has pointed out that the longterm outlook with and without surgery is poor and this is supported by the series of Buckley *et al.* (1976) and Trusler *et al.* (1976). The difficult decision is whether surgery should be undertaken at all. The infants can be helped initially by balloon septostomy and maintaining patency of the ductus with prostaglandins (p. 173). If then, after careful assessment of the angiograms, surgery is feasible, then a combination of a systemic-pulmonary artery shunt and a pulmonary valvotomy will improve the immediate survival rate. Right heart hypoplasia and tricuspid valve abnormalities limit the possibility of surgical correction later in life.

TRICUSPID ATRESIA

Incidence

Tricuspid atresia accounts for about 2 per cent of all congenital deformities and is the next most common cyanotic lesion to the tetralogy of Fallot after the first year of life.

Definition

The tricuspid valve is absent and there is no direct communication between the right atrium and right ventricle. Survival depends on there being an open foramen ovale or atrial septal defect for right atrial blood to empty into the left side of the heart, which is well developed. The development of the right side of the heart varies with the size of the ventricular septal defect and the degree of pulmonary stenosis. Most commonly there is pulmonary stenosis and the ventricular septal defect is small and some blood from the left ventricle passes through this into a very small right ventricle and then through a narrowed outflow tract into a small pulmonary artery. The blood flow to the lungs is reduced (*Figure 9.9*).

Occasionally, there is only mild or no pulmonary stenosis and the ventricular septal defect is large. Blood flows into a well developed ventricular infundibulum and into a pulmonary artery of good size, producing an increased flow of blood to the lungs (*Figure 9.9*). As the child grows the ventricular septal defect becomes relatively smaller and may eventually close. This causes a deterioration in the child's condition with increasing cyanosis.

Rarely, there is no ventricular septal defect and there is associated pulmonary valve atresia. The only way blood can reach the lungs in this group is through a patent ductus arteriosus or bronchial arteries.

Natural history

Half the patients will die before six months if help is not given. It is rare for patients with a small ventricular septal defect and diminished blood flow to the lungs to survive more than one year.

The prognosis is best in cases where the pulmonary stenosis is mild, the ventricular septal defect is large and there is an adequate flow of blood to the lungs. The expectation of life for this group without treatment is 8–10 years.

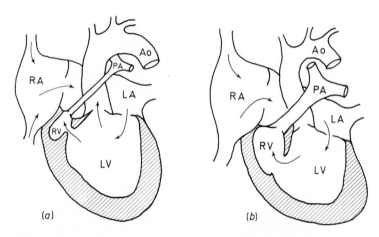

Figure 9.9. Tricuspid atresia. (*a*) With pulmonary stenosis and small ventricular septal defect. (*b*) With no pulmonary stenosis and increased pulmonary blood flow. RA: right atrium; RV: diminutive right ventricle; LA: left atrium; LV: left ventricle; PA: pulmonary artery; Ao: aorta

Clinical presentation

When there is diminished pulmonary blood flow, cyanosis is present at birth and the less the pulmonary blood flow, the greater the degree of cyanosis. There is dyspnoea and the infant feeds poorly and fails to thrive normally. Heart failure does not occur. A systolic thrill is unusual but, unless pulmonary atresia is present, a systolic murmur can be heard along the left sternal edge. The second sound is single.

When there is an adequate or excessive flow of blood to the lungs, there may be only a mild degree of cyanosis and the physical signs in the heart are those of ventricular septal defect with a systolic thrill and pansystolic murmur in the third and fourth left interspace. Heart failure may occur in this group.

Radiology

The heart size is not increased. There is little cardiac shadow to the right of the spine. The configuration resembles tetralogy of Fallot but the left border assumes a more 'square shape' and the apex is not tilted upwards. The vascularity of the lungs is diminished except in the group with a large ventricular septal defect.

Electrocardiography

Left axis deviation is the most common finding and its occurrence in a *cyanotic* infant makes tricuspid atresia by far the most likely lesion. The precordial leads show evidence of left ventricular hypertrophy. The deep S waves in V_4R and V_1 are more impressive than the tall R waves in V_5 and V_6. There are tall P waves in lead 2, indicating right atrial hypertrophy.

Echocardiography

The presence of a single atrioventricular valve is confirmed and, by its continuity with a semilunar valve, that it is the mitral valve. Usually only a single ventricle is shown, but when there is a well-developed outflow chamber this too may be demonstrated. Two-dimensional studies, angling the transducer up from the apex, will show the detailed anatomy.

Investigation

Infants with oligaemic lung fields usually require surgical help; cardiac catheterization and angiography are indicated to confirm the anatomical arrangement and to demonstrate the size of the pulmonary arteries.

The right ventricle cannot be entered but the catheter passes easily into the left atrium and left ventricle where the blood is desaturated. Injection of contrast into the right atrium shows obstruction of the tricuspid valve; the contrast often refluxes into the hepatic veins. A dimple is visible in the anteroposterior view at the level of the tricuspid valve. Selective angiography with the catheter tip in the left ventricle demonstrates the size of the ventricular septal defect, right ventricle and pulmonary arteries.

Treatment

In the newborn or young infant in whom the foramen ovale is small and obstructive there will be some improvement from atrial septostomy at the time of diagnostic catheterization. When the pulmonary arteries are small and the infant is moderately or severely cyanosed a shunt operation of some sort is required, either a Blalock–Taussig or Waterston. There was some enthusiasm for the Glenn operation which is an anastomosis between the superior vena cava and right pulmonary artery. This is unsatisfactory in young infants however because the pulmonary arteries are too small. Other disadvantages of the Glenn operation are thrombosis of the superior vena cava and gradual decrease in the perfusion of the lung because of the development of collateral vessels between the superior and inferior vena cava.

When the pulmonary blood flow is excessive and heart failure occurs, banding of the pulmonary artery may be the only way in which the heart failure can be controlled.

A more definitive operation has now become possible—the Fontan operation, in which a conduit is placed between the right atrium and pulmonary artery directly. The right atrium is then being used as the pumping chamber (*Figure 9.10*). Some surgeons use valves in the conduit and may also place a valve at the IVC–right atrial junction to limit regurgitation of blood into the IVC. The fate of the valves is uncertain, but some reports indicate that they fail to retain their function and may actually produce obstruction. The best results are obtained when the patient has a good pulmonary valve and the right atrium can be joined into the outlet chamber below it.

Mair *et al.* (1980) had an overall mortality of 14 per cent but in their last 29 cases the mortality is down to 7 per cent and the results have been excellent or good. Patients have to be carefully selected and many have already had shunt operations earlier in life. The

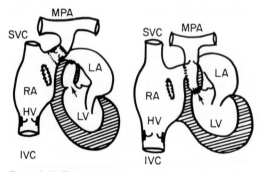

Figure 9.10. Fontan operation for tricuspid atresia. *Left:* the right atrium is connected to the main pulmonary artery. *Right:* patient's own pulmonary valve is normal; the right atrium is connected to the outflow chamber and the VSD (arrowed) closed. The homograft valves (HV) in the IVC are sometimes omitted

pulmonary resistance must be low and the artery of a reasonable size for anastomosis and there must be good left ventricular function.

EBSTEIN'S ANOMALY WITH RIGHT-TO-LEFT INTERATRIAL SHUNT

The abnormality of the tricuspid valve known as Ebstein's anomaly is discussed in detail in the section on lesions causing right heart obstruction (p. 153). Although about one-fifth of patients with this condition are acyanotic, the remainder present with cyanosis due to a right-to-left shunt through a patent foramen ovale or an atrial septal defect. In its most severe form, the lesion causes cyanosis and heart failure in infancy.

The radiograph shows a large globular heart with oligaemic lung fields and it must be differentiated from pulmonary stenosis with a right-to-left shunt through an atrial septal defect. This may be difficult clinically because both conditions may cause murmurs of tricuspid incompetence and in both the second heart sound may be single or widely split with a very soft second element. The electrocardiogram is of great value in differentiation, for in Ebstein's disease there is usually complete right bundle branch block with small R waves and gross right atrial hypertrophy, the P waves being often taller than the QRS complexes. Sometimes, however, cardiac catheterization is necessary to exclude severe pulmonary stenosis with a reversed shunt, which is an operable condition.

Treatment

Treatment may not be required for many cases of Ebstein's disease. If however cyanosis is severe or heart failure cannot be controlled, then in older children either tricuspid valve replacement or closure of the tricuspid annulus followed by a Fontan operation (*see* p. 182) is possible.

BIBLIOGRAPHY AND REFERENCES

Tetralogy of Fallot
Abbott, M. E. (1936). *Atlas of Congenital Cardiac Disease.* p. 46. New York: American Heart Association
Bertranon, E. G., Blackstone, E. H., Hazelrig, J. B., Turner, M. E. and Kirklin, J. W. (1978). Life expectancy without surgery in tetralogy of Fallot. *Am. J. Cardiol.* **42**, 458–466
Bristow, J. D., Kloster, F. E., Lees, M. H., Menashe, V. D., Griswood, H. E. and Starr, A. (1970). Serial cardiac catheterisations and exercise hemodynamics after correction of tetralogy of Fallot. *Circulation* **41**, 1057

184   CYANOTIC LESIONS WITH DIMINISHED PULMONARY FLOW

Burnell, R. H., Woodson, R. D., Lees, M. H., Bristow, J. D. and Starr, A. (1969). Results of correction of tetralogy of Fallot in children under four years of age. *J. thorac. cardiovasc. Surg.* **57**, 153

Cumming, G. R. (1970). Propranolol in tetralogy of Fallot. *Circulation* **41**, 9

Eriksson, B. O., Thorén, C. and Zetterqvist, P. (1969). Long term treatment with propranolol in selected cases of Fallot's tetralogy. *Br. Heart J.* **31**, 37

Gotsman, M. S., Beck, W., Barnard, C. N., O'Donovan, T. G. and Shrire, V. (1969). Results of repair of tetralogy of Fallot. *Circulation* **40**, 803

Gunteroth, W. G., Mortan, B. C., Mullins, G. L. and Baum, D. (1968). Venous return with knee–chest position and squatting in tetralogy of Fallot. *Am. Heart J.* **75**, 313

Haworth, S. G. and Macartney, F. J. (1980). The intrapulmonary arterial circulation in pulmonary atresia with ventricular septal defect and major aortopulmonary collateral arteries: how the anatomy determines treatment. Abstract. World Congress on Paediatric Cardiology

Haworth, S. G., Rees, P. G., Taylor, J. F. N., deLeval, M., Stark, J. and Macartney, F. J. (1980). Pulmonary atresia with ventricular septal defect and major aortopulmonary collateral arteries: angiographic assessment of the pulmonary circulation before and after a systemic-pulmonary anastomosis. Abstract. World Congress on Paediatric Cardiology

Levy, J., Tripp, M. and Kahn, D. (1980). Optimal surgical management for minimal mortality for tetralogy of Fallot. Abstract. World Congress on Paediatric Cardiology

Lincoln, C., Shinebourne, E., Treasure, T., Leijala, M. and Lane, I. (1980). Direct surgical management of right ventricular outflow tract obstruction in children with diminutive pulmonary arteries. Abstract. World Congress on Paediatric Cardiology

Martelle, R. R. and Linde, L. M. (1961). Cerebrovascular accidents with tetralogy of Fallot. *Am. J. Dis. Child.* **101**, 206

Norwood, W. I., Keane, J. F., Borrow, K. and Castaneda, A. R. (1980). Repair of tetralogy of Fallot in infancy: early and late results. Abstract. World Congress on Paediatric Cardiology

Radley-Smith, R., Ilsley, C., Reid, C. and Yacomb, M. (1980). Late clinical and haemodynamic results after primary correction of tetralogy of Fallot. Abstract. World Congress on Paediatric Cardiology

Silove, E. D., Coe, J. Y., Page, A. J. F. and Mitchell, M. D. (1979). Long term oral prostaglandin E_2 maintains patency of ductus arteriosus. (Abstr.) *Circulation* **60**, 11

Singh, S. P., Astley, R. and Rigby, M. (1980). Wider experience with pulmonary vein angiography and indirect measurement of pulmonary artery pressure. Abstract. World Congress on Paediatric Cardiology

Starr, A., Bonchek, L. I. and Sunderland, C. O. (1973). Total correction of tetralogy of Fallot in infancy. *J. thorac. cardiovasc. Surg.* **65**, 45

Taussig, H. B., Crocetti, A., Eshagpour, E., Keinonen, R. and others (1971). Long-term observations of the Blalock–Taussig operation. *Johns Hopkins Med. J.* **129**, 243

Pulmonary atresia with ventricular septal defect

Kouchoukos, N. T., Barcia, A., Bargeron, L. M. and Kirklin, J. W. (1971). Surgical treatment of congenital pulmonary atresia with ventricular septal defect. *J. thorac. cardiovasc. Surg.* **61**, 70

Macartney, F., Deverall, P. and Scott, Olive (1973). Haemodynamic characteristics of systemic arterial blood supply to the lungs. *Br. Heart J.* **35**, 28

Miller, W. M., Nadas, A. S., Bernhard, W. F. and Gross, R. E. (1968). Congenital pulmonary atresia with ventricular septal defect. Review of the clinical course of fifty patients with assessment of the results of palliative surgery. *Am. J. Cardiol.* **21**, 673

Moller, J. H., Girod, G., Amplatz, K. and Varco, R. L. (1970). Pulmonary valvotomy in pulmonary atresia with hypoplastic right ventricle. *Surgery, St Louis* **68**, 630

Somerville, J. (1970). Management of pulmonary atresia. *Br. Heart J.* **32**, 641

Pulmonary atresia and stenosis

Benton, J. W. Jr., Elliott, L. P., Adams, P. Jr., Anderson, R. C., Hong, C. T. and Lester, R. G. (1962). Pulmonary atresia and stenosis with intact ventricular septum. *Am. J. Dis. Child.* **104**, 161

Bowman, F. O., Malm, J. R., Hayes, C. J., Gersony, W. M. and Ellis, K. (1969). Pulmonary atresia with intact ventricular septum. *J. thorac. cardiovasc. Surg.* **61**, 85

Dhanavaravibul, S., Nora, J. J. and McNamara, D. G. (1970). Pulmonary valvular atresia with intact ventricular septum. Problems in diagnosis and results of treatment. *J. Pediat.* **77**, 1010

Gamboa, R., Gersony, W. R. and Nadas, A. S. (1966). The electrocardiogram in tricuspid atresia and pulmonary atresia with intact ventricular septum. *Circulation* **34**, 24

Gersony, W. M., Bernhard, W. F., Nadas, A. S. and Gross, R. E. (1967). Diagnosis and surgical treatment of infants with critical pulmonary outflow obstruction. *Circulation* **35**, 765

Khoury, G. H., Gilbert, E. F., Chang, C. H. and Schmidt, R. (1969). The hypoplastic right heart complex: clinical hemodynamic, pathological and surgical considerations. *Am J. Cardiol.* **23**, 792

Mustard, W. T., Jain, S. C. and Trusler, G. A. (1968). Pulmonary stenosis in the first year of life. *Br. Heart J.* **30**, 255

Shams, A., Fowler, R. S., Trusler, G. A., Keith, J. D. and Mustard, W. T. (1971). Pulmonary atresia with intact interventricular septum. *Pediatrics, Springfield* **47**, 370

Pulmonary atresia with intact ventricular septum

Buckley, L. P., Dooley, K. J. and Fyler, D. C. (1976). Pulmonary atresia and intact ventricular septum in New England. *Am. J. Cardiol.* **37**, 124

Kachener, J. (1979). The assessment and medical management of newborn infants with pulmonary atresia and intact ventricular septum. In *Paediatric Cardiology.* pp. 297–304

Trusler, G. A., Yamamoto, N., Williams, G. W., Izukawa, T., Rowe, R. D. and Mustard, W. T. (1976). Surgical treatment of pulmonary atresia with intact ventricular septum. *Br. Heart J.* **38**, 957–960

Zuberbuhler, J. R., Fricker, F. J., Park, S. C., Anderson, R. H., Lennox, C. C., Neches, W. H. and Mathews, R. A. (1979). Pulmonary atresia with intact ventricular septum — morbid anatomy. *Paediatric Cardiology.* Vol. 2. pp. 285–295. *Heart Disease in the Newborn.* Eds M. J. Godman and R. M. Marquis. London: Churchill Livingstone

Tricuspid atresia

Edwards, S. W. and Bergeron, L. M. Jr. (1968). The superiority of the Glenn operation for tricuspid atresia in infancy and childhood. *J. thorac. cardiovasc. Surg.* **55**, 60

Mair, D. D., Danielson, G. K., Puga, F. J. and McGoon, D. C. (1980). The Fontan procedure for tricuspid atresia: criteria for patient selection and late results. Abstract. World Congress on Paediatric Cardiology

Morgano, B. A., Riemenschneider, T. A., Ruttenberg, H. D., Goldberg, S. J. and Gyepes, M. (1969). Tricuspid atresia with increased pulmonary blood flow. *Circulation* **40**, 398

Subramanian, S., Carr, I., Waterston, D. J. and Bonham Carter, R. E. (1965). Palliative surgery in tricuspid atresia. *Circulation* **32**, 977

CHAPTER 10

Cyanotic Lesions with Increased Pulmonary Blood Flow

TRANSPOSITION OF THE GREAT ARTERIES

Incidence

Complete transposition of the great arteries is the second most common cyanotic congenital heart lesion and accounts for about 5 per cent of all congenital heart lesions.

Definition

The term 'transposition' is used because the aorta and pulmonary artery have changed places. The aorta lies anterior to the pulmonary artery instead of posterior to it and the pulmonary artery lies posterior to the aorta instead of anterior to it. Regardless of any abnormality which may also exist, the term 'transposition' is used to describe this change in the position of the two great arteries. The term 'complete transposition' is used to describe the situation in which the aorta receives systemic venous blood and the pulmonary artery receives pulmonary venous blood. In these cases the heart has undergone normal looping to the right in its development; that is, there is a dextro-loop, and because of this the term 'D-transposition' is used. This also indicates that the aortic valve is to the right of the pulmonary valve in the anteroposterior view. It is also possible to describe transposition in the general terms used for complex anomalies described in Chapter 11. Using this terminology trans-

186

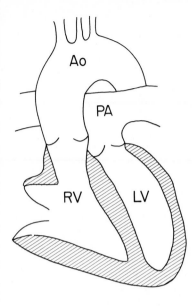

Figure 10.1. Complete transposition of the great arteries. The aorta (Ao) arises from the right ventricle (RV) above anterior and to the right of the pulmonary artery (PA) which arises from the left ventricle (LV)

position becomes 'situs solitus, atrioventricular concordance ventriculoarterial discordance' indicating that the atria and ventricles are normally situated and connected but that the great arteries are wrongly (discordantly) connected to the ventricles.

In complete transposition (synonymous with D-transposition), therefore, the aorta lies anterior to the pulmonary artery and receives desaturated systemic venous blood from the right ventricle; the aortic valve lies to the right of the pulmonary valve (*Figure 10.1*). As a result of the abnormality, two separate circulations are produced (*Figure 10.2*): the *systemic circulation*, consisting of venae cavae, right atrium, right ventricle and aorta; and the *pulmonary circulation*, consisting of pulmonary veins, left atrium, left ventricle and pulmonary artery.

Clinical presentation

During intrauterine life, transposition is of little consequence since the lungs are bypassed and the small difference in oxygen saturation between pulmonary artery and aortic blood is unimportant. After birth the clinical picture is influenced by the degree of communication between the two circulations. Patients may be divided into three groups.

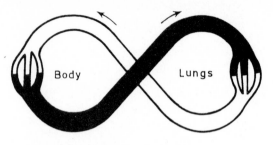

Normal circulation

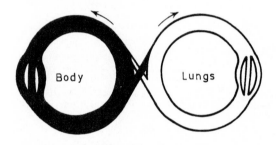

Transposition

Figure 10.2. Complete transposition of the great arteries. In the normal circulation right and left sides of the heart are connected in series; in the transposition they are in parallel and the effective flow to the lungs for gas exchange is the small amount of cross-over at, for example, an atrial septal defect

1. Those in whom the only communication between the two circulations is a patient foramen ovale and a small patent ductus arteriosus and where there is poor mixing between the two circulations. This type has been termed 'simple' transposition or 'isolated' transposition. The pulmonary blood flow is normal or slightly increased.
2. Those in whom there is a significant ventricular septal defect or large patent ductus arteriosus, and in whom there is a high pulmonary blood flow.
3. Those in whom there is pulmonary stenosis of a significant degree, resulting in a low pulmonary blood flow and oligaemic lung fields.

ISOLATED TRANSPOSITION

Patients in the first group present in the first week of life. The infant may appear relatively well at birth but cyanosis gradually becomes obvious and increases, the infant becoming acidotic. Feeding becomes more difficult and breathlessness and heart failure follow. There are usually no murmurs but the second sound is loud due to the anterior position of the aorta.

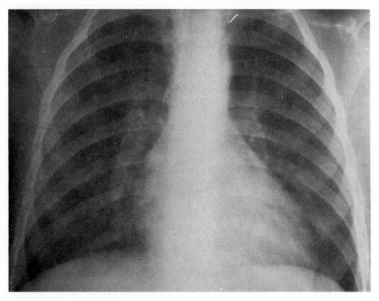

Figure 10.3. Radiograph of transposition of the great arteries. There is a narrow vascular pedicle and the shape of the heart resembles an egg on its side. Pulmonary vasculature is normal or slightly increased

Radiology

Radiology gives most help in making the diagnosis. The pedicle of the heart is narrow and the heart itself looks like an egg on its side, the pointed part of the 'egg' forming the apex of the heart (*Figure 10.3.*). The lung fields may appear normal in the early days of life but later they become plethoric. If the thymus is large the narrow pedicle is obscured and the film is then not so helpful.

Electrocardiography

The electrocardiogram shows the normal neonatal pattern of right ventricular hypertrophy at first and this persists, or increases with age (*Figure 10.4*).

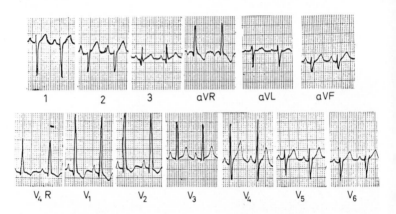

Figure 10.4. Electrocardiogram of a 2-year-old boy with transposition of the great arteries. (Balloon atrial septostomy in infancy). There is right atrial and right ventricular hypertrophy. The electrical axis is $-160°$ (extreme right axis deviation in this case) and the q waves in $V_4 R$ to V_2 are due to right atrial enlargement

Echocardiography

It is difficult to make the diagnosis of transposition directly by echocardiography as the aortic and pulmonary valves give the same type of echo. Modern two-dimensional techniques may enable the branching of the main pulmonary artery to be shown and therefore identified as the posterior great artery. However, by excluding conditions such as pulmonary atresia and tricuspid atresia, which can be done readily, echocardiography enables a diagnosis of exclusion in transposition.

Investigation

Investigation is a matter of urgency. The acidosis is corrected and the diagnosis is confirmed by catheterization and angiography as quickly as possible, avoiding hypothermia. The left ventricular pressure can usually be measured by passing the catheter through the foramen ovale and then into the left ventricle. The pulmonary artery pressure is usually not recorded in the sick infant. Right and left ventricular angiograms will exclude the presence of a ventricular septal defect and patent ductus arteriosus (*Figure 10.5*). The aorta is seen arising anteriorly from the right ventricle and the pulmonary artery fills when dye is injected into the left ventricle. The pulmonary venous blood is usually fully saturated with oxygen but the aortic blood oxygen saturation may be as low as 16 per cent. The left atrial pressure is high when there is a very small communication between the two atria.

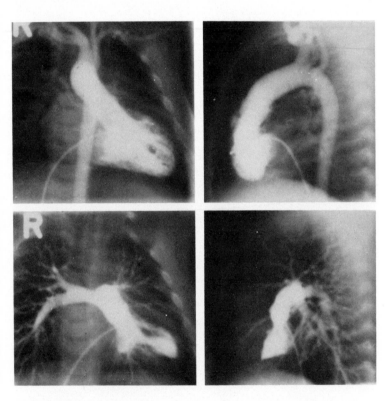

Figure 10.5. Transposition of the great arteries and no ventricular septal defect. Upper films are of a right ventricular injection, lower ones of a left ventricular injection. Anteroposterior films are on the right and lateral ones on the left

Treatment

After the diagnosis is confirmed a Rashkind balloon catheter is inserted and passed through the foramen ovale into the left atrium

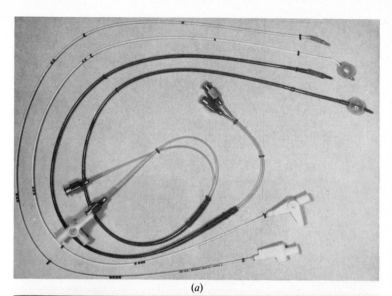

(a)

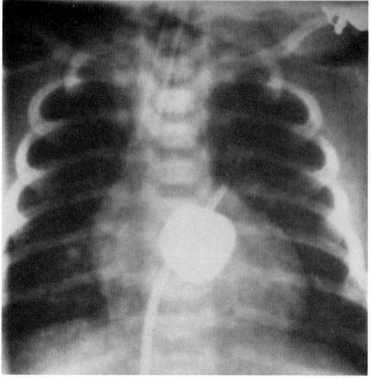

(b)

(*Figure 10.6*). The balloon is then filled with radio-opaque dye and pulled back through the foramen rapidly so as to tear the atrial septum around the foramen. The procedure is repeated several times until there is no resistance when the balloon is pulled through the atrial septum and until the gradient between the two atria is abolished. The results of this balloon septostomy are variable and in some infants the result seems disappointing initially but the infant gradually improves after two or three days. In others there is a marked improvement immediately and the oxygen saturation rises by 20–30 per cent.

The procedure carries a risk. Care is necessary to ensure that the catheter is lying in the left atrium when the balloon is filled with dye and not in the right ventricle, otherwise damage to the tricuspid valve may result if the balloon is pulled through it. In experienced hands, however, the risks are small. Some patients may require a further septostomy after some weeks if their condition deteriorates. In a few, a satisfactory result is not achieved following septostomy and the creation of an atrial septal defect by operation is required. Alternatively an early Mustard operation (*see below*) is performed.

Medical treatment with digoxin and diuretics is often required and chest infections must be prevented if possible or treated early if they occur. The initial procedures are palliative and a definitive operation is advised when the patients are bigger. This is called a Mustard operation after the surgeon who described it. An intra-atrial cardiac baffle of pericardium or Dacron is placed in such a way as to route the systemic venous return into the left atrium and so into the left ventricle to reach the lungs (*Figure 10.7*). The pulmonary venous blood is directed into the right atrium and so to the right ventricle and into the aorta. The time at which corrective surgery is advised depends on the progress made following palliative treatment, but most centres aim to carry out corrective surgery between 1 and 2 years of age. The immediate results of this operation are good but there has not been sufficient time for longterm follow-up.

The Mustard operation is not strictly a corrective operation, and worry about the longterm ability of the right ventricle and tricuspid valve to support the systemic circulation has led surgeons to attempt alternative methods of treatment.

Figure 10.6. (a). Atrioseptostomy catheters. Outer pair: Foggarty catheters (by Edwards Laboratories). Inner pair: Rashkind double-lumen type (USCI). One of each pair has been partially inflated (*see also (b)*). (*b*). Double-lumen Rashkind catheter partially inflated in the left atrium

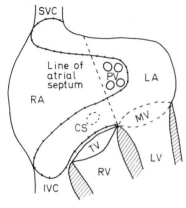

Figure 10.7. Mustard's operation for transposition of the great arteries. The blood from the superior vena cava (SVC) and the inferior vena cava (IVC) is routed by the patch into the left atrium (LA), through the mitral valve (MV) into the left ventricle (LV). Blood from the pulmonary veins (PV) passes to the right atrium (RA), through the tricuspid valve (TV) into the right ventricle (RV). The atrial septum is removed prior to insertion of the patch. The blood from the coronary sinus (CS) is, in this instance, drained into the left ventricle, but this means putting the patch close to the atrioventricular node and some surgeons prefer to allow this small amount of desaturated blood to drain into the systemic circulation

Additionally, about 7–10 per cent of children who have had Mustard's operation require a subsequent operation to correct obstruction to the various venous pathways within the atria, usually from shrinkage of the pericardial patch.

A direct 'switch' of the aorta and pulmonary artery is initially an attractive operation, since it does produce a true correction, but there are two major snags. Firstly, the coronary arteries have to be moved with the aorta and this produces technical problems. Secondly, if definitive operation is deferred by more than about one month, the left ventricle has adapted to its role of pumping blood into the lungs by thinning its muscle wall, and it cannot thereafter take over the higher pressure load of the systemic circulation.

Recently, attempts have been made to overcome these problems (Yacoub *et al.*, 1977). As soon as the diagnosis of transposition is made, the infant has a preliminary operation in which the pulmonary artery is 'banded' (to keep the pressure high in the left ventricle) and a shunt is made from aorta to pulmonary artery distal to the band to increase mixing between the two circulations and relieve cyanosis. At the age of about 2 years, the aorta and pulmonary artery are transected just above their valves. The aorta can then be anastomosed to the left ventricle and a graft put from the right ventricle to pulmonary artery. The coronary arteries have to be re-anastomosed to the aorta, either directly or by grafts of saphenous vein. The overall mortality of the operative approach is considerably higher than that of balloon septostomy followed by Mustard's operation, and most cardiologists and surgeons still feel that Mustard's operation is the most satisfactory for routine use.

TRANSPOSITION WITH VENTRICULAR SEPTAL DEFECT

About one-third of patients with transposition of the great arteries have a ventricular septal defect of variable size. When the defect is small the patients are similar to those in group 1 except that a systolic murmur is heard. The management is the same as in group 1.

When there is a large ventricular septal defect the picture is different. The onset of cyanosis is often delayed but is usually obvious by the end of the first month of life. The murmur is the same as in a simple ventricular septal defect but is well conducted to the apex of the heart and the left axilla. Dyspnoea increases and congestive cardiac failure develops.

Radiology

Radiology shows cardiac enlargement and pulmonary plethora and the pedicle of the heart is narrow.

Electrocardiography

The electrocardiogram shows right ventricular hypertrophy, but there is also left ventricular hypertrophy which increases in later childhood as pulmonary vascular disease develops.

Investigation

Investigation by cardiac catheterization usually shows equal pressures in both ventricles and the oxygen saturation in the aorta is much higher than in the first group. There may be a gradient between the left ventricle and the pulmonary artery when there is marked increase in pulmonary flow.

Angiography demonstrates the ventricular septal defect (*Figure 10.8*). The left atrial pressure is usually raised.

Treatment

Balloon septostomy is usually advised as this further improves the mixing between the two circulations and lowers the left atrial pressure. When the pulmonary flow is very high, banding of the pulmonary artery may be necessary to control the heart failure, and it also prevents a rapid rise in pulmonary vascular resistance.

When the patient is older, total correction is carried out either by using the Mustard operation and closing the ventricular septal defect or by using the Rastelli procedure. In this latter operation the pulmonary artery is closed off completely from the left ventricle, a

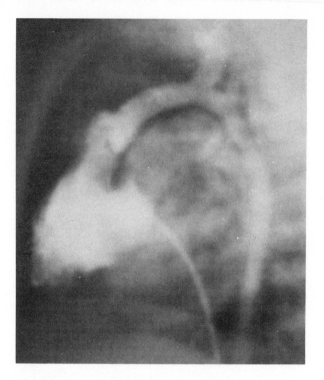

Figure 10.8. Transposition with ventricular septal
defect. Right ventricular angiogram viewed from
the left side. The aorta is anterior to the pulmonary
artery, which fills through the ventricular septal
defect. The pulmonary artery is much larger than
the aorta as there is a high pulmonary blood flow.
Note also that the aortic valve is higher than, as
well as anterior to, the pulmonary valve

patch is placed from the lower margin of the ventricular septal
defect to the anterior wall of the right ventricle, directing the left
ventricle blood into the aorta, and a homograft of aortic valve and
aorta is connected from the right ventriculotomy to the distal portion
of the pulmonary artery, establishing a channel for the systemic
venous blood to be carried to the lungs (*Figure 10.10*, p. 200). Early
reports suggest that the homograft frequently calcifies, but provided
the pulmonary vascular resistance is low, it functions satisfactorily.
    Since the left and right ventricles have equal pressures and equally
thick walls, patients with transposition plus VSD may also be

suitable for the 'switch' operation described on p. 194, the ventricular septal defect being closed at the same time.

There is clearly some overlap between patients suitable for each procedure. At the moment, in view of the greater complexity of the Rastelli procedure and the switch operation, opinion favours closure of the ventricular septal defect and a Mustard operation where this is feasible.

TRANSPOSITION WITH VENTRICULAR SEPTAL DEFECT AND PULMONARY STENOSIS

The clinical picture depends upon the size of the ventricular septal defect and the severity of the pulmonary stenosis. Patients with a large ventricular septal defect and moderate pulmonary stenosis have the best prognosis untreated of all patients with transposition, and live into teenage or adult life. Cyanosis is moderate and cardiac failure unusual. Clinical examination reveals evidence of moderate cardiac enlargement, usually involving both ventricles, and a loud systolic murmur due to the pumonary stenosis. When pulmonary flow is greatly reduced due to tight pulmonary stenosis, a systemic–pulmonary artery shunt may be required in infancy. Definitive surgery is usually by a Rastelli type of operation which avoids the difficulty of relieving the pulmonary stenosis but the condition has also been treated with a combination of a Mustard operation, closure of the ventricular septal defect and a conduit from left ventricle to pulmonary artery (Singh *et al.*, 1976).

TRUNCUS ARTERIOSUS

Incidence

Truncus arteriosus is a rare defect, occurring in less than 0.5 per cent of cases.

Definition

There is no division of the primitive truncus arteriosus into aorta and pulmonary artery. Instead a common trunk arises from both ventricles. According to the way in which the pulmonary arteries arise from the truncus, three types are described (*Figure 10.9*).

In type 1 there is a short pulmonary trunk arising from the posterior aspect of the truncus. Type 2 has the two pulmonary arteries arising separately from the posterior aspect of the truncus and in type 3 the pulmonary arteries arise from the lateral aspects. A fourth type, in which the pulmonary arteries arise from the descending aorta was formerly included but this is now considered to be a form of pulmonary atresia in which the 'pulmonary arteries' are actually well developed bronchial collateral vessels.

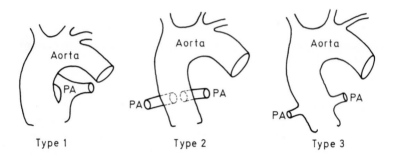

Figure 10.9. Types of truncus arteriosus. The pulmonary arteries (PA) arise from the truncus with a common stem in type 1, separately from the back of the truncus in type 2, and separately from the sides of the truncus in type 3. Type 1 is the most suitable for surgery and type 3 the most difficult

The single truncal valve may have three or four cusps, and often these are malformed and either stenosed or incompetent. There is always a ventricular septal defect occupying the portion of the interventricular septum normally formed from the conotruncal septum immediately below the truncal valve. The right ventricle is hypertrophied. In older children the pulmonary arteries show hypertensive pulmonary vascular disease.

Clinical presentation

In infancy, the low pulmonary vascular resistance allows a large pulmonary blood flow, so that cardiac failure is common, but frank cyanosis unusual. Over the age of 1 year the pulmonary vascular resistance rises so that cyanosis increases progressively.

When there is a high pulmonary blood flow there is little cyanosis and the pulses are bounding. Otherwise there is variable cyanosis and the pulses are normal. The heart is enlarged, usually both right and left ventricular pulsation being increased. There is usually a loud ejection systolic murmur at the base and an ejection click is common. A continuous murmur is unusual, but may occur when there is constriction at the orifice of the pulmonary arteries. The second heart sound is loud and single, and in about half of the patients an early diastolic murmur due to regurgitation through the truncal valve is heard at the left sternal edge. When the pulmonary blood flow is high, a diastolic flow murmur is heard in the mitral area.

Radiology

Chest films show moderate cardiac enlargement involving both ventricles, and a prominence in the region of the ascending aorta. The main pulmonary artery is not visible and there is often a hollow in the region of the main pulmonary artery. The peripheral lung fields indicate the state of the pulmonary vascular resistance, being plethoric when this is low and showing peripheral oligaemia when it is high.

Electrocardiography

The electrical axis is usually normal but occasionally shows moderate or extreme left axis deviation (-90 to -120 degrees). When pulmonary flow is high there is biventricular hypertrophy. When a high pulmonary vascular resistance reduces pulmonary flow the picture changes to one of right ventricular hypertrophy. (The electrocardiographic patterns are similar to those found with large ventricular septal defects in different stages of hypertensive pulmonary vascular disease.)

Ultrasound cardiography

Only one semilunar valve is shown with a great artery usually straddling the interventricular septum. High quality two-dimensional studies may enable the origin of the pulmonary trunk from the truncus to be demonstrated.

Cardiac catheterization and angiography

As the ventricular septal defect is high it is unusual to determine much shunting of blood in either direction until the truncus is entered. Right and left ventricular pressures are, obligatorily, the same. Usually the pressures in the pulmonary arteries are the same as that in the truncus, but, particularly when there is a high flow, gradients as high as 30–40 mmHg may be detected.

Angiography performed from either ventricle demonstrates the truncus, but occasionally streaming of blood or overlying of structures makes it difficult to interpret the pictures and a separate injection in the truncus is necessary.

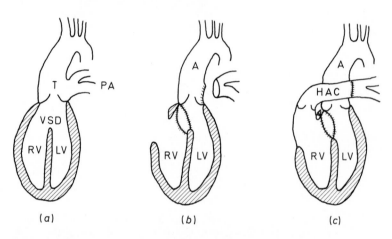

(a)   (b)   (c)

Figure 10.10. Rastelli operation for type 1 truncus, viewed from the left. (*a*) Preoperative. (*b*) The pulmonary trunk (PA) has been detached from the truncus (T) which is then repaired. Through a right ventriculotomy the ventricular septal defect (VSD) is patched to the base of the truncus so as to direct the left ventricular (LV) blood into aorta (Ao). (*c*) A homograft aortic conduit (HAC), bearing the aortic valve (which now becomes the recipient's pulmonary valve), is inserted to direct the blood from the right ventricle (RV) into the pulmonary artery

Diagnosis

Clinically, the condition in infants resembles a large patent ductus arteriosus and in older children the situation is similar to the Eisenmenger syndrome.

The hyperoxia test is useful in distinguishing infants with minimal cyanosis from those with acyanotic lesions such as patent ductus arteriosus or large ventricular septal defect.

Prognosis

Without surgical intervention about three-quarters of the patients die in infancy with congestive heart failure. If infancy is survived, many children are well and virtually asymptomatic until adolescence, when increasing cyanosis, effort intolerance and complications of hypertensive pulmonary vascular disease such as haemoptysis occur. The lesion is rare in adult life.

Treatment

Vigorous antifailure treatment should be given to those patients presenting in infancy with breathlessness and heart failure. About one-quarter can be kept reasonably well in this way, and surgery deferred.

In the remaining 75 per cent a decision has to be made between attempting early correction or carrying out a palliative operation. If the pulmonary trunk arises as a single vessel from the truncus, it may be possible to 'band' this (*see* p. 53) but the mortality is still high—about 50 per cent. The Rastelli procedure (*see below*) has been used in infancy but, particularly under the age of 1 month, there have been very few reported survivors, and subsequent operation to replace a graft that the patient has outgrown will be required. The dilemma is still unsolved.

Those children who survive the early years of life, with or without palliation, can be treated by the Rastelli procedure (*Figure 10.10*) but it is essential to carry this out before hypertensive pulmonary vascular disease occurs in those patients with high pulmonary artery pressures (i.e. most of those who have not previously been 'banded').

ORIGIN OF ONE PULMONARY ARTERY FROM THE AORTA

The origin of one pulmonary artery from the aorta is a rare anomaly. Usually the right pulmonary artery is the one involved. Over half the patients have other defects, including ventricular septal defect, patent ductus arteriosus and tetralogy of Fallot.

Patients usually present with cardiac failure within the first two months of life. The clinical picture simulates that of a large patent ductus arteriosus, the pulses are bounding and the left ventricle is enlarged. A loud systolic murmur is heard in the aortic area and a diastolic flow murmur at the apex. The chest radiographs show pulmonary plethora, localized to the side involved. Diagnosis is by angiocardiography.

Surgical treatment is usually required to control the cardiac failure. Re-anastomosis of the anomalous pulmonary artery to the main pulmonary artery has been performed either with or without cardiopulmonary bypass, or a palliative banding of the anomalous vessel can be performed.

ORIGIN OF BOTH GREAT ARTERIES FROM THE RIGHT VENTRICLE
(double outlet right ventricle)

An uncommon condition, origin of both great arteries from the right ventricle is best considered as a partial form of transposition. As the term implies, both the aorta and the pulmonary artery arise from the right ventricle (*Figure 10.11*). Except in rare instances, incompatible with survival, there is an associated ventricular septal defect. The diagnosis is made only by angiography. Three haemodynamic situations are possible.

1. Large ventricular septal defect with no pulmonary stenosis. This simulates a large ventricular septal defect with pulmonary hypertension.
2. Large ventricular septal defect with pulmonary stenosis. This is clinically indistinguishable from Fallot's tetralogy.
3. Small ventricular septal defect causing obstruction to left ventricular outflow and simulating aortic stenosis.

The Taussig–Bing malformation is another variant of the condition in which the ventricular septal defect is immediately below the pulmonary valve.

Treatment of most of these abnormalities is now possible by the creation of intracardiac tunnels but operation must be carried out in the first and third groups before irreversible pulmonary vascular disease develops.

The most straightforward type to deal with by operation is that in which the ventricular septal defect is large and immediately below the aortic valve. A relatively simple patch across the subaortic outlet isolates this from the rest of the right ventricle.

When the ventricular septal defect lies below the pulmonary valve it is not possible to connect the VSD with aorta without obstructing the pulmonary outflow. One possibility is to connect the VSD with

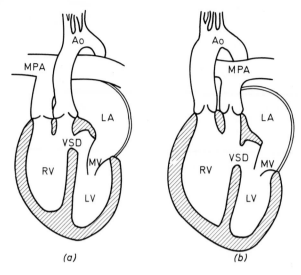

Figure 10.11. Origin of both great arteries from the right ventricle. Both the aorta (Ao) and the pulmonary artery (MPA) arise from the right ventricle (RV) and neither is contiguous with the mitral valve (MV). (Compare with *Figure 9.1* page 160 showing overriding of the aorta, but contiguity of mitral and aortic rings.) In (*a*) the ventricular septal defect (VSD) is directly below the aorta so that oxygenated blood from left atrium (LA) and left ventricle (LV) flows preferentially into the aorta and the patient is not cyanosed. Repair is more simple than in (*b*) (sometimes called the Taussig–Bing complex) where the pulmonary artery is close to the defect and the aorta receives mainly desaturated blood

the pulmonary artery, producing effectively complete transposition, and then correcting this with a Mustard operation. The alternative is to close off the VSD and place a valved conduit from LV to aorta. (It is not necessary to close the patient's aortic valve, as the higher aortic pressure should keep this closed.)

TOTAL ANOMALOUS PULMONARY VENOUS CONNECTION

Definition

In total anomalous pulmonary venous connection all the pulmonary veins drain by abnormal routes directly or indirectly into the right atrium. Anomalous pulmonary venous *drainage* is the physiological result of the anatomical abnormality termed anomalous pulmonary venous *connection*.

Incidence

The defect is uncommon, accounting for about 1 per cent of all cases of congenital heart disease.

TABLE 10.1
Types of total anomalous pulmonary venous connection

Type	Variety	Obstruction	Incidence*
Supracardiac	Left innominate vein	±	36
	Superior vena cava	−	11
Cardiac	Right atrium	−	15
	Coronary sinus	−	16
Infracardiac	Portal vein	+ +	6
	Ductus venosus	+	4
	Inferior vena cava	+	2
	Hepatic vein	+	1

*Data from Burroughs and Edwards, 1960.

Anatomy and physiology

The sites of anomalous venous connection are usually divided into supracardiac, cardiac and infracardiac (*see Table 10.1* and *Figure 10.12*).

With the non-obstructive forms there is a large flow of arterialized blood into the right atrium which mixes with the systemic venous blood. Most of the mixed blood then flows into the right ventricle and pulmonary artery. The amount which enters the left atrium depends upon the size of the interatrial communication (Burrows and Edwards 1960). With a large defect, about one-third to one-quarter of the total blood entering the right atrium is shunted into the left atrium; with a patent foramen ovale, as little as one-sixth to one-tenth. The right ventricle is greatly dilated and moderately hypertrophied and the pulmonary artery is large. The pulmonary arteries show mild hypertensive changes and the lungs are relatively normal histologically. The left side of the heart is normal-sized or small. When the drainage is into the coronary sinus the oxygenated blood streams preferentially through the tricuspid valve and the

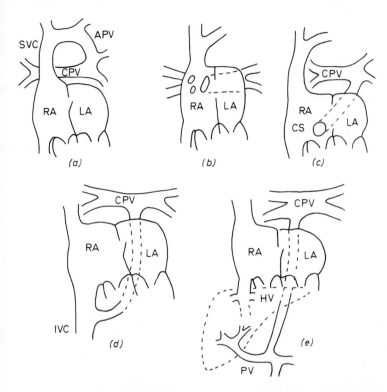

Figure 10.12. Types of total anomalous pulmonary venous connection. (*a*) Supracardiac via ascending pulmonary vein and left innominate vein. (*b*) Cardiac, direct to right atrium. (*c*) Cardiac into coronary sinus. (*d*) Infracardiac into inferior vena cava. (*e*) Infracardiac into portal vein. APV: ascending pulmonary vein; RA: right atrium; LA: left atrium; SVC: superior vena cava; CPV: confluence of pulmonary veins; IVC: inferior vena cava; CS: coronary sinus; PV: portal vein; HV: hepatic vein

caval blood streams into the left atrium so that the arterial blood is less saturated than that in the pulmonary artery.

When there is pulmonary venous obstruction the pulmonary blood flow is not greatly increased and therefore the amount of oxygenated blood returning to the right atrium is small. Hence the patient is clearly cyanosed. The pulmonary venous hypertension produces secondary pulmonary arterial hypertension and the small pulmonary arteries show severe hypertensive vascular disease, the lungs are oedematous, and on section show dilatation of lymphatics and the presence of 'heart failure' cells (haemosiderin-laden macrophages) in the alveoli. The right ventricle is only slightly dilated but more hypertrophied than in the non-obstructed form.

Associated defects

About 40 per cent of patients with total anomalous pulmonary venous connection have other cardiovascular defects, particularly dextrocardia, abnormalities of systemic venous return, ventricular septal defect and endocardial cushion defects. Transposition and pulmonary atresia have also been reported. Apart from dextrocardia the presence of other defects has a profound effect on the clinical presentation.

Clinical presentation

The infant with obstructed anomalous pulmonary venous connection presents in the first few days of life with cyanosis and evidence of pulmonary venous congestion—cough, respiratory difficulty and sometimes, frank pulmonary oedema. Clinical examination reveals

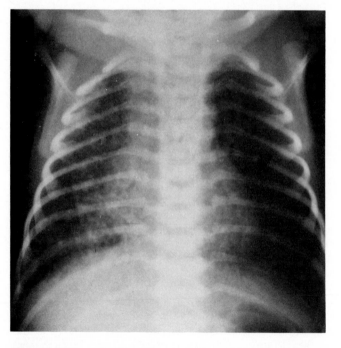

Figure 10.13. X-ray showing miliary appearance of the lungs (particularly on right side) in patient with total anomalous pulmonary venous drainage to the portal vein

obvious central cyanosis, poor pulses and a rapid respiratory rate with marked lower costal and intercostal incession. There are no murmurs but the second heart sound is loud and usually not audibly split. Fine rales may be heard over the lungs. The chest radiograph shows pulmonary venous obstruction and often a miliary or reticular pattern due to pulmonary oedema. (*Figure 10.13*). The electrocardio-gram is normal or shows right ventricular hypertrophy.

Non-obstructive forms do not usually produce symptoms for the first two to three months of life and occasionally not until the second or third year. The symptoms are usually respiratory difficulty and failure to gain weight. A respiratory infection may precipitate referral to hospital. Examination typically reveals an undernourished infant with a tinge of cyanosis on feeding or crying but little or none at rest. The respiratory rate is raised and there is moderate lower costal incession. The heart rate is fast, the right ventricular pulsation easily palpable at the left sternal border and a fairly loud systolic ejection murmur is heard in the pulmonary area, due to the high right ventricular output. The second heart sound is usually clearly split without obvious variation over the different phases of respiration and there is usually a diastolic murmur due to high tricuspid blood flow. This murmur is usually best heard at the lower left sternal border but may be heard further laterally when right atrial enlargement rotates the heart in a clockwise direction, displacing the tricuspid valve laterally.

Radiology

The chest radiograph shows right atrial and right ventricular enlargement (best seen on lateral views) and obvious pulmonary plethora (*Figure 10.14*). The characteristic 'cottage loaf' appearance of the type with connection via the left innominate vein is rarely seen in infancy.

Electrocardiography

The standard leads show right axis deviation and usually right atrial hypertrophy. In precordial leads there is evidence of right ventricular hypertrophy with either a qR or an rR pattern in leads V_1 and V_2.

Diagnosis

The *obstructed* form of total anomalous pulmonary venous connection should be suspected in any newborn infant with cyanosis and severe

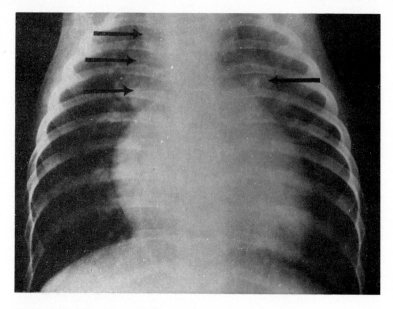

Figure 10.14. Radiograph of 3-month-old patient with supracardiac
type of total anomalous pulmonary venous connection. The right
ventricle is enlarged and the lungs pleonaemic. The ascending
pulmonary vein is faintly seen on the left of the upper mediastinum and
the superior vena cava is prominent on the right

respiratory difficulty, particularly if the chest radiographs show a
normal-sized heart. Other causes of pulmonary venous hypertension
such as the hypoplastic left heart syndrome, present similarly but
with a much larger heart on plain X-ray. The lung opacities may
simulate respiratory disease but the cyanosis is not relieved by
oxygen.

In the infant with *non-obstructed* total anomalous pulmonary
venous connection the differential diagnosis includes large ventricular septal defect or patent ductus arteriosus. The wide, fixed
splitting of the second heart sound is uncommon in either of these
conditions but is found in patients with endocardial cushion defects
and mitral insufficiency who have a similar clinical picture.
(However, the characteristic electrocardiographic pattern of endocardial cushion defect with left axis deviation should enable it to be
distinguished.) In older children the signs are those of an atrial
septal defect with mild cyanosis but the radiograph shows increased
heart size in total anomalous pulmonary venous connection, which
should be a helpful pointer.

Cardiac catheterization

The characteristic finding in the *non-obstructed* form is a large shunt of oxygenated blood into the right atrium. The exact site of the shunt can be determined by careful sampling in the venae cavae and in different parts of the atrium, coupled with samples, if necessary, from both innominate veins. There is moderate elevation of right ventricular and pulmonary artery pressures. The pulmonary wedge pressure is normal or slightly elevated. The left atrial pressure is lower than the right atrial if there is only a patent foramen ovale. Arteral blood is nearly fully saturated except when the pulmonary venous return is through the coronary sinus, when the arterial saturation is usually only about 80 per cent, whereas it may be 90 per cent in the pulmonary artery.

In the *obstructed* form the right atrial blood is less highly saturated but the shunt can still be readily detected. The right ventricular and pulmonary artery pressures are markedly elevated and the wedge pressure, if it can be obtained, is elevated.

The catheter can usually be passed into the confluence of the pulmonary veins in the supracardiac and cardiac forms, and angiography can be performed either from this site or by injecting into the right ventricle or pulmonary artery and following the contrast round into the pulmonary veins (*Figure 10.15*).

Confusion may occur with the types of anomalous pulmonary venous connection draining into the right atrium or coronary sinus where the findings resemble those of an uncomplicated atrial septal defect, but infants and small children with uncomplicated atrial septal defect are virtually never symptomatic and the presence of desaturated blood in the left atrium and left ventricle, together with a right atrial pressure a little higher than left, should make the true diagnosis clear.

Prognosis

In the *obstructed* type, death usually occurs any time from the first day to the end of the second month. Without surgery, most patients with the *unobstructed* form have symptoms in infancy and even in those who survive the first year of life the prognosis is poor.

Treatment

Medical therapy is ineffectual in the obstructed form and in the unobstructed form at best produces only a temporary improvement, once symptoms have occurred. Surgical treatment is therefore

210

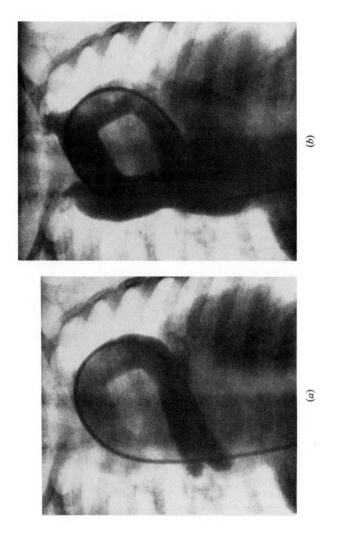

Figure 10.15. Total anomalous pulmonary venous drainage to superior vena cava. The catheter has been passed into the collecting vein. (*a*) The radio-opaque dye demonstrates the dilated vein which causes the 'cottage loaf' appearance in the upper, mediastinum on the plain X-ray. (*b*) The dye has entered the superior vena cava and right atrium

urgent. Although there are a few reports of successful closed operations, most surgeons prefer an open technique with either profound hypothermia or cardiopulmonary bypass. When the anomalous pulmonary venous connection joins the coronary sinus, operation is carried out within the heart to open the coronary sinus widely into the left atrium (along whose posteroinferior border it runs). The opening of the coronary sinus into the right atrium and the atrial septal defect (if present) are then closed with a patch. (This leaves the coronary sinus blood draining into the left atrium but the small right-to-left shunt so produced is not symptomatically important.) In patients with pulmonary veins draining directly into the right atrium, a patch of pericardium or Teflon is used to divert the pulmonary veins through the atrial septal defect, which is enlarged if necessary. In all other forms a wide, direct anastomosis is made between the confluence of pulmonary veins and the posterior wall of the left atrium. Usually this is performed behind the heart but occasionally through an incision opening both atria. The anomalous venous connections are then ligated. The symptomatic result is usually excellent. In theory there is a risk of subsequent narrowing of the anastomotic site but this has not been generally reported. In a few reports available of postoperative catheter studies the pulmonary artery pressures have usually fallen to normal or near normal.

Congenital absence of pulmonary venous connection

Occasional cases have been described in which pulmonary veins connect neither to the left atrium nor any other part of the circulation. These patients present within the first day of life, as extremely dyspnoeic, blue and with poor cardiac output. In many, the ductus arteriosus remains patent, so that a persistent fetal circulation occurs. Since the flow through the lungs is very poor, it is almost impossible to diagnose the condition angiographically, but it is suspected in an infant with radiological features of obstructed total anomalous pulmonary venous obstruction. If time permits, surgical exploration is worthwhile as there is usually a confluence of pulmonary veins suitable for anastomosis to the left atrium, but occasionally there are no pulmonary veins at all to be found.

BIBLIOGRAPHY AND REFERENCES

Transposition
Aberdeen, E., Waterston, D. J., Carr, I., Graham, G., Bonham Carter, R. E. and Subramanian, S. (1965). Successful 'correction' of transposed great arteries by Mustard's operation. *Lancet* **1**, 1233

Blalock, A. and Hanlon, C. R. (1950). The surgical treatment of complete transposition of the aorta and pulmonary artery. *Surg. Gynec. Obstet.* **90**, 1

Sillard, D. H., Mohri, H., Merendino, K. A., Morgan, B. C., Baum, D. and Crawford, E. W. (1969). Total surgical correction of transposition of the great arteries in children less than six months of age. *Surg. Gynec. Obstet.* **129**, 1258

Ferencz, C. (1968). Transposition of the great vessels; pathophysiological considerations based upon a study of the lungs. *Circulation* **33**, 232

Gutgesell, H. P., Garson, A. and McNamara, D. G. (1979). Transposition of the great arteries; Longterm follow-up after balloon atrial septostomy in 112 patients. *Paediat. Cardiol.* **1**, 88–89

Haller, J. A., Crisler, C., Bawley, R. and Cameron, J. (1969). Mustard operation for transposition of the great vessels. Technical considerations. *J. thorac. cardiovasc. Surg.* **58**, 296

Imamura, E. S., Morikawa, T., Tatsuno, K., Konno, S., Arai, T. and Sakakibara, S. (1971). Surgical considerations of ventricular septal defect associated with complete transposition of the great arteries and pulmonary stenosis. *Circulation* **44**, 914

Jordan, S. C. and McCarthy, C. (1967). Haemodynamic consequences of atrial septostomy in an infant with transposition of the great arteries. *Lancet* **1**, 310

Mair, D. D., Rutter, D. G., Danielson, G. K., Wallace, R. B. and McGoon, D. C. (1976). The palliative Mustard operation: rationale and results. *Am. J. Cardiol.* **37**, 762

Mustard, W. T. (1964). Successful two-stage correction of transposition of the great vessels. *Surgery, St. Louis* **55**, 469

Parsons, C. G., Astley, R., Burrows, F. G. O. and Singh, S. P. (1971). Transposition of great arteries. A study of 65 infants followed for 1 to 4 years after balloon septostomy. *Br. Heart J.* **33**, 725

Rashkind, W. J. (1971). Transposition of the great arteries. *Pediat. Clins. N. Am.* **18**, 1075

Rashkind, W. J. and Miller, W. W. (1966). Creation of an atrial septal defect without thoracotomy; a palliative approach to complete transposition of the great vessels. *J. Am. med. Ass.* **196**, 991

Rastelli, G. C., McGoon, D. C. and Wallace, R. B. (1969). Anatomic correction of transposition of the great arteries with ventricular septal defect and subpulmonary stenosis. *J. thorac. cardiovasc. Surg.* **58**, 545

Shumacker, H. B. Jr. and Girod, D. A. (1969). Transposition of the great vessels. Long-term follow-up of corrected case. *J. thorac. cardiovasc. Surg.* **57**, 747

Singh, A. K., Stark, J. and Taylor, J. F. N. (1976). Left ventricle to pulmonary artery conduit in the treatment of transposition of great arteries, restrictive ventricular septal defect and acquired pulmonary atresia. *Br. Heart J.* **38**, 1213

Tynan, M. (1972). Haemodynamic effects of balloon atrial septostomy in infants with transposition of great arteries. *Br. Heart J.* **34**, 791

Venables, A. W. (1970). Balloon atrial septostomy in complete transposition of the great arteries in infancy. *Br. Heart J.* **32**, 61

Viles, P. H., Ongley, P. A. and Titus, J. L. (1969). The spectrum of pulmonary vascular disease in transposition of the great arteries. *Circulation* **40**, 31

Yacoub, M. H., Radley-Smith, R. and MacLaurin, R. (1977). Two-stage operation for anatomical correction of transposition of the great arteries with intact interventricular septum. *Lancet* **1**, 1275

Truncus arteriosus
Wallace, R. B., Rastelli, G. C., Ongley, P. A., Titus, J. L. and McGoon, D. C. (1969). Complete repair of truncus arteriosus defects. *J. thorac. cardiovasc. Surg.* **57**, 95

Origin of both arteries from right ventricle

Hightower, B. M., Barcia, A., Bargeron, L. M. and Kirklin, J. W. (1969). Double-outlet right ventricle with transposed great arteries and subpulmonary ventricular septal defect. The Taussig–Bing malformation. *Circulation* **39**, Suppl. 1, 207

Neufeld, H. N., DuShane, J. W. and Edwards, J. E. (1961). Origin of both great vessels from the right ventricle. II. With pulmonary stenosis. *Circulation* **23**, 603

Neufeld, H. N., Wood, E. H., Kirklin, J. W. and Edwards, J. E. (1961). Origin of both great vessels from the right ventricle. I. Without pulmonary stenosis. *Circulation* **23**, 399

Total anomalous pulmonary venous connection

Bonham Carter, R. E., Capriles, M. and Noe, Y. (1969). Total anomalous pulmonary venous drainage: a clinical and anatomical study of 75 children. *Br. Heart J.* **31**, 45

Burroughs, J. T. and Edwards, J. E. (1960). Total anomalous pulmonary venous connection. *Am. Heart J.* **59**, 913

Clarke, D. R., Stark, J., De Leval, M., Pincott, J. R. and Taylor, J. F. N. (1977). Total anomalous pulmonary venous drainage in infancy. *Br. Heart J.* **39**, 436

Dillard, D. H., Mohri, H., Jessel, E. A., Anderson, H. N., Nelson, R. J., Crawford, E. W., Morgan, B. C., Winerscheid, L. C. and Merendino, K. A. (1967). Correction of total anomalous pulmonary venous drainage in infancy utilizing deep hypothermia with total circulatory arrest. *Circulation* **36**, Suppl. 1, 105

Duff, D. F., Nihill, M. R. and McNamara, D. G. (1977). Infradiaphragmatic total anomalous pulmonary venous return. Review of clinical and pathological findings and results of operation in 28 cases. *Br. Heart J.* **39**, 619

Gatham, G. E. and Nadas A. S. (1970). Total anomalous pulmonary venous connections. Clinical and physiologic observations of 75 pediatric patients. *Circulation* **42**, 143

CHAPTER 11

Complex Lesions, Malposition and Malconnection

With improved surgical techniques it has proved possible to correct or palliate a number of complex defects such as single ventricle, formerly regarded as inoperable. Cardiologists and surgeons have needed to make much more detailed study of the anatomy of such conditions, and this has led to the need for a more comprehensive terminology (Tynan *et al.*, 1979). Basically, this terminology is used to determine the *connections* of the various parts of the heart, and to add to this descriptions of *positions* and of *additional lesions*. This avoids the confusion that arises with such terms as 'dextrocardia' (which can mean the pushing or pulling of the heart into the right chest by pulmonary disease, the rotation of the apex of the heart or complex malconnection of the heart chambers) or the use of eponyms such as 'Holmes heart'.

MALPOSITION OF THE HEART

It is unfortunate, in this context, that we have for centuries used such terms as right and left ventricle. In the normal heart there is no problem, as the ventricle on the right always has the same morphology—a tricuspid inlet valve, small papillary muscles, a heavily trabeculated septum and a prominent ridge of muscle (the conus septum) separating inlet and outlet portions, while the ventricle to its left has a bicuspid (mitral) inlet valve, large papillary muscles, a finely trabeculated septal surface and continuity between

214

inlet and outlet valves. However, in complex hearts the ventricles may occupy unusual positions, and we have to decide whether we define a ventricle as a 'right ventricle' if it occupies a position to the right of the other ventricle or if it has the anatomical features of a normal right ventricle. The agreed convention is to use the latter terminology and thus define a right ventricle as a ventricle with the anatomy of a normal right ventricle, irrespective of the position it occupies. Right and left atria are similarly defined.

Position of the viscera and atria

The position of the viscera is important in complex heart disease, mainly because the right atrium nearly always occupies the same side (situs) as the liver.

The terms used are first defined:

Solitus: usual or normal.

Situs solitus: normal place.

Situs solitus of the viscera: the viscera are in their normal place.

Situs solitus of the atria: the atria are in their normal place.

Inversus: the opposite side to normal.

Situs inversus of the viscera: the viscera are on the opposite sides to normal — i.e. liver on the left, stomach on the right.

Situs inversus of the atria: the atria are on the opposite sides to normal, i.e. right atrium on left.

Ambiguous: not clearly related to one side or other.

Situs ambiguous of viscera: liver and stomach not clearly related to one side (midline liver)

Atrial situs ambiguous: either a common atrium or two identical atria (usually right) one on either side.

Clinical and radiological determination of visceral and atrial situs

It may be possible to determine the side of the liver clinically, but nearly always a radiograph showing not only the chest but the upper abdomen is necessary. A small amount of swallowed contrast is useful in demonstrating the stomach, but often the gastric air bubble is sufficient.

Although the liver is a good guide to atrial situs, a more accurate method is to study the bronchial anatomy (Van Mierop, Eisen and Schiebler, 1970). Usually a slightly penetrated film will be adequate,

216

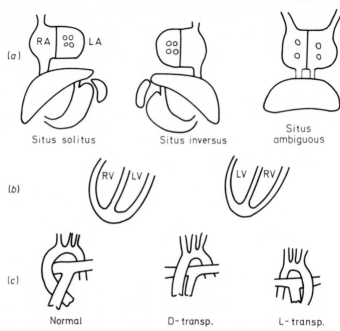

(a) Situs solitus

RA ∘∘ LA
    ∘∘

Situs inversus

    ∘∘
    ∘∘

Situs
ambiguous

∘   ∘
∘   ∘

(b)

RV / LV

LV / RV

(c)

Normal

D-transp.

L-transp.

Figure 11.1. Varieties of dextrocardia. In row (*a*) are shown the three types of visceral and atrial situs. Note that the anatomical 'right atrium' (RA) is always on the same side as the liver. Row (*b*) shows the ventricular situs. RV and LV refer to ventricles which have the anatomical characteristics of the normal right and left ventricles respectively. Row (*c*) represents the three possible arrangements of the great arteries. In theory, 18 different combinations are possible

TABLE 11.1
Types of connection

Atrial situs:	Situs solitus
	Situs inversus
	Situs ambiguous
Atrioventricular connection	Concordant
	Discordant
	Absence of one A-V valve
	Double inlet ventricle
	Ambiguous
Ventriculo- arterial connection	Concordant
	Discordant
	Double outlet ventricle
	Single outlet

but occasionally tomograms will be required. The right main bronchus is more vertical than the left, and the distance to its first (eparterial) bronchus is shorter. If it can be determined which is the right bronchus, then the right atrium will lie on that side. If there is ambiguous atrial situs with two right atria, then there will be two equally short ('right') main bronchi.

Asplenia is usually associated with 'right sided isomerism', that is to say that normal right sided structures are found in a mirror image condition on the left side as well. There are then 2 right lungs (with 3 lobes) and bilateral superior venae cavae, usually with a single atrium.

A similar, but rarer syndrome of polysplenia, associated with left sided isomerism and complex anomalies is also described (Moller et al., 1967).

Attempts have been made to explain the various abnormalities of position and connection in complex anomalies on an embryological basis (Van Praagh et al., 1964), in particular with reference to the early looping of the primitive cardiac tube. The normal loop is towards the right (D- or dextrolooping). Looping to the left (L- or laevolooping) is thought to cause 'corrected' transposition, while failure to develop any loop is associated with the syndromes of asplenia and polysplenia.

ABNORMALITIES OF CONNECTION OF THE CARDIAC CHAMBERS

Atrioventricular connection

Such connections can be: concordant (i.e. left atrium to left ventricle as in the normal heart), discordant (i.e. left atrium to right ventricle); with one A-V connection missing (as in tricuspid atresia); with two valves entering one ventricle, or ambiguous with single atrium or single atrioventricular valve common to both ventricles.

Ventricular great artery connection

Again this can be concordant (aorta from left ventricle), discordant (as in transposition), double outlet from one ventricle (usually the right), or a single great artery as in truncus arteriosus.

The value of such a system is that it enables complex anomalies to be specified. In the less complex conditions, the pre-existing names such as tricuspid atresia, are more likely to be retained. The various possibilities of situs and connection can be seen from *Figure 11.1* and *Table 11.1*.

Atrial anomalies

Besides abnormal position (situs) of the atria in patients with situs inversions and situs ambiguous, other anomalies of the atria may occur.

Bilateral right atria occur with asplenia as part of the right sided isomerism. The condition is recognized by angiography as both atria have short wide appendages. The corresponding condition of *bilateral left atria* occurs with greater rarity.

Juxtaposition of the atrial appendages usually occurs on the left side and the morphologically right one is superior to the left. The condition is only diagnosed at angiography (or autopsy) and its only real importance is that it implies complex malformation of atria, ventricles and atrioventricular valves.

Diagnosis of complexes associated with malposition

It will be clear that a complete diagnosis cannot be made without cardiac catheterization, and frequently two or more investigations are required to establish all the abnormalities. Echocardiography prior to catheterization is often helpful in establishing whether there is a single ventricle and whether one or two atrioventricular valves are present (Solinger, Elbi and Minhas, 1975). The diagnosis is then built up in a sequential fashion, as indicated in *Figure 11.1* or by determining the connections as described earlier in this chapter.

CORRECTED TRANSPOSITION (OR L-TRANSPOSITION) OF THE GREAT ARTERIES

Definition

As in complete transposition, the great arteries have changed places so that the aorta lies anterior and the pulmonary artery posterior, but in addition the aorta and pulmonary artery have changed places in a right-to-left direction so that the aorta lies to the left of the pulmonary artery instead of to the right of it and the pulmonary artery is to the right of the aorta instead of to its left. The primitive heart tube has looped to the left instead of the right and the aorta occupies the left or laevo-position, that is, L-transposition (*Figure 11.2*).

The ventricles with their appropriate atrioventricular valves do not occupy their normal positions. The anatomical right ventricle lies on the left and the anatomical left ventricle lies on the right.

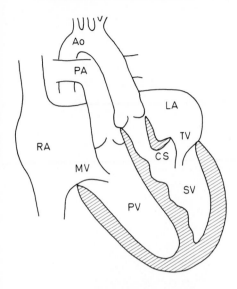

Figure 11.2. Corrected or L-transposition. The
aorta arises from the systemic ventricle (SV)
which resembles the normal right ventricle,
having a tricuspid valve (TV) and crista supraventricularis (CS) separating the tricuspid and
aortic valves. The pulmonary artery (PA) arises
behind and to the right of the aorta (Ao) from the
pulmonary ventricle (PV) which has a mitral
valve (MV) which is in direct continuity with the
pulmonary valve. The right atrium (RA) and left
atrium (LA) are normally situated

In the terminology described previously, this condition represents
'atrioventricular discordance with ventriculoarterial discordance'—
that is connection of right atrium to anatomical left ventricle (with
left atrium to right ventricle) and anatomical left ventricle to
pulmonary artery (with right ventricle to aorta).

The result therefore in corrected transposition is that systemic
venous blood enters the normal right atrium and then passes through
a *mitral* valve into the smooth walled, morphological 'left' ventricle,
which supplies the pulmonary artery lying posterior and to the right
of the aorta. The pulmonary venous blood comes back to a normal
left atrium and passes through a *tricuspid* valve into a trabeculated,
morphological 'right' ventricle which supplies the aorta and which
lies anterior and to the left of the pulmonary artery. Clearly, then,
the oxygenated blood reaches the aorta and the deoxygenated blood
reaches the lungs. If there were no other defects the only functional

abnormality would be that the morphological right ventricle supplied the aorta and the morphological left ventricle supplied the pulmonary artery.

It is, however, very rare for corrected transposition to occur without associated abnormalities. Ventricular septal defect and pulmonary stenosis are the most common abnormalities and frequently the left atrioventricular valve (the tricuspid) is abnormal and allows regurgitation into the left atrium. Heart block of all degrees is common, and other arrhythmias may occur.

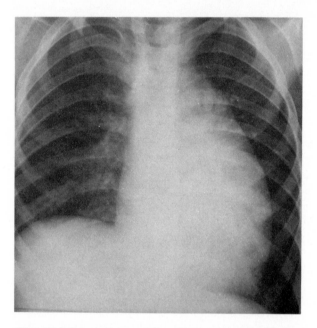

Figure 11.3. Corrected transposition. Plain radiograph. The upper part of the left border of the heart is made up of the ascending aorta. Compare with angiogram in *Figure 11.5* from the same patient. A right sided Blalock operation has been performed which accounts for the increased vasculature and elevation of the diaphragm on the right side

Natural history

The overall prognosis without surgery is poor. Infants may die from arrhythmias or congestive heart failure. The patients most likely to survive without therapy are those with ventricular septal defect and pulmonary stenosis.

Clinical presentation

It is the associated defects which determine the way in which the lesion presents. The ventricular septal defects are usually large and the symptoms and signs are like those described for this lesion in its uncomplicated form. Corrected transposition is suspected, however, if there is atrioventricular block or paroxysmal atrial tachycardia, and is also likely if there is clinical evidence of 'mitral' regurgitation. When there is a ventricular septal defect and pulmonary stenosis the presentation is similar to a tetralogy of Fallot.

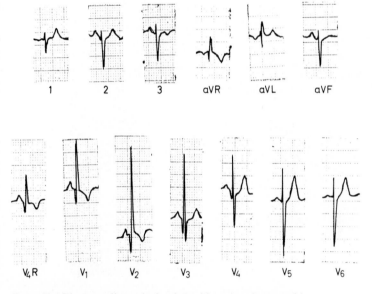

Figure 11.4. Electrocardiograph of patient with corrected transposition, ventricular septal defect and pulmonary stenosis. There are q waves in V_4R to V_3 but not in V_{5-6} and also (not due to corrected transposition) left axis deviation and right ventricular hypertrophy

Radiology

There is a long bulge on the left cardiac border formed by the aorta, which is not visible in the usual place (*Figure 11.3*). The lung fields may be plethoric or oligaemic, depending on whether ventricular septal defect or pulmonary stenosis is the dominant lesion.

Electrocardiography (*Figure 11.4*)

Atrial arrhythmias are common. In 75 per cent of the patients there is a qR pattern in leads V_4R and V_1 and an absence of the normal q wave in V_5 and V_6. This is due to the fact that the interventricular septum is depolarized in the opposite direction to that of the normal heart. Heart block varying from first to third degree occurs in at least one-third of the patients.

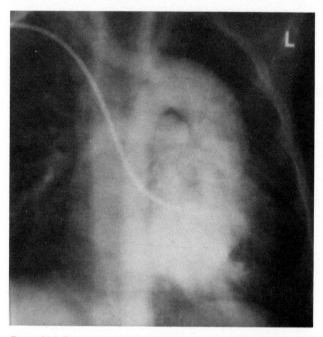

Figure 11.5. Pre-operative angiogram of patient with corrected transposition, single ventricle and pulmonary stenosis whose plain radiograph is shown in *Figure 11.3*. The aorta is seen arising on the left of, and slightly above, the pulmonary artery

Investigation

Cardiac catheterization and angiography show the abnormal position of the aorta and confirm the associated lesions (*Figure 11.5*). It is easier to enter the aorta through a ventricular septal defect than to enter the pulmonary artery from the venous ventricle. Arrhythmias, both heart block and tachycardia, are common during catheterization.

Treatment

Medical treatment is given to control arrhythmias or heart failure. Palliative operations such as banding of the pulmonary artery for associated ventricular septal defect or a shunt operation for severe pulmonary stenosis with ventricular septal defect are of benefit. Corrective procedures are difficult because of the abnormal course of the coronary arteries (as they come off the abnormally placed aorta) which interferes with the ventriculotomy, the abnormal left atrioventricular valve and the risk of arrhythmias.

SINGLE OR PRIMITIVE VENTRICLE

Single ventricle is uncommon, but is particularly associated with malposition of the heart. The term primitive ventricle arises from the belief that it represents an arrested form of development of the ventricular system. The most usual type consists of a main chamber with a shape similar to the normal left ventricle, and a rudimentary chamber opening from it. Usually the pulmonary artery arises from the main ventricular chamber and the aorta from the rudimentary chamber. There may be one or two atrioventricular valves entering the main cavity. Pulmonary stenosis or atresia are present in about half the cases.

Other forms of single ventricle are described but about 80 per cent fit into the above classification. A single ventricle in which both right and left ventricular components are equally represented is most uncommon. (It should be pointed out that tricuspid atresia, too, can be regarded as a form of single ventricle.)

The clinical picture depends upon whether or not there is obstruction to flow into the pulmonary circulation. If there is severe pulmonary stenosis or atresia the patient presents with severe cyanosis within the first day or two of life. Without pulmonary obstruction cyanosis is minimal, but breathlessness and heart failure develop, mainly at about one to two weeks of age.

The electrocardiogram commonly shows left ventricular hypertrophy, or absence of the normal right ventricular dominance. The QRS axis is variable and may be superior ('left') or inferior ('right'). Echocardiography is useful in demonstrating not only the absence of an interventricular septum but also in demonstrating whether there are one or two atrioventricular valves (*Figure 11.6*).

A near correction of some patients with single ventricle can be obtained, provided there are two atrioventricular valves, by septating the primitive ventricle, but the mortality is still very high. Those who only have one atrioventricular valve and a low pulmonary artery pressure may be suitable for the Fontan operation (*see* p. 182).

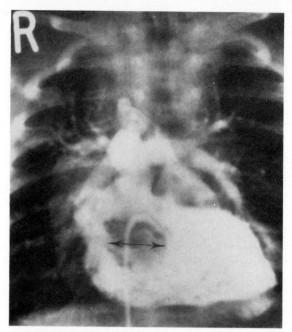

(a)

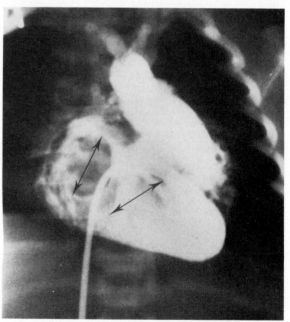

(b)

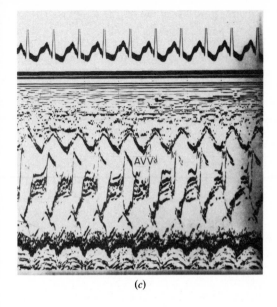

(c)

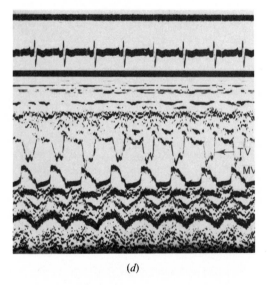

(d)

Figure 11.6. Single (primitive) ventricle. Angiograms
with (a) a single A-V valve and (b) with two A-V valves
(arrowed). The corresponding echocardiograms are
shown in (c) and (d). AVV: common atrioventricular
valve; TV: tricuspid valve; MV: mitral valve

Careful assessment of the possibilities and discussion with parents is therefore essential at an early stage, if palliative surgery is being considered. Such surgery consists of increasing the pulmonary flow, if it is low, by a Blalock or Waterston's shunt, or banding the pulmonary artery if it is too high.

ASPLENIA

Congenital heart disease may be associated with asplenia, when the spleen is absent, or polysplenia, when there are multiple small spleens. The heart lesion is usually a complicated one, causing cyanosis. There is often pulmonary atresia, a functionally common atrium and a common atrioventricular valve. The ventricular septum is always defective. Anomalies of systemic and pulmonary venous drainage are common. There is often malposition of the abdominal viscera.

Examination of the peripheral blood is helpful in diagnosing the condition and should be carried out in cyanotic infants. There is an increase in the number of nucleated red cells and target cells, and Howell–Jolly bodies are seen. Infants with asplenia are prone to infections. Many die early in life from severe infections. Otherwise the prognosis is that of the congenital heart lesion which is of a complex nature.

TABLE 11.2
Anomalies of systemic venous connection

Physiologically normal
Left superior vena cava—coronary sinus with or without right SVC
Inferior vena cava—azygos vein
Inferior vena cava—hemi-azygos vein—left SVC—coronary sinus
Coronary sinus—left SVC—left innominate vein—right SVC
Coronary sinus—IVC

Producing cyanosis
Left SVC—left atrium with or without right SVC
Coronary sinus—left atrium
IVC—left atrium
IVC + SVC—left atrium

ANOMALIES OF SYSTEMIC VENOUS CONNECTION

Anomalous systemic venous connections are comparatively unimportant in cardiology except for the technical problems which they introduce in investigation and surgery. They may be divided into those where the return is to the right atrium, where there is no physiological disturbance, and those in which there are one or more systemic veins draining into the left heart, which produces mild or moderate cyanosis without any other physical signs (*Table 11.2*). Usually there are associated severe defects, including common ventricle, which are responsible for the clinical picture; the anomalous venous drainage is an incidental finding. Asplenia is commonly associated.

BIBLIOGRAPHY AND REFERENCES

Corrected transposition
de la Cruz, M. V., Anselmi, C., Cisneros, F., Reinhold, M., Portillo, B. and Espino-Vela, J. (1959). An embryologic explanation for corrected transposition of the great vessels; additional description of the main anatomic features of this malformation and its varieties. *Am. Heart J.* **57**, 104
Dekker, A. (1965). Corrected transposition of the great vessels with Ebstein malformation of left atrioventricular valve. *Circulation* **31**, 119
Fernandez, F., Laurichesse, J., Seebat, L. and Lenegre, J. (1970). Electrocardiogram in corrected transposition of the great vessels of the bulboventricular inversion type. *Br. Heart. J.* **32**, 165
King, H., Kilman, J. N., Petry, E. L. and Shumaker, H. B. Jr. (1964). Surgical correction for 'mitral' incompetence in corrected transposition of the great vessels. *J. thorac. cardiovasc. Surg.* **47**, 769
Van Praagh, R. and Van Praagh, S. (1966). Isolated ventricular inversion with a consideration of the morphogenesis, definition and diagnosis of non-transposed and transposed great arteries. *Am. J. Cardiol.* **17**, 395

Single ventricle; malposition of the heart; asplenia
Lev, M., Liberthson, R. R., Kirkpatrick, J. R., Eckner, F. A. O. and Arcilla, R. A. (1969). Single (primitive) ventricle. *Circulation* **39**, 577
Moller, J. H., Nakib, A., Anderson, R. C. and Edwards, J. E. (1967). Congenital cardiac disease associated with polysplenia. A developmental complex of bilateral 'left sidedness'. *Circulation* **36**, 789
Ruttenberg, H. D., Neufield, H. N., Lucas, R. L. Jr., Carey, L. S., Adams, P. Jr., Anderson, R. C. and Edwards, J. E. (1964). Syndrome of congenital cardiac disease with asplenia. *Am. J. Cardiol.* **13**, 387
Solinger, R., Elbi, F. and Minhas, K. (1975). Deductive echocardiographic analysis of infants with congenital heart disease. *Circulation* **50**, 1072
Tynan, M. J., Becker, A. E., Macartney, F. J., Jiminez, M. Q., Shinebourne, E. A. and Anderson, R. H. (1979). Nomenclature and classification of congenital heart disease. *Br. med. J.* **41**, 544
Van Praagh, R., Ongley, P. A. and Swan, H. J. C. (1964). Anatomic types of single or common ventricles in men. Morphological and geometric aspects of 60 necropsied cases. *Am. J. Cardiol.* **13**, 367
Van Praagh, S., Vlad, P. and Keith, J. D. (1964). Anatomic types of congenital dextrocardia. Diagnostic and embryologic implications. *Am. J. Cardiol.* **13**, 510
Von Mierop, L. H. J., Eisen, S. and Schiebler, E. S. (1970). The radiographic appearance of the tracheobronchial tree as an indication of visceral situs. *Am. J. Cardiol.* **26**, 432

CHAPTER 12

Miscellaneous Congenital Abnormalities

DISEASES OF THE CORONARY ARTERIES

Anomalous coronary artery

All diseases of the coronary arteries are rare in infancy and childhood. Anomalous origin of one of the coronary arteries from the pulmonary artery is probably the most important since it can be cured. The left coronary artery is the most commonly affected.

Definition

One coronary artery, usually the left, arises from the pulmonary artery, the other normally from the aorta.

Natural history

The degree and rapidity of onset of symptoms are related to the extent of distribution of the anomalous coronary artery, but symptoms are unusual in the first few weeks of life as the pulmonary artery pressure initially remains high enough to perfuse the anomalous vessel. When the anomalous vessel is the left and this is dominant, symptoms begin at 3–4 weeks of age. When the right coronary artery is anomalous there may be no important symptoms in childhood and the lesion may only be found at autopsy in adult life. Basically three physiological situations may develop. In the first, the commonest, the pulmonary artery pressure is low and anastomotic channels develop between the normal and anomalous arteries which carry blood into the territory of the anomalous vessel and thence retrogradely into the pulmonary artery. There is thus a 'steal' of blood from the territory of the normal coronary artery in addition. In the second group the pulmonary artery pressure is moderately raised, blood flows from collaterals into the anomalous vessel but there is only a small retrograde flow into the pulmonary artery and hence no significant 'steal'. In the third group the pulmonary artery pressure is high enough to perfuse the anomalous vessel with desaturated blood. Surprisingly, this latter group are the most ill (Perry and Scott, 1970).

Clinical presentation

Cough and breathlessness due to left heart failure are the commonest symptoms, followed by vomiting due to right heart failure. A few patients have screaming attacks, thought to be due to ischaemic pain. Examination reveals evidence of cardiac enlargement involving mainly the left ventricle and a loud gallop rhythm (third heart sound). About one-third of patients have functional mitral regurgitation due to left ventricular dilatation and papillary muscle dysfunction. In older children who have a high flow through anastomotic vessels there is a continuous murmur, usually to the left of the sternum.

Investigations

When the left coronary artery is involved the chest radiograph shows moderate or marked cardiac enlargement and pulmonary venous congestion. The electrocardiogram classically shows deep Q waves and inverted T waves over the territory supplied by the anomalous vessel, but less than half the patients show this pattern, more common patterns being generalised T wave inversion or a pattern of left ventricular hypertrophy. Occasionally the electrocardiogram may be normal (Perry and Scott, 1970).

Cardiac catheterization demonstrates a left-to-right shunt into the pulmonary artery in group 1 patients. Aortography is the definitive investigation and usually shows retrograde filling of the anomalous vessel (*Figure 12.1*). In group 3, however, it may also be necessary to make an injection of contrast in the pulmonary artery.

Treatment

Preliminary treatment of cardiac failure with digoxin and diuretics should be followed by surgery at the time indicated by the severity of the symptoms. Patients in group 3 with perfusion from the

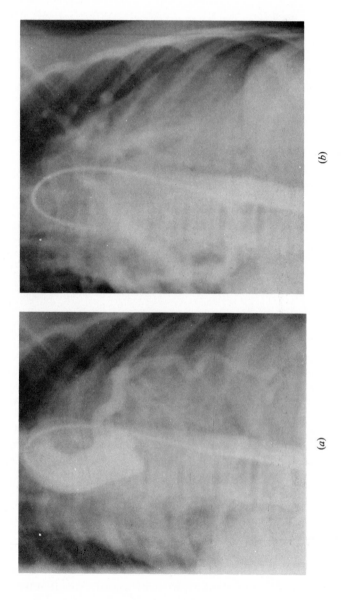

Figure 12.1. Anomalous right coronary artery. Aortogram of a 12-year-old girl with no symptoms but a continuous murmur. (*a*) Early phase showing a large left coronary artery arising normally from the aorta. (*b*) Later phase. The anomalous right coronary artery has filled through collateral channels and is seen draining upwards into the pulmonary artery, the left branch of which is clearly opacified

(*a*)

(*b*)

pulmonary artery can only be treated by reimplantation in the aorta, using hypothermia or cardiopulmonary bypass. Few patients have survived to date. When there is a large retrograde flow in the anomalous vessel, ligature near the pulmonary artery stops the 'steal' and allows adequate perfusion of the whole heart from the normal artery. However, these patients are usually less ill and somewhat older and will usually stand reimplantation, which is favoured as allowing a normal circulation less at risk from coronary atheroma in later life. Various plastic operations have been described to incorporate the part of the pulmonary artery giving rise to the anomalous vessel into the aortic root.

Coronary artery fistula

A rare anomaly consists of a fistula from one of the coronary arteries into a chamber of the heart or into a coronary vein. Patients do not usually have symptoms in childhood and the lesion is suspected when a soft continuous murmur is heard along the left or right sternal edge. It must be differentiated from other causes of continuous murmurs and is demonstrated by aortography. Attempts at resection may damage the blood supply to the part of the heart supplied by the affected vessel and are not generally advised unless there is evidence of important haemodynamic abnormality, such as cardiac enlargement, or a large shunt on cardiac catheterization. Now that surgeons are experienced in using grafts to bypass coronary artery disease in adults, they can use this technique to place a graft into the coronary artery distal to the fistula and then ligate the artery proximally.

Coronary artery aneurysm

A rare lesion, coronary artery aneurysm, is only detected clinically if it is large enough to cause a continuous or diastolic bruit. The aneurysm may develop a secondary communication with a coronary vein or rupture into a cardiac chamber and then act as a coronary artery fistula. Treatment is the same as for coronary artery fistula.

Coronary artery narrowing

The coronary arteries may be narrowed by arterial disease such as fibromuscular hyperplasia, generalized arterial calcification and as part of the hypercalcaemia syndrome. In Japan, Kawasaki disease or mucocutaneous lymph node syndrome (Kawasaki et al., 1974) produces an intense coronary arteritis with occlusion and aneurysm formation: Landing and Larson (1977) reported a similar syndrome in North America under the name of infantile periarteritis nodosa. They are also involved in systemic diseases such as xanthoma tuberosum, progeria and Friedreich's ataxia and, in adolescence, in familial hypercholesterolaemia. Symptoms of heart failure are more common than chest pain and are usually progressive. Successful surgical treatment has not yet been reported.

ANEURYSM OF A SINUS OF VALSALVA

A congenital weakness of one or more sinuses of Valsalva can lead to progressive dilatation with two important consequences. Firstly an aneurysm develops which eventually bursts either, rarely, into the pericardial cavity or, more commonly, into one of the cardiac chambers, usually the right atrium. A large shunt is produced which causes cardiac failure. Irrespective of the site of communication the pulse is collapsing and a loud murmur is heard. This is diastolic only when the rupture is into the left ventricle, but continuous when it is into any other cavity. Aortography demonstrates the lesion which can be repaired under cardiopulmonary bypass. This situation is more common in adult life. Bacterial endocarditis is a frequent complication.

The second consequence of aneurysmal dilatation of the sinus of Valsalva is the production of aortic incompetence by depriving the aortic valve of its support. Although repair is theoretically possible, in practice it is difficult and replacement of the aortic valve is frequently required. For this reason attempts at repair should be postponed, if at all possible, until the patient is fully grown.

AORTO – LEFT VENTRICULAR TUNNEL

This is a rare lesion presenting as aortic regurgitation. The tunnel arises at right-angles from the aorta (unlike a sinus of Valsalva aneurysm; and enters the left ventricle. Surgical repair is possible once the condition has been demonstrated by angiography (Somerville, English and Ross, 1974) but older patients with the condition frequently have additional valvar aortic regurgitation.

ARTERIOVENOUS ANEURYSM OF THE LUNG

In arteriovenous aneurysm of the lung, a branch of the pulmonary artery containing desaturated blood communicates with a pulmonary vein without passing through the alveoli. Hence desaturated blood reaches the left side of the heart, and the patient becomes cyanosed. Patients present with cyanosis, clubbing of fingers and toes and polycythaemia. There are usually no murmurs over the heart but a continuous murmur is audible over the aneurysm in the lung. It is important to listen over the whole of the chest routinely or this condition may be overlooked.

Lesions may be single or multiple, and occur in one or both lungs. Shadowing in the lung may be seen on a plain radiograph and pulmonary angiography will demonstrate the abnormal communication. Treatment is to remove the affected lobe or segment and is then curative, but when there are multiple aneurysms this may not be possible.

SEQUESTRATED SEGMENT OF THE LUNG

During the development of the lung, vessels in the lung parenchyma join up to the developing pulmonary trunks. Occasionally a segment of lung fails to develop a vascular connection with the pulmonary artery, but retains instead a major communication with the systemic arterial circulation. This sequestrated segment of lung is usually overvascularized and does not expand properly. It tends to be the seat of recurrent infection and on the plain radiograph appears collapsed. There is often a continuous murmur over the affected area, almost always in one or other of the lower lobes (usually the right), but if this is not heard the usual clinical diagnosis is basal bronchiectasis. If there is doubt, an arteriogram will settle the diagnosis. Removal of the segment is advised because of the risk of recurrent infection, but care is necessary to secure the supplying artery, which usually enters the segment from below and frequently originates from the aorta below the diaphragm.

A similar condition, sometimes called an intralobar sequestration, may occur in which there are both normal pulmonary arteries and an anomalous supply to a segment of lung (*Figure 12.2*). If the condition is diagnosed early and the segment of lung otherwise healthy, the anomalous artery can be ligated and the lung segment left in place.

SCIMITAR SYNDROME

A rare syndrome given much prominence in radiological textbooks, the scimitar syndrome consists of an anomalous connection of the right pulmonary veins to the inferior vena cava. The lung is smaller

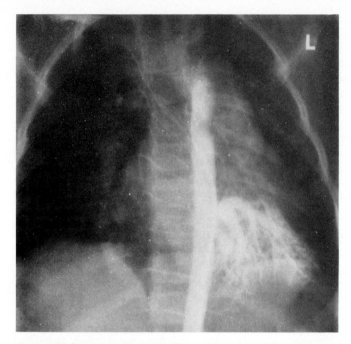

Figure 12.2. Sequestrated segment of lung. A large branch from the aorta supplies a segment of the left lower lobe

than normal so that the ribcage is reduced in size and the heart displaced to the right. The arterial supply derives from one or more branches from the descending thoracic aorta, with or without a normal pulmonary artery, and there is a single vein which descends towards the right cardiophrenic angle, and is clearly seen on the chest radiograph, its resemblance to a scimitar being responsible for the name. Occasionally only the right lower lobe is involved. Where there is a normal pulmonary artery supply as well as the anomalous one it may be possible to ligate the anomalous arteries and divert the venous drainage. The latter is carried out by first anastomosing the pulmonary vein to the right atrium and then building a tunnel within the right atrium to carry the blood to the left atrium. However, the condition rarely produces symptoms and is usually best left alone.

PULMONARY ARTERY SLING

In this rare anomaly the left pulmonary artery arises from the right pulmonary artery and winds backwards round the trachea and right bronchus. The ductus (or ligamentum) keeps it pulled tight around the trachea. It may occur on its own or in association with other anomalies, mainly tetralogy of Fallot. Although not producing any haemodynamic abnormality it causes constriction of the trachea or right main bronchus and presents as a stridor or right sided obstructive emphysema. Surgical treatment consists usually of reimplantation into the main pulmonary artery, but sometimes division of the ligament of the ductus provides relief of symptoms.

BIBLIOGRAPHY AND REFERENCES

Diseases of the coronary arteries
Barnes, R. J., Cheung, A. C. S. and Wu, R. W. Y. (1969). Coronary artery fistula. *Br. Heart J.* **31**, 299
Cafferky, E. A., Crawford, D. W., Turner, A. F., Lau, F. Y. K. and Blankenhorn, D. H. (1969). Congenital aneurysm of the coronary artery with myocardial infarction. *Am. J. med. Sci* **257**, 320
Kawasaki, T., Kokasi, F., Okawa, S., Shigematsu, I. and Yangagawa, H. (1974). A new infantile acute muco-cutaneous lymph node syndrome (MLNS) prevailing in Japan. *Pediatrics* **54**, 271
Landing, B. H. and Larson, E. J. (1977). Are infantile periarteritis nodosa with coronary artery involvement and fatal mucocutaneous lymph node syndrome the same? Comparison of 20 patients from North America with patients from Hawaii and Japan. *Pediatrics* **59**, 651
MacMahon, H. E. and Dickinson, P. C. T. (1967). Occlusive fibroelastosis of coronary arteries in the newborn. *Circulation* **35**, 3
Perry, L. W. and Scott, L. P. (1970). Anomalous left coronary artery from pulmonary artery. Report of 11 cases. Review of indication for and results of surgery. *Circulation* **41**, 1043.
Somerville, J., English, T. and Ross, D. N. (1974). Aorto-left ventricular tunnel. Clinical features and surgical management. *Br. Heart J.* **36**, 321

Scimitar syndrome
Neill, C. A., Ferencz, C., Sabiston, D. C. and Sheldon, H. (1960). The familial occurrence of hypoplastic right lung with systemic arterial supply and venous drainage: scimitar syndrome. *Bull. Johns Hopkins Hosp.* **107**, 1

SPECIAL PROBLEMS

CHAPTER 13

Heart Disease in the Newborn Infant

INTRODUCTION

Of all the infants admitted to hospital in the first year of life, about half are admitted in the first month and about half of these will die before their first birthday (*Report of New England Regional Infant Cardiac Program*, 1980). Nevertheless there has been continuing improvement in the life expectancy of newborns (Izukawa *et al.*, 1979). They are transferred earlier to centres with the appropriate facilities and this alone lessens the risks of investigation and surgery.

Although some of the defects presenting in the newborn are multiple, complex and inoperable, others which cause severe symptoms are amenable to treatment. Investigation is quicker and safer, there has been miniaturization of equipment and most cardiac catheterizations are done by direct puncture; radio-opaque dyes are safer. Echocardiography has proved a very useful guide to diagnosis in the newborn period. It can be performed within a few minutes of the infant arriving at the specialist centre and, in conjunction with the clinical picture, allows a provisional diagnosis to be made and treatment started while arrangements are made for cardiac catheterization. In the cyanotic baby it is usually possible to distinguish conditions such as pulmonary or tricuspid atresia which may benefit from prostaglandin infusion from transposition, where the need for catheterization and balloon septostomy is urgent. In the patient with heart failure it can usually indicate complex lesions such as single ventricle, truncus arteriosus and common atrioventricular canal. Hypoplastic left heart syndrome can be diagnosed with sufficient accuracy to make cardiac catheterization unnecessary in most cases (Godman, Tham and Langford-Kidd, 1974). Surgical techniques have improved, deep hypothermia is being used again with greater success and new methods of cardioplegia give improved myocardial protection. Continuous positive airway pressure helps to wean patients off ventilators more safely.

The clinical diagnosis is more difficult in this age group than at any other time, yet correct definitive diagnosis without delay is essential for effective treatment. Severe heart disease usually presents with either cyanosis or heart failure or there may be a combination of the two.

CYANOSIS

The younger the infant, the more difficult it is to be certain that the cyanosis is due to heart disease, and the following causes of cyanosis have to be excluded.

Peripheral cyanosis of the hands and feet is commonly observed in the newborn and must be differentiated from true central cyanosis.

Mechanical purpura. If there is delay in delivery of the body after the birth of the head, mechanical purpura on the face may make the infant appear cyanotic, but the lips are pink.

Polycythaemia. Some infants may have polycythaemia due to delayed clamping of the cord or the fetal transfusion syndrome.

Racial. Apparent cyanosis of the lips is seen in infants with pigmented skin.

Respiratory diseases causing cyanosis may cause difficulty, but in the respiratory distress syndrome, dyspnoea develops in the first 6 hours of life and the child has an expiratory grunt; cyanosis occurs only when the dyspnoea is severe and is usually promptly relieved by oxygen. The chest radiograph shows bilateral diffuse reticulogranular pattern and a well-defined tracheobronchogram.

Lung disease can cause cyanosis and dyspnoea but there may be localizing signs in the chest and a good chest radiograph will show neonatal pneumonia, the massive aspiration syndrome, pneumothorax, lobar emphysema, pleural effusion or diaphragmatic hernia. The oxygen test (Jones *et al.*, 1976) is helpful in differentiating primary lung disease from cyanotic heart disease. If the arterial oxygen tension rises over 150 mm when the infant is breathing 80 per cent oxygen, primary lung disease is likely and cardiac catheterization can be avoided.

Persistent fetal circulation, see p. 256.

Myocardial ischaemia in the newborn, see p. 258.

Choanal atresia, when bilateral, causes severe cyanosis and respiratory distress but it is obvious that the infant can breathe only through his mouth. Symptoms are present from birth and the diagnosis is confirmed by the inability to pass a catheter through either nostril into the nasopharynx.

Brain damage, with or without haemorrhage, often causes cyanosis but there are usually periods of apnoea rather than dyspnoea and there may be twitching or convulsions, a high-pitched cry, changes in muscle tone and reflexes and a bulging fontanelle

Sepsis may cause peripheral cyanosis but is then accompanied by evidence of peripheral circulatory collapse.

After careful examination the paediatrician may still be in doubt. *There may be no heart murmurs in some of the most severe cyanotic lesions which are nevertheless correctable* and this leads to delay in referral. If an infant is cyanosed in the first few days of life and *particularly if that cyanosis does not improve with oxygen*, it is useless to adopt a 'wait and see' attitude. He must be referred to a special centre for paediatric cardiology. If heart disease is not present, no harm will have resulted. The worst that can happen is that an unnecessary cardiac catheterization is performed and when the heart is normal this is a very low risk procedure. The condition which is very difficult to differentiate from cyanotic congenital heart disease is Persistent Fetal Circulation (*see* p. 256).

HEART FAILURE

In recognizing the early signs of heart failure in the newborn, frequent and careful observation is more valuable than anything else. The signs are:

tachycardia	heart rate more than 180/minute at rest
tachypnoea	respiratory rate more than 60/minute persistently when the infant is at rest
excessive weight gain	gain of more than 1 oz/day even though feeding is poor
liver enlargement	liver palpable 2 or more cm below the right costal margin in the midclavicular line
wheezing respirations and a dry cough	occur when there is left ventricular failure and moist sounds can be heard over both lungs

There may be no cyanosis and no murmurs at this stage, but heart disease may be suggested by feeling abnormal or unequal peripheral pulses. The earlier in life the signs of heart failure develop, the more serious is the lesion causing it. *Any infant developing heart failure in the first month of life should be referred for investigation immediately.* Heart failure in the first month of life can rarely be treated medically for any length of time. Simple lesions such as patent ductus arteriosus and ventricular septal defect rarely cause heart failure as early as the first month of life (*Figure 13.1*). It is usually caused by a lesion requiring surgery or is due to a complex inoperable lesion.

TRANSPORT

The general care of the newborn is of paramount importance and the following complications must be avoided before and during transport.

1. Hypothermia

Cyanosed infants will readily become hypothermic and if hypothermia is allowed to occur, it is extremely difficult to correct and increases the hazards of investigation. The baby must be transported in an incubator with extra layers of cotton wool and aluminium foil to prevent heat loss.

2. Acidosis

Metabolic acidosis occurs rapidly in cyanosed infants and must be corrected by intravenous bicarbonate before transfer. (*See* p. 289.)

3. Metabolic disturbances

Hypoglycaemia, hypocalcaemia and hypovolaemia should be corrected.

4. Severe hypoxia

If this can be improved by ventilation then it should be established before the journey begins.

DIAGNOSIS OF LESION

Having established that heart disease is present because of the existence of cyanosis or heart failure, or both, it then remains to diagnose the precise lesion. The classic signs found in older children are often absent in the newborn. Auscultation is surprisingly unhelpful unless diastolic murmurs are present or unless one can be

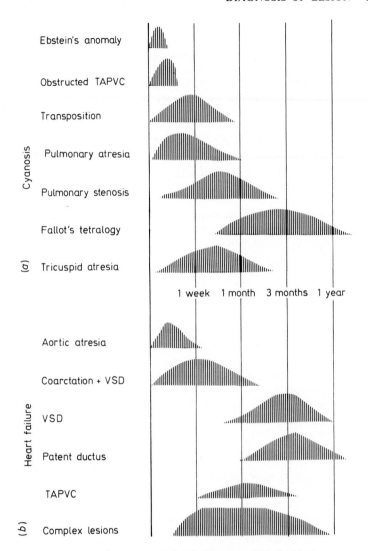

Figure 13.1. Onset of symptoms during the first year of life. TAPVC:
total anomalous pulmonary venous connection; VSD: ventricular
septal defect. The shaded areas represent the variation in onset of
symptoms, not the duration of symptoms

certain whether the second heart sound is single or split. Diastolic
murmurs are heard in absent pulmonary valve (p. 151) and with the
systolic murmur gives a to-and-fro rhythm. An early diastolic

murmur occurs in some infants with Type I persistent truncus arteriosus due to an incompetent truncal valve. A scratchy diastolic murmur is heard at the lower left sternal edge in Ebstein's anomaly. It is helpful for the paediatrician to know what time in life individual lesions most commonly cause severe distress. Lambert, Canent and Hohn (1966) and Varghese and co-workers (1969) found that the commonest *in the first week of life* are:

1. Hypoplasia of the left heart
2. Transposition of the great arteries
3. Coarctation of the aorta syndrome
4. Multiple major cardiac defects

In making a diagnosis it is simplest first to consider the group which present primarily with *severe cyanosis* and, secondly, the group which present primarily with *heart failure*—although clearly there is some overlap between these two groups. *It is valuable to remember that patients who have lesions associated with a reduced supply of blood to the lungs, rarely develop heart failure.*

Group 1: Patients presenting with severe cyanosis

1. Transposition of the great arteries (with inadequate mixing between the two circulations).
2. Pulmonary atresia or severe pulmonary valve stenosis with intact ventricular septum.
3. Pulmonary atresia or severe pulmonary stenosis with ventricular septal defect.
4. Total anomalous pulmonary venous drainage *with obstruction* to the venous return.
5. Tricuspid atresia.
6. Ebstein's anomaly of the tricuspid valve.

Group 2: Patients presenting with heart failure

1. Hypoplasia of the left heart.
2. Coarctation of the aorta syndrome.
3. Severe aortic stenosis.
4. Persistent truncus arteriosus.
5. Double outflow right ventricle without pulmonary stenosis.
6. Common atrioventricular canal.
7. Cor triatriatum.
8. Complex, combined lesions.
9. Large arteriovenous fistula.

A chest radiograph should first be taken to look at the heart shape and the amount of blood flowing to the lungs. The film must be straight, taken during inspiration and of the correct penetration to assess pulmonary vascularity. The classic findings are listed in *Table 13.1*. Unfortunately the classic shape is not always present or may be masked by an enlarged thymus gland or the presence of a left superior vena cava. A film taken very early in life may fail to show an increase in pulmonary vascularity which will become obvious later and similarly pulmonary venous congestion in total anomalous pulmonary venous drainage may not be obvious initially. Serial films are of great help, but it is unwise to wait for the classic findings to develop while the infant's condition deteriorates. It is better to make the wrong diagnosis and refer the infant for investigation than to make the correct diagnosis when the infant is moribund.

The next helpful investigation is an electrocardiogram. This tells us which ventricle is dominant and whether there is atrial hypertrophy. Again, serial electrocardiograms are helpful but when cyanosis is severe it is better to send the infant to a special unit so that cardiac catheterization and angiography can be carried out at any time.

A few lesions have characteristic electrocardiograms; for example tricuspid atresia will always show left axis deviation and left ventricular dominance (*Table 13.1* lists the usual findings).

It is important to stress that although ventricular septal defect and patent ductus are common causes of heart failure, they rarely cause heart failure in the first month of life except in premature infants where the fall in pulmonary vascular resistance is more rapid than in the fullterm baby (*see* Patent ductus in premature infant, p. 70). Atrial septal defect results in a left-to-right shunt in the newborn period only if there is some obstruction to flow from the left ventricle as well, or a mitral valve lesion.

Many of the lesions which present in infancy are discussed in detail elsewhere in this book. It remains to discuss hypoplasia of the left heart and atresia of the aortic arch which are seen only in the newborn and to describe the problems of persistent fetal circulation and myocardial ischaemia in the newborn.

HYPOPLASIA OF THE LEFT HEART

As the name suggests, in hypoplasia of the left heart there is underdevelopment of the whole of the left side of the heart. In the most severe form there is atresia of the aortic valve, the left ventricle is rudimentary and represented by a mere slit, and there is atresia or

TABLE 13.1

Differential diagnosis of heart disease in the newborn infant—main findings

Lesion	Cyanosis	Heart failure	Heart shape	Pulmonary vascularity	Electrocardiogram
Pulmonary atresia with VSD	Severe	None	Hollow pulmonary arc; uptilted apex	Reduced	RAD RVH
Pulmonary atresia with intact septum	Severe	Occurs when RV very small	RA+	Reduced	Normal axis LVH or decreased right ventricular activity for age
Tricuspid atresia	Severe	None	Square heart. RA+ Pulmonary arc hollow	Reduced	LAD LVH RAH
Tricuspid atresia with high pulmonary flow	Slight or moderate	Frequently	RA + Pulmonary arc +	Increased	LAD LVH RAH

			Heart shape	Pulmonary vascularity	ECG
Severe pulmonary stenosis with ASD	Slight initially, gradually increasing	Rare in first month	Large RA	Reduced	RAH++ RVH
Ebstein's disease	Moderate	Rare in first month	Large RA	Reduced	RAH Right bundle branch block
Transposition with intact septum	Rapidly becomes severe	Second to fourth week	Narrow pedicle Egg-shaped heart	Normal or increased	RVH
Total anomalous PVD with obstruction	Rapidly becomes severe	Liver enlarged if drainage below diaphragm	Normal size	Pulmonary venous congestion	RAH RVH
Hypoplasia of left heart	Slight at first, increasing by third day	First few days of life and is severe	General enlargement	Increased + pulmonary venous congestion	RVH RAD

Table 13.1 – continued

Lesion	Cyanosis	Heart failure	Heart shape	Pulmonary vascularity	Electrocardiogram
Coarctation of aorta	Slight	In first week; left heart failure frequent	General enlargement	Increased + pulmonary venous congestion	RVH RAD
Truncus	Slight or moderate	In first few weeks	Pulmonary arteries high up or not seen	Increased	RVH but may be LVH or combination of RV+LV
Atrioventricular canal	None	In first few weeks	RA+PA+ RV+LV+	Increased	LAD. rsR pattern in V_3R+V_1. Usually combined ventricular hypertrophy
Normal heart with enlarged thymus	None	None	Broad pedicle	Normal	Normal

severe hypoplasia of the mitral valve. The left atrium empties through a foramen ovale or atrial septal defect to the right atrium and right ventricle (*Figure 13.2*). If there is a small communication between the two atria, the left atrial pressure and consequently the pulmonary venous pressure become markedly elevated and pulmonary oedema results. The only way that blood can reach the aorta is by retrograde flow through the patent ductus arteriosus. The ascending aorta is markedly hypoplastic, as are the coronary arteries arising from it, and blood flows down the aorta in a retrograde manner from the patent ductus.

In the less severe form the aortic valve is narrowed and the ascending aorta and its arch are small and form an obstruction to outflow from the left ventricle. The mitral valve ring is also small so there is a high left atrial pressure which predisposes to pulmonary hypertension.

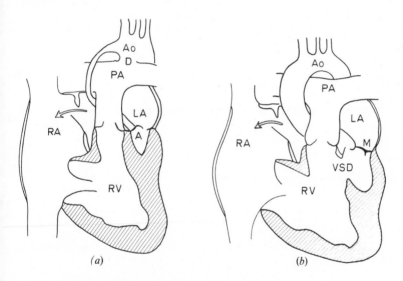

Figure 13.2. Types of left heart hypoplasia. (*a*) Aortic atresia. Ao: aorta; A: atretic aortic valve; LA: left atrium; PA: pulmonary artery; D: ductus arteriosus; RA: right atrium; RV: right ventricle. (*b*) Mitral atresia. M: atretic mitral valve; VSD: ventricular septal defect

Natural history

Patients with this condition become critically ill in the first few hours or days of life. The symptoms occur earlier than with any other heart lesion and it is the commonest cause of heart failure in the first two to three *days* of life. The majority die in the first week of life although, surprisingly, a few patients survive for two or three months on medical treatment.

Clinical presentation

The patient may appear normal at birth but then becomes progressively cyanosed and pulmonary oedema and right-sided heart failure quickly follow. As the ductus closes, the peripheral pulses become difficult to feel and the infant is pale and shocked; there is preferential flow into the descending aorta and the femoral pulses may be easier to feel than the brachial pulses. The respirations are very rapid. There may be no systolic murmur or only a faint one heard along the left sternal border. The second heart sound is single and loud. The blood pressure is low in both the arms and the legs. The liver is greatly enlarged. There is usually oliguria or anuria due to the low arterial pressure.

Radiology

Radiology shows generalized cardiac enlargement in the first 24–48 hours and there is evidence of pulmonary venous congestion or frank oedema.

Electrocardiography

The electrocardiogram usually shows right axis deviation and right ventricular hypertrophy with very little left ventricular activity.

Echocardiography

The investigation is usually diagnostic, showing the hypoplastic aorta and small, slit-like left ventricle, with enlargement of the right ventricle and pulmonary artery (*Figure 13.3*).

Cardiac catheterization

The mortality of cardiac catheterization in this lesion is higher than in any other because of the severity of the lesion, most infants dying in the first 3 days of life. Echocardiography is so reliable now that cardiac catheterization is no longer necessary.

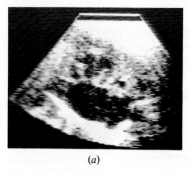
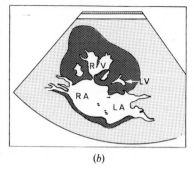

(a)   (b)

Figure 13.3. (*a*) Two dimensional echocardiogram of hypoplastic left heart (4 chamber view). (*b*) Diagram of (*a*). RA: right atrium; LA: left atrium; RV: right ventricle; LV: diminutive left ventricle (arrowed)

Treatment

There is no effective surgical treatment. Some surgeons have tried enlarging the atrial septal defect, but this carries a high risk and is of little lasting benefit. Enthusiastic medical treatment will sometimes prolong life for two or three months.

MITRAL ATRESIA

A less common variety of left heart hypoplasia is associated with mitral valve atresia (*Figure 13.2b*). Left atrial blood passes to the right atrium and from the right ventricle a hypoplastic left ventricle fills. The aortic valve is frequently stenosed. The presentation is similar to that of aortic atresia.

ATRESIA OF THE AORTIC ARCH
(Interrupted aortic arch)

A rare condition is that in which there is absence or atresia of part of the aortic arch. In one type the atresia begins after the origin of the left subclavian artery, so that both arms receive their blood from the aorta above the atresia, and the supply to the legs is through a patent ductus arteriosus which supplies the descending aorta. In another type the atresia begins before the origin of the left subclavian artery and that vessel arises from the descending aorta opposite the patent ductus. In a third type the right subclavian artery also arises from the descending aorta below the atretic segment (*Figure 13.4*). There are usually associated intracardiac abnormalities such as ventricular septal defect.

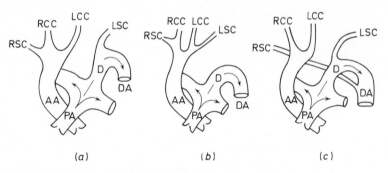

Figure 13.4. Types of aortic arch atresia. (*a*) Between left common carotid (LCC) and left subclavian (LSC). (*b*) Beyond left subclavian. (*c*) Between left common carotid and left subclavian with anomalous right subclavian (RSC). AA: ascending aorta; DA: descending aorta; PA: pulmonary artery; D: ductus; RCC: right common carotid

Natural history

Death usually occurs in the first three to four weeks of life and survival beyond 1 year of age is very rare.

Clinical presentation

The patient usually presents with mild cyanosis which may be more marked in the legs than in the right arm, but such differential cyanosis is often difficult to detect. The pulses distal to the atretic segment are difficult to feel, and in the type where the atretic segment is proximal to both subclavian arteries pulsation can only be felt in the neck. Usually there are no cardiac murmurs. The second sound is loud and single. Heart failure occurs early and the patient gradually deteriorates despite medical treatment. The clinical presentation resembles the hypoplastic left heart syndrome.

Radiology

The radiograph shows an enlarged heart with pulmonary congestion.

Electrocardiography

The electrocardiogram may be normal or show combined ventricular hypertrophy.

Investigation

Cardiac catheterization and angiography are required to demonstrate the exact site and extent of the atresia and to show other intracardiac lesions, particularly ventricular septal defect.

Treatment

The only effective treatment is surgical. When the atresia is localized and occurs distal to the left subclavian artery, the atretic segment can be resected and the subclavian artery used in the anostomosis with the descending aorta after the ductus has been divided. This is done using deep hypothermia and a short period of cardiopulmonary bypass. When the atretic segment is proximal to the left subclavian artery, surgery carries a very high risk and is technically very difficult even though a graft is theoretically possible.

THE MURMURLESS HEART

One of the greatest problems with the sick infant is deciding whether heart disease is present or not. There are a surprising number of lesions which may not produce a heart murmur in infancy, and these are listed in *Table 13.2*. They are divided into acyanotic and cyanotic groups, but it must be remembered that when heart failure and respiratory difficulty occur, the patient may appear cyanotic even though the underlying lesion is an acyanotic one.

TABLE 13.2
Murmurless heart in the newborn infant

A. CYANOTIC

Lesion	Radiology		Electrocardiography
	Vascularity of lungs	*Heart shape*	
Transposition of great arteries	Normal or increased	Narrow pedicle and 'egg-shaped' heart	RAD RVH
Total anomalous pulmonary venous drainage with obstruction	Reticular appearance of pulmonary venous congestion	Normal size and shape	RAD RAH RVH
Hypoplasia of left heart	Increased and pulmonary venous congestion	General cardiac enlargement with broad pedicle	RAD RVH
Pulmonary atresia with VSD	Decreased	Boot shape with long left cardiac border and uptilted apex	RAD RVH
Pulmonary atresia with intact ventricular septum	Decreased	Large right atrium; left cardiac border normal	Normal axis. LVH or diminished right ventricular activity for age
Tricuspid atresia ± pulmonary atresia	Decreased	Square shape with prominent right atrium	LAD RAH LVH or poor RV activity

255

B. ACYANOTIC

Lesion	Radiology		Electrocardiography
	Vascularity of lungs	Heart shape	
Normal heart and pulmonary disease	Normal or pulmonary venous congestion	Normal	Normal or RVH
Coarctation of aorta syndrome	Increased and pulmonary venous congestion	General cardiac enlargement	RAD RVH
Cor triatriatum	Pulmonary venous congestion	Normal	LAH RAD RVH
Myocarditis	Pulmonary venous congestion	General cardiac enlargement	Low voltage record with abnormal T waves
Endocardial fibroelastosis	Normal	General cardiac enlargement	LVH T waves in LV leads usually inverted
Common ventricle with L-transposition	Increased	Prominent left cardiac border	S waves in all precordial leads. q waves in V_4R and V_1
Anomalous coronary artery	Pulmonary venous congestion	General cardiac enlargement	Inverted T waves in leads 1, 2, 3. Deep Q waves in leads 1 and aVL. QS or QR waves in leads V_{2-4}

PERSISTENCE OF THE FETAL CIRCULATION
(TRANSITIONAL CIRCULATION)

This refers to a situation in which the haemodynamics of the fetal circulation persist after birth. There is constriction of the pulmonary vascular bed and if the pulmonary vascular resistance is higher than the systemic resistance then shunting will take place from the pulmonary artery through a persistent ductus arteriosus to the aorta and through the foramen ovale from the right atrium to the left atrium. The infant will then be cyanosed. Pulmonary vascular resistance may be high, secondary to some congenital heart lesion, but the term persistence of the fetal circulation refers to the primary form unassociated with any anatomical cardiac defect. The cause is unknown but it has been shown that the small pulmonary arteries have an abnormally thick muscular coat (Haworth and Reid, 1976; Haworth, 1979). Clinically the infant presents within 24 hours of birth with respiratory distress and cyanosis and there is usually a history of some perinatal hypoxia. The mother may be a diabetic. Resuscitation may have been required after delivery. There is marked heaving of the right ventricle. A systolic murmur due to tricuspid regurgitation may be present at the lower left sternal border. The ECG shows right ventricular hypertrophy. X-ray shows cardiomegaly and variable lung vascularity. The haematocrit is unusually high. Since there is right-to-left shunting occurring, the child will remain blue in 100 per cent oxygen and cyanotic heart disease is suspected. Echocardiography is useful in that it will show the presence of 4 cardiac chambers and 2 A-V valves in transitional circulation and thus exclude complex abnormalities. If however there is any doubt that the child may have transposition of the great arteries or total anomalous pulmonary venous drainage, then catheterization is necessary. Some patients who have myocardial ischaemia secondary to anoxia, present in a similar way but have poor left ventricular function on the echocardiogram.

Treatment

The infant should be kept well oxygenated and mechanical ventilation may be required. Acidosis and hypoglycaemia should be corrected and if there is severe polycythaemia blood should be withdrawn and replaced by plasma. In patients with severe cyanosis, acidosis, and hypoxaemia, a vicious circle of events may occur with severe pulmonary vasoconstriction and myocardial dysfunction. Digoxin and diuretics help this group and tolazoline has been used to dilate the pulmonary vascular bed (Goetzman *et al.*, 1976). Abbott *et al.* (1978) used nitroprusside for its direct vasodilator effect. Tolazoline however does have a 30 per cent incidence of side-effects, particularly haemorrhage and renal abnormalities.

Recently Fiddler *et al.* (1980) have used dopamine in a medium dose range 2–10 µg/kg per minute intravenously. In that dose it has a direct effect on the beta-adrenergic cardiac receptors causing an increase in cardiac output. It gives immediate inotropic support to the hypoxic failing myocardium and by dilating peripheral vascular beds reduces some of the afterload on the heart. Their experience suggests that it hastens the resolution of the myocardial dysfunction. There is a significant mortality in this condition between 25 and 30 per cent (Levin *et al.*, 1976).

PERSISTENT
FETAL CIRCULATION WITH CLOSED DUCTUS
(Partial PFC, persistent neonatal pulmonary hypertension).

Occasionally a rather different syndrome is seen, in which the pulmonary vascular resistance remains high but the ductus closes. Here the pressure load in the right ventricle causes it to dilate and fail, so that the shunt occurs entirely through the foramen ovale. The infant is blue, has a large liver and a murmur due to functional tricuspid regurgitation. The chest X-ray shows a large heart (right ventricle and right atrium) and the ECG right atrial and right ventricular hypertrophy.

Clinical distinction from patients with premature intrauterine closure of ductus (*see below*) and those with Ebstein's anomaly of the tricuspid valve (p. 183) is usually impossible, but the treatment is in any case the same and consists of treatment for persistent fetal circulation plus digoxin.

PREMATURE CLOSURE OF DUCTUS ARTERIOSUS

If the ductus closes before birth, when the pulmonary vascular resistance is high the right ventricle dilates and triscupid regurgitation occurs. This seems to be extremely rare. There is a clinical picture of heart failure and cyanosis and the X-ray often shows an enormous heart, almost filling the chest. As the pulmonary vascular resistance falls after the birth the infant's condition improves and the heart size gradually diminishes over the first year of life. Apart from oxygen to speed the fall in pulmonary artery pressure, no specific treatment is required.

MYOCARDIAL ISCHAEMIA IN THE NEWBORN

It has recently been recognized that some infants with transient tachypnoea and heart failure in the neonatal period, show electrocardiographic (and sometimes echo or angiographic) evidence of myocardial ischaemia (Rowe and Hoffman, 1972; Rowe *et al.*, 1979).

Incidence and aetiology

Minor degrees with rapid resolution are probably fairly common but symptoms severe enough to warrant treatment or raise suspicion of more serious disease are uncommon. Even in severe cases the coronary arteries are structurally normal (Rowe *et al.*, 1979). Most infants have a history of perinatal distress and asphyxia which may cause myocardial damage. Myocardial glycogen may be reduced when there is fetal hypoxaemia (Dawes *et al.*, 1960), and the myocardium of the newborn is dependent on glucose.

Clinical picture

Seventy per cent of affected infants have a history of fetal distress or asphyxia. Tachypnoea, a variable degree of cyanosis and enlargement of the liver are the most constant signs. A murmur due to mitral regurgitation is occasionally heard and râles may be heard over the back of the chest. In severe cases there is a 'shock' syndrome with diminished peripheral pulses and metabolic acidosis. The chest X-ray shows mild or moderate cardiac enlargement and, in severe cases, venous congestion and pulmonary oedema.

Electrocardiography

The ECG changes are still the subject of debate, but are generally regarded as indicative of myocardial ischaemia, with ST depression and T wave inversion mainly in left ventricular leads V5–V6 but sometimes seen in inferior leads (III and AVF) or anterior leads V2–V3 (Rowe *et al.*, 1979). Usually the abnormalities regress over a period of a week or two but some persist for up to 6 months.

Treatment and prognosis

Mild cases require no specific treatment. Digoxin, diuretics and oxygen, with the correction of hypoglycaemia and acidosis usually produce prompt improvement in those with more obvious signs and symptoms. Death has been reported but is rare in mature infants with no other problems. Most survivors make a complete recovery, although persistent mitral regurgitation may occur and it has been postulated that late onset arrhythmia from myocardial fibrosis may be a cause of 'cot death' (Keeton *et al.*, 1977).

NEONATAL HYPOCALCAEMIA

Low serum calcium concentration is an uncommon, but treatable cause of heart failure in the newborn. Usually there are other, central nervous system, signs of hypocalcaemia but it is worth checking the serum calcium of any newborn baby with unexplained heart failure or cardiomegaly. The condition responds to elevation of serum calcium by intravenous infusion followed by Parathormone and vitamin D analogues. Ideally the diagnosis should be made and treatment started before digoxin has been given, as there is a risk of arrhythmias when intravenous calcium is given to a digitalized patient. ECG monitoring should, in any case, be employed.

REFERENCES

Abbott, T. R., Rees, G. J., Dickinson, D., Reynolds G. and Lord D. (1978). Sodium nitroprusside in idiopathic respiratory distress syndrome. *Br. Med. J.* **1**, 1113–1114
Dawes, G. S., Jacobson, H. N., Mott, J. C. and Shelley, J. J. (1960). Some observations on fetal and newborn rhesus monkeys. *J. Physiol.* **152**, 271
Fiddler, G. I., Chatrath, R., Williams, G. J., Walker, D. R. and Scott, Olive (1980). Dopamine infusion for the treatment of myocardial dysfunction associated with a persistent transitional circulation. *Archs Dis. Childh.* **55**, 3. 194–198
Godman, M. J., Tham, P. and Langford-Kidd, B. S. (1974). Echocardiography in the evaluation of the cyanotic newborn infant. *Br. Heart J.* **36**, 154
Goetzman, B. W., Sunshine, P., Johnson, J. D., Wennberg, R. P., Hakel, A., Merton, D. F., Bartoletti, A. L. and Silverman, N. H. (1976). Neonatal hypoxia and pulmonary vascular response to tolazaline. *J. Pediat.* **89**, 617–621
Izukawa, T., Mulholland, H. C., Rowe, R. D., Cook, D. H., Bloom, K. R., Trusler, G. A., Williams, W. G. and Chance, G. W. (1979). Structural heart disease in the newborn. Changing profile; comparison of 1975 with 1965. *Archs Dis. Childh.* **54**, 281–285
Jones, R. W. A., Baumer, J. H., Joseph, M. C. and Shinebourne, E. A. (1976). Arterial oxygen tension and response to oxygen breathing in differential diagnosis of congenital heart disease in infancy. *Archs Dis. Childh.* **51**, 667–673
Keeton, B. R., Southall, E., Rutter, N., Anderson, R. H., Shinebourne, E. A. and Southall, D. P. (1977). Cardiac conduction disorders in six infants with 'near miss' sudden death. *Br. Med. J.* **2**, 600

Lambert, E. C., Canent, R. V. and Hohn, A. R. (1966). Congenital cardiac anomalies in the newborn. *Pediatrics, Springfield* **37**, 343

Report of New England Regional Infant Cardiac Program (1980). *Pediatrics* **65**, 2 part 2. Suppl.

Rowe, R. D. and Hoffman, T. (1972). Transient myocardial ischaemia of the newborn infant. A form of severe cardiorespiratory distress in full term infants. *J. Pediat.* **81**, 243

Rowe, R. D., Finley, J. P., Gilday, D. L., Dislche, M. R., Jimenez, C. L. and Chance, G. W. (1979). Myocardial ischaemia in the newborn. In *Paediatric Cardiology*. Vol. 2. *Heart Disease in the Newborn*. Eds M. J. Goodman and R. M. Marquis. London: Churchill Livingstone

Sinha, S. N., Kardatyke, B. A., Cole, R. B., Muster, A. J., Vesser, H. V. and Paul, M. H. (1969). Coarctation of the aorta in infancy. *Circulation* **60**, 385

Varghese, P. J., Celermajer, J., Izukawa, T., Haller, J. A. and Rowe, R. D. (1969). Cardiac catheterization in the newborn. *Pediatrics, Springfield* **44**, 24

CHAPTER 14

Heart Failure in Infancy and Childhood

Heart failure occurs more commonly in the first three months of life than in any other period of childhood. Hypoplasia of the left heart is the commonest cause of heart failure in the first week of life, coarctation of the aorta causes failure most commonly in the first month of life and transposition of the great arteries with ventricular septal defect in the first two months of life. Ventricular septal defect or patent ductus arteriosus rarely cause heart failure before 6 weeks of age unless they occur together or with other lesions (*see Figure 13.1*, p. 243).

After 1 year of age, heart failure due to congenital heart disease is rare and the possibility that it has been precipitated by bacterial endocarditis or anaemia should be considered.

ASSESSMENT OF SYMPTOMS AND SIGNS

It is often difficult to separate the symptoms and signs of the underlying cardiac disease from those due to heart failure but assessment of the following signs is helpful.

Tachycardia

When the rate is greater than 180/minute in infants, and 150/minute in older children, heart failure is usually present. (If the rate is greater than 200/minute in infants, or 180/minute in older children, supraventricular tachycardia is probably present and should be looked for on the electrocardiogram.)

Gallop rhythm

A third heart sound is frequently heard at the cardiac apex in childhood but it is faint and not easy to hear. If there is a very obvious third sound causing gallop rhythm, heart failure is likely.

Tachypnoea and dyspnoea

The respiratory rate in heart failure is greater than 60/minute in infants and greater than 40/minute in older children. Such rapid rates, however, and difficult breathing may occur when there is respiratory disease alone and they are not of value in differentiation.

Enlargement of the liver

Enlargement of the liver is a very valuable sign in heart failure and if the liver is 2 cm or more below the right costal margin in the midclavicular line, then failure is present.

Cardiomegaly

Cardiomegaly is usually present in heart failure but enlargement may be present without failure. The only time that the heart remains small in the presence of heart failure is when there is obstructed pulmonary venous return.

Cough

A persistent irritating cough is common in lesions causing left heart failure.

Sweating

Sweating is a frequent and often overlooked sign of early heart failure. There may be profuse sweating at inappropriate ambient temperatures. Patients whose defects are associated with large left-to-right shunts, such as ventricular septal defect and patent ductus arteriosus, are particularly prone to profuse sweating. They sweat for two reasons: they have a high metabolic rate and a diminished peripheral blood flow and the only way that they can maintain a normal body temperature is by excessive sweating. Kinnaird (1971) has shown that sweating is significantly associated with overt heart failure or that the infant is on the verge of developing heart failure.

Pulmonary signs

Moist sounds in the chest may be due to infection but may alternatively be due to left ventricular failure. Differentiation is difficult but when there is associated wheezing and the rales are bilateral, left ventricular failure should be considered. The rapid improvement of the patient and disappearance of the rales in the lungs following an intramuscular dose of frusemide are further indications that they are caused by left ventricular failure.

Left ventricular failure is most commonly seen in coarctation of the aorta, endocardial fibroelastosis and aortic stenosis.

Oedema

Oedema is a late manifestation of heart failure, but a gain in weight in an infant, who is not taking his feed adequately, suggests fluid retention due to heart failure.

TREATMENT

The most important part of the treatment of congestive heart failure is rapid and adequate digitalization. Most paediatric cardiologists are agreed that the best preparation for routine use is the solution of digoxin marketed by Burroughs Wellcome as Lanoxin Paediatric Elixir. It is a stable solution which is easily administered using the dropper provided and the dose can be measured accurately. Lanoxin can also be given intramuscularly and intravenously but the latter route is rarely required and should *never* be used without electrocardiographic control. Its action begins 2 hours after oral administration and reaches its full effect after 6–8 hours (Robinson, 1960). It is rapidly excreted; Batterman and DeGraff (1947) found that 3 days after discontinuing Lanoxin, 87 per cent of the initial dose had gone.

This is advantageous if toxic doses are given. The duration of its effect varies from 4 to 7 days.

An electrocardiogram should be recorded before digitalization begins and again after 24 hours. *Rapid digitalization should always be carried out in hospital because close observation is necessary.* Digitalization is best carried out over 24 hours. A single large dose, especially if given intramuscularly, may cause a high blood level before distribution can occur. If vomiting is present the drug should be given intramuscularly, otherwise the oral route is adequate in most cases. There is an individual variation in the response to digoxin and the therapeutic dose approximates to the toxic dose more closely than with any other drug. Dosage schedules related to weight are given in *Table 14.1.* In premature and newborn infants, where renal function may be inadequate, a lower dosage schedule is desirable than that used for infants over 1 month old (Neill, 1965). This is because of the dangers of toxicity in the small infant.

TABLE 14.1

Dosage scheme for digitalization using lanoxin (Burroughs and Wellcome)

Age of patient	Total digitalizing dose given over 24 hours		Maintenance dose/24 hours	
	Oral	Intramuscular	Oral	Intramuscular
Premature or less than 1 month	0.04 mg/kg	0.03 mg/kg	0.010 mg/kg	0.010 mg/kg
1 month to 2 years	0.06 mg/kg	0.04 mg/kg	0.020 mg/kg	0.015 mg/kg
2 years to 10 years	0.04 mg/kg	0.03 mg/kg	0.010 mg/kg	0.010 mg/kg

After the age of 10 years adult doses may be used.

 The digitalizing dose should be given in three doses. Half the total digitalizing dose is given immediately, then a quarter of the total dose after 8 hours and the remaining quarter of the total dose after a further 8 hours.

 The maintenance dose should be given in two divided doses at 12-hourly intervals.

Von Bernuth *et al.* (1979) found that newborns tend to have higher plasma and tissue digoxin concentrations than older children and adults. They found that a relatively low digoxin dose in newborns is effective and safe. The clinical manifestations of toxicity in newborns are poor feeding and persistent vomiting (Krasula *et al.*, 1974) and these are symptoms which have many other causes. If in doubt plasma concentrations should be measured. Von Bernuth *et al.* (1979) concluded that plasma digoxin concentrations in newborns of 5 ng/ml and higher are highly suggestive of digoxin toxicity and values below 3 ng/ml are unlikely to be associated with toxicity. The lower limit of therapeutic serum concentration is not known. As in adult hypokalaemia, hypoxia and acidosis increase the tendency to digoxin intoxication at any given plasma concentration. The work of Nyberg and Wettrell (1978) suggests that even lower loading doses than in *Table 14.1* are effective and recommend a loading dose of 0.025 mg/kg followed by 0.01 mg/kg after 12 hours.

Digoxin should not be used in heart disease when heart failure is not present. It may do harm in lesions such as tetralogy of Fallot by further obstructing the outflow tract from the right ventricle.

After digitalization has begun, the following additional measures should be taken.

1. *Oxygen* should be given in a concentration of 30 per cent. This is best done in a tent or incubator.
2. *Position.* The child should be propped up; a small chair is useful for this in older infants and if it does not fit into the incubator, a tent should be used.
3. *Infection.* The presence of any infection, particularly chest infection, should be looked for and treated.
4. *Sedation* should be given only if the child is very restless. Phenobarbitone is best. Respiratory depressants should be avoided, particularly in cyanosed infants.
5. *Feeding.* Clear fluids should be given initially and in young infants this is best given by oesophageal tube if they are very distressed. As improvement occurs milk feeds by bottle can be given. There is no necessity to give low-sodium milk or low-sodium diets with the potent diuretics now available.
6. *Temperature control.* Infants who have large shunts and high metabolic rates must be nursed in a relatively cool environment or their metabolic rates will increase further and put an additional strain on their metabolism.
7. *Diuretics.* Since a stable oral preparation of frusemide is now available, other diuretics are rarely used in paediatric practice. It is a safe, potent diuretic and is easily administered. It acts quickly and lacks toxicity. The intramuscular route is more reliable and should be used initially, then followed by the oral preparation. The dose is 1 mg/kg twice daily i.m., and 1–2 mg/kg twice daily orally. Hypokalaemia is uncommon in infants but potentiates the action of digoxin and increases the tendency to toxicity so it is wise to check the electrolytes and give potassium supplements orally, if required. Potassium chloride 2 mmol/kg per day is used.
8. Aldosterone antagonists such as spironolactone may be added to the treatment when heart failure is difficult to control or potassium loss is a problem. The dose is 1.5–3.0 mg/kg per day in 3 divided doses.

It must be stressed that in congenital heart disease, the treatment of heart failure is only a first step in management and the child should be referred to a paediatric cardiologist with a view to establishing the diagnosis and deciding whether surgical treatment is advisable. Heart failure in the first four weeks of life *demands urgent investigation*, as does heart failure at any age which does not respond *promptly* to digoxin and frusemide.

Digoxin toxicity

Digoxin toxicity is most commonly due to overdosage but may occur in accidental poisoning, usually when a child takes tablets prescribed for a parent or grandparent. The presence of a low potassium level in the blood potentiates the arrhythmogenic (but not the inotropic) action of digoxin, and toxic effects such as arrhythmias occur. Care must be taken therefore when diuretics which cause potassium depletion are being given, or when the patient has diarrhoea or vomiting, or is given steroids.

Although nausea, vomiting and diarrhoea are early symptoms of toxicity, they do not always occur and a cardiac arrhythmia may be the first evidence of toxicity. There may be ventricular ectopic beats or pulsus bigeminus or bradycardia and atrioventricular dissociation. In newborn infants bradycardia, supraventricular arrhythmias and second and third degree heart block are the commonest. Paroxysmal atrial tachycardia with atrioventricular block may occur and if this is not recognized more digoxin may be administered to correct the rapid rate with disastrous results. If in doubt, further doses of digoxin should be withheld, an electrocardiogram recorded and the serum digoxin estimated.

Treatment of intoxication

1. Stop the digoxin. In many cases this may be sufficient and, after two or three days, treatment can be resumed using a lower dosage.
2. Check serum electrolytes.
3. Check digoxin levels in blood. Values more than 5 ng/ml are found in digoxin toxicity, levels between 3 and 5 ng/ml may be toxic in some circumstances.
4. If intoxication is severe, the administration of potassium is required and constant electrocardiographic monitoring is essential. Older children can be given 1 g of potassium chloride orally every 8 hours. Intravenous potassium is only given in desperate cases and only when there is a good urinary output. It should be

given slowly over 1 hour using a solution of 40 mmol of potassium chloride in 500 ml of dextrose in water. The total dose should not exceed 2 mmol/kg body weight and it should be discontinued when the arrhythmia disappears or peaked T waves appear on the electrocardiogram (Neill, 1965).

REFERENCES

Batterman, R. C. and DeGraff, A. C. (1947). Comparative study on the use of purified digitalis glycosides, digoxin and lanatoside C, for the management of ambulatory patients with congestive heart failure. *Am. Heart J.* **34**, 663

Kinnaird, D. L. (1971). Personal communication

Krasula, R., Yanagi, R., Hastreiter, A. R., Levitsky, S. and Soyka, L. F. (1974). Digoxin intoxication in infants and children; correlation with serum levels. *J. Pediat.* **84**, 265–269.

Neill, C. A. (1965). Recognition and treatment of congestive heart failure in infants. *Prog. cardiovasc. Dis.* **7**, 399

Nyberg, L., Wettrell, G. (1978). Digoxin dosage schedules for neonates and infants based on pharmacokinetic considerations. *Clin. Pharmacokinetics* **3**, 453–461

Robinson, S. J. (1960). Digitalis therapy in infants and children. *J. Pediat.* **36**, 536

Von Bernuth, G. V., Lang, D. and Hofstetter, R. (1979). Digoxin in the newborn infant. In *Paediatric Cardiology.* Vol. 2, p. 413. Eds M. J. Godman and R. M. Marquis, London: Churchill Livingstone.

CHAPTER 15

Pulmonary Hypertension, Cor Pulmonale and the Eisenmenger Syndrome

PULMONARY HYPERTENSION

The term 'pulmonary hypertension' (strictly, pulmonary arterial hypertension) refers to an elevation of the pressure above the normal in the pulmonary artery. *In utero* and in the few days following birth pulmonary hypertension is normal. At other times it may take one of three forms.

1. *Passive pulmonary hypertension* is due simply to a back pressure transmitted through the pulmonary capillaries from raised pulmonary venous and left atrial pressure.
2. *Hyperdynamic pulmonary hypertension* is caused by high flow of blood in the pulmonary system. The pulmonary vessels can normally dilate to take an increase of 100–200 per cent in flow without any actual increase in pulmonary artery pressure, as occurs on exercise and in uncomplicated atrial septal defects.
3. *Reactive pulmonary hypertension* represents an increase in the vascular resistance of the lungs, brought about by constriction of the small, muscular pulmonary arteries. The rise in resistance may in some circumstances be temporary and reversible, in others permanent. The only physiological stimulus which consistently produces a rise in pulmonary vascular resistance is hypoxia, and the sensing area of the lungs appears to be the pulmonary venous system. A rise in carbon dioxide tension or a fall in pH in the

pulmonary venous system may also have an effect on pulmonary vascular resistance, particularly when occurring with hypoxia.

Although three types of pulmonary hypertension are described, it is unusual to find either passive or hyperdynamic forms in isolation. Patients with raised left atrial pressure from left heart obstruction usually have both passive and reactive pulmonary hypertension, and patients with large ventricular septal defects have both hyperdynamic and reactive components, and, if associated with left ventricular failure, all three types.

Hypertensive pulmonary vascular disease

Patients with pulmonary hypertension which has been present since birth have main pulmonary arteries which are similar in structure to the aorta, showing a thick medial coat with abundant elastic tissue. This is never seen in acquired pulmonary hypertension.

In both congenital and acquired forms, the small muscular pulmonary arteries show the most striking changes, which have been classified by Heath and Edwards (1958) into six grades of severity.

Grade 1	Muscular hypertrophy of the media and development of longitudinal muscle fibres.
Grade 2	Cellular intimal proliferation.
Grade 3	Intimal fibrosis, with narrowing of the lumen.
Grade 4	Dilatation, with thinning of the vessel wall.
Grade 5	Plexiform vascular lesion (possibly due to thrombosis and recanalization or to attempts at formation of anastomotic vessels).
Grade 6	Fibrinoid necrosis of the interna and media.

Muscular hypertrophy is regarded as a result of the stimulus causing the arterial contriction and the other lesions are the result of the high intravascular pressure. Grade 1 lesions are reversible. Grade 2 and 3 lesions are associated with reversible pulmonary hypertension and may themselves regress. Grades 4, 5 and 6 are uncommon but in general indicate irreversible pulmonary hypertension (as in primary pulmonary hypertension).

In addition to the arterial lesions the pulmonary arterioles develop a muscle coat which in health they do not possess.

Much has been written about the value of assessment of pulmonary vascular disease by lung biopsy in the selection of patients for surgery of ventricular septal defect and other lesions. Although patients with grade 4–6 lesions are not suitable for surgery, this is usually clear from their clinical state, and in most cases careful clinical and haemodynamic assessment is at least as reliable.

Signs of pulmonary hypertension

In severe pulmonary hypertension, not associated with intracardiac defects, the pulse has a small volume and there is peripheral and frequently slight central cyanosis, the latter being due to ventilation–perfusion inequality in the lungs. The jugular venous pressure shows a large 'a' wave when the condition is chronic and the mean level of pressure may be raised when the condition is acute or subacute. The right ventricular pulsation to the left of the sternum is increased and the second heart sound is very loud and palpable. Pulmonary artery dilatation gives rise to an ejection click and a soft ejection systolic murmur and there may be a pulmonary diastolic murmur due to functional pulmonary regurgitation.

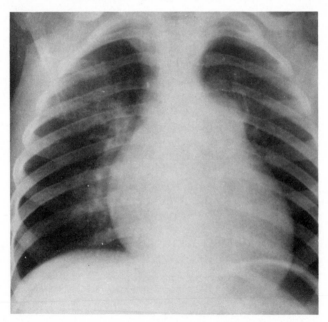

Figure 15.1. Pulmonary hypertension. Chest radiograph of a 4-year-old girl who had had a Pudenz valve inserted for infantile hydrocephalus. The tip of the valve is seen in the superior vena cava. Note the right atrial and right ventricular hypertrophy, the prominent main pulmonary artery and the 'pruning' of the pulmonary vessels peripherally

Radiology, electrocardiography and echocardiography

Chest radiographs (*Figure 15.1*) show dilatation of the main pulmonary artery and its left and right branches, but the peripheral branches are small ('pruned' or 'pollarded' pulmonary arteries). The electrocardiogram in chronic pulmonary hypertension shows right ventricular hypertrophy, but in acute forms may show a right bundle branch block pattern or deep inversion of T waves in right ventricular leads (3, aVF and V_{2-3}). P waves are usually peaked in leads 2 and V_1 in either acute or chronic forms, due to right atrial hypertrophy.

Echocardiography shows an absence of the usual presystolic opening movement of the pulmonary valve and prolongation of the right ventricular ejection time. The hypertrophy of the right ventricular wall can also be demonstrated.

Causes of pulmonary hypertension

Passive ($\pm$ reactive) pulmonary hypertension:

Left ventricular failure
Mitral valve disease
Cor triatriatum
Pulmonary veno-occlusive disease
Obstructed total anomalous pulmonary venous connection

Hyperdynamic ($\pm$ reactive) pulmonary hypertension:

Patent ductus arteriosus
Ventricular septal defect
Atrial septal defect (rarely in childhood)
Total anomalous pulmonary venous connection (non-obstructed)
Transposition of the great arteries
Truncus arteriosus
Common or single ventricle
High output states
Carcinoid syndrome

Pure reactive pulmonary hypertension:

Cor pulmonale
Eisenmenger syndrome
Primary pulmonary hypertension

Most of the conditions mentioned are dealt with in other sections of the book. The remainder are discussed in this chapter.

Pulmonary veno-occlusive disease

Generalized obstruction to pulmonary veins by clot or constriction is extremely rare but has been reported in children with liver disease and as a result of ingestion of certain plants, usually in the form of 'bush tea'. Patients complain of cough and breathlessness and have signs of pulmonary arterial hypertension. Cardiac catheterization shows pulmonary arterial hypertension and a raised 'wedge' pressure with normal left atrial pressure. Specific therapy is not available and the condition is fatal.

Thromboembolic pulmonary hypertension

Embolization to the lungs is a complication of ventriculoatrial drains used in the treatment of hydrocephalus and the emboli may be infected. Embolization from the heart occurs in endomyocardial fibrosis, myxoma of the right atrium and right sided endocarditis. Embolization from systemic veins is rare in childhood but has been reported from hepatic veins in patients with liver disease.

Thrombosis *in situ*

Thrombosis *in situ* occurs in patients with a generalized clotting tendency, in those with a low pulmonary flow (as in Fallot's tetralogy) and those with pre-existing pulmonary hypertension.

Schistosomiasis

In Africa and South America schistosomiasis is the commonest cause of pulmonary hypertension but is unusual in those under the age of 10 years since emboli of the ova do not reach the lungs until hepatic involvement has produced portal hypertension and collateral channels bypassing the liver.

Primary pulmonary hypertension

Pulmonary hypertension occurring with no detectable cause is rare at any age and particularly so in children. The condition usually progresses to right heart failure and death within a year from diagnosis, but occasional patients remain static for many years. No specific therapy is known to affect the disease.

High altitude pulmonary hypertension

Inhalation of air with a low oxygen tension causes acute or chronic elevation of pulmonary artery pressure. In people living constantly at moderate altitude this is well tolerated but at very high levels or in subjects brought rapidly to moderate levels, right heart failure may occur. Restoration to sea level produces cure in acute cases and amelioration in chronic cases but the latter are then unable to return to the higher levels since rapid deterioration occurs.

COR PULMONALE

Heart disease due to malfunction of the lungs is known as pulmonary heart disease or cor pulmonale. The condition is recognized either because of symptoms and signs of right heart failure or from clinical or electrocardiographic evidence of right ventricular hypertrophy. The basic cause of cor pulmonale, irrespective of the underlying disease, is pulmonary hypertension caused by constriction of pulmonary arteries due to hypoxia.

Hypoventilation (Pickwickian syndrome)

Chronic hypoventilation, from severe obesity, central nervous system disease or from respiratory paralysis, causes pulmonary hypertension and right heart failure. In addition, the rise in arterial carbon dioxide tension is responsible for the drowsiness which is characteristic of the condition.

Kyphoscoliosis

Children with severe chest deformities become hypoxic partly due to pure ventilatory difficulty and partly due to ventilation–perfusion inequalities. The condition rarely causes heart failure before adult life.

Fibrocystic disease

Of all the chronic respiratory diseases, fibrocystic disease (mucoviscidosis) is most likely to produce pulmonary hypertension and right heart failure, although usually not before the early teens. When right heart failure does occur it is a bad prognostic sign and few patients survive much more than two years from its occurrence.

Asthma

In severe episodes some degree of acute right heart failure may occur, but chronic cor pulmonale is most unusual in childhood.

Upper airways obstruction

Choanal atresia, or stenosis, in infancy usually causes obvious respiratory obstruction but occasional patients present with unexplained right heart failure. Large tonsils and adenoids have also been described as a cause of acute and subacute cor pulmonale. Characteristically the patients are under 2 years of age and present with somnolence and right heart failure. Respiration may be obviously obstructed but sometimes is shallow and not always noisy, and cyanosis is moderate or severe. Examination of the heart shows evidence of pulmonary hypertension. Chest radiographs show considerable cardiomegaly and the electrocardiogram indicates right heart strain (Macartney, Panday and Scott, 1969.) This situation is also seen in achondroplasia when the postnasal space is particularly small.

Treatment is urgent and consists of intubation followed by tonsillectomy

THE EISENMENGER SYNDROME

The Eisenmenger syndrome has been mentioned in the sections on ventricular septal defect, patent ductus arteriosus and atrial septal defect and is now described in further detail.

Eisenmenger in 1897 described a patient who gave a history of cyanosis and breathlessness since infancy and who developed heart failure at 32 years and died following a large haemoptysis. A large ventricular septal defect was found at autopsy and the aorta 'overrode' both ventricles. Eisenmenger stated that the pulmonary vascular resistance had been increased but did not realize that this caused the right-to-left shunt and cyanosis. Since his description, patients with large ventricular septal defects with right-to-left shunts producing cyanosis have been said to have 'the Eisenmenger complex'.

Paul Wood (1958) rightly pointed out that there were other lesions in which an increase in pulmonary vascular resistance to a level greater than the systemic vascular resistance resulted in a right-to-left shunt and cyanosis. He noted that such cases were often indistinguishable from one another if they were first seen when the patient had a right-to-left shunt. He therefore redefined the condition and called it 'the Eisenmenger syndrome'. Any condition in which there is 'pulmonary hypertension at systemic level, due to a high pulmonary vascular resistance, with a reversed or bidirectional shunt at aortopulmonary, ventricular or atrial level' may be given this name. It may occur in patent ductus arteriosus, aortopulmonary window, ventricular septal defect and atrial septal defect. The term has also been applied to other more complex defects when a very high pulmonary vascular resistance causes a dominant right-to-left shunt, such as persistent truncus, transposition (D- or L-) with ventricular septal defect and without pulmonary stenosis, single ventricle, single atrium, atrioventricular canal and total anomalous pulmonary venous connection.

When the Eisenmenger syndrome occurs the *defect between the two circulations is large*. Yet some patients with large defects do not develop a high pulmonary vascular resistance. There is still argument as to whether in some cases the high resistance is present from birth. Certainly in the majority of patients there is evidence of a large left-to-right shunt prior to the development of the Eisenmenger syndrome. It is rarely seen before 2 years of age in ventricular septal defect alone but occurs earlier, often by 1 year of age, when there is associated transposition of the great arteries. Children with Down's syndrome and ventricular septal defect or common A-V canal are particularly liable to develop pulmonary hypertension and reversal of shunt at an early age. The probable reason is that they tend to hypoventilate and become hypoxic. The Eisenmenger syndrome occurs much later in life in atrial septal defect than in patent ductus arteriosus and ventricular septal defect.

Natural history and prognosis

There is a gradual increase in cyanosis over many years and ultimately heart failure develops. Many patients die suddenly from haemoptysis associated with pulmonary artery thrombosis or dilated angiomatous lesions arising from small pulmonary arteries. Other complications are chest infections, bacterial endocarditis and cerebral abscess. Death usually occurs in the fourth or fifth decade (Wood, 1958).

Clinical picture

In patients who are minimally cyanosed, symptoms are few, and breathlessness and fatigue are noted only on strenuous exertion. Apart from cyanosis and finger clubbing, the signs are those of pulmonary hypertension. The pulse is generally of normal volume, but the jugular venous pulse shows an exaggerated 'a' wave. Increased right ventricular pulsation is palpable at the left sternal border, and closure of the pulmonary valve is palpable. Auscultation reveals a short ejection systolic murmur (due to ejection of blood into the dilated pulmonary artery), often preceded by an ejection click, and a very loud second heart sound in the pulmonary area. Splitting of the second heart sound is close or undetectable when the communication is at ventricular or aortopulmonary level, but may be wide when the communication is at atrial level. There may also be a soft early diastolic murmur in the pulmonary area and at the left sternal border, due to functional pulmonary incompetence. This is rather more common when the underlying defect is a patent ductus arteriosus.

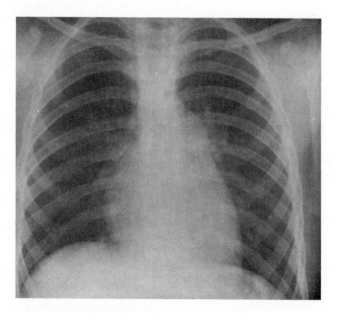

Figure 15.2. Eisenmenger syndrome. Plain radiograph showing normal-sized heart, prominent main pulmonary arteries and peripheral pruning, which is less marked than in *Figure 15.1*

Radiology

The heart shows little or no overall enlargement but the right ventricle is prominent in the lateral view. The main pulmonary artery and its branches are dilated, but the peripheral vessels are small ('pruning' of the pulmonary artery) (*Figure 15.2*). The radiograph may also be helpful in indicating the site of the intracardiac communication. With an atrial septal defect the pulmonary artery and its main branches are usually greatly enlarged; with a ventricular septal defect they are only slightly or moderately so. With a patent ductus arteriosus not only is the main pulmonary artery considerably dilated but the aortic arch may also be dilated.

Electrocardiography

Standard leads usually show strong right axis deviation. The P waves are peaked, indicating right atrial hypertrophy. Moderate or marked right ventricular hypertrophy is indicated by tall R waves in leads V_4R and V_1.

Cardiac catheterization

Some authorities feel that cardiac catheterization is not indicated when the diagnosis of the Eisenmenger syndrome can be made clinically, on the grounds that no treatment can be indicated from the information obtained. Although undoubtedly catheterization is not without risk in the presence of severe pulmonary hypertension, few cardiologists or paediatricians would be happy to watch the gradual downhill course of such patients without knowing for certain that the diagnosis is correct.

The essential findings at catheterization are: identical aortic and pulmonary artery pressures (and identical pressures in the two ventricles) when the communication is at ventricular or aortopulmonary level, no significant left-to-right shunt but a right-to-left shunt at the site of the defect, or defects (occasionally more than one is present).

Since the defect is large the catheter can usually be directed through it. Angiography is certainly contraindicated because it may be followed by a severe rise in pulmonary vascular resistance. When the presence or position of a defect is in doubt, injection of a green dye in different chambers of the heart and recording of dye-dilution curves will demonstrate the site of the right-to-left shunt.

Treatment

Surgical treatment is not possible when there is a right-to-left shunt and there is no known medical treatment which will influence the pulmonary vascular resistance. Anoxia from any cause should be avoided. Chest infections must be treated early and enthusiastically, and care must be taken to avoid anoxia during any anaesthesia. Pregnancy carries a high risk and should be avoided or terminated if it occurs. Oral contraceptives have been reported to cause rapid deterioration. Recently it has been suggested that excessive physical exertion in those patients with few symptoms, may cause rapid deterioration.

BIBLIOGRAPHY AND REFERENCES

Pulmonary hypertension and cor pulmonale
Ainger, L. E. (1968). Large tonsils and adenoids in small children with cor pulmonale. *Br. Heart J.* **30**, 356
Bristow, J. D., Morris, J. F. and Kloster, F. E. (1969). Haemodynamics of cor pulmonale. *Prog. cardiovasc. Dis.* **9**, 239
Goldring, R. M., Fishman, A. P., Turino, G. M., Cohen, H. I., Denning, C. R. and Anderson, D. H. (1964). Pulmonary hypertension and cor pulmonale in cystic fibrosis of the pancreas. *J. Pediat.* **65**, 501
Heath, D. (1971). Dietary pulmonary hypertension. *Br. Heart J.* **33**, 616
Heath, D. and Edwards, J. E. (1958). The pathology of hypertensive pulmonary vascular disease. A description of six grades of structural changes in pulmonary arteries with special reference to congenital cardiac septal defects. *Circulation* **18**, 533
Macartney, F. J., Panday, J. and Scott, O. (1969). Cor pulmonale as a result of chronic naso-pharyngeal obstruction due to hypertrophied tonsils and adenoids. *Archs Dis. Childh.* **44**, 585
Noonan, J. A. (1971). Pulmonary heart disease. *Pediat. Clins N. Am.* **18**, 1255
Penaloza, D., Arias-Stella, J., Sime, F., Recauarreu, S. and Marticorena, E. (1964). The heart and pulmonary circulation in children at high altitudes—physiological, anatomical and clinical observations. *Pediatrics, Springfield* **34**, 568
Rao, B. N. S., Moller, J. and Edwards, J. E. (1969). Primary pulmonary hypertension in a child; response to pharmacologic agents. *Circulation* **40**, 583
Robertson, N. R. C., Hallidie-Smith, K. A. and Davis, J. A. (1967). Severe respiratory distress syndrome mimicking cyanotic heart disease in term babies. *Lancet* **2**, 1108

The Eisenmenger syndrome
Brammell, H. L., Vogel, J. H. K., Prior, R. and Blount, S. G. Jr. (1971). The Eisenmenger syndrome. A clinical and physiologic reappraisal. *Am. J. Cardiol.* **28**, 679
Wood, P. (1958). The Eisenmenger syndrome. *Br. med. J.* **2**, 708, 755
Young, D. and Mark, H. (1971). Fate of the patient with the Eisenmenger syndrome. *Am. J. Cardiol.* **28**, 658

CHAPTER 16

Complications of Congenital Heart Disease

THROMBOSIS AND EMBOLISM

Thrombosis is a common complication of cyanotic congenital heart disease. It is most often seen in the early years of life, particularly when the oxygen saturation of the arterial blood is less than 50 per cent. It is the polycythaemia and high haematocrit which make clotting more likely, rather than the actual haemoglobin content of the blood. Indeed, the cyanotic infant who has an iron deficiency anaemia and normal, or lowered, haemoglobin level but a high haematocrit, is most at risk from thrombosis. Dehydration from any cause such as gastroenteritis or sweating following pyrexia will further aggravate the tendency for thrombosis to occur.

Thrombosis is most serious when it occurs in the cerebral circulation. Its onset is often insidious and in young children the presence of malaise and headache may be overlooked. Vomiting often occurs and there may be visual defects. Often the first realization that something is wrong is the occurrence of monoplegia or hemiplegia. The hemiplegia may improve gradually over a day or two but there is usually some permanent disability, a tragic happening in a child already handicapped by cyanotic congenital heart disease.

Treatment

The condition should be prevented as far as possible. Surgery should be performed whenever practicable to relieve the stimulus for a high haematocrit; iron deficiency anaemia should be corrected. Dehydration should be prevented or treated promptly if it occurs. Anticoagulant therapy has been advocated by some but there is a danger that cerebral infarction will be converted to a cerebral haematoma. Physiotherapy for the affected limbs should be started at once.

DIFFUSE INTRAVASCULAR THROMBOSIS AND CONSUMPTION COAGULOPATHY

Under some circumstances, particularly when dehydration increases the haematocrit and therefore the viscosity of the blood, a few infants and children develop silent intravascular clotting. Blood clotting factors, particularly platelets and prothrombin, are consumed to such an extent that a haemorrhagic state ensues, with haematuria, gastrointestinal bleeding and uncontrollable haemorrhage from surgical wounds. The bleeding and clotting times are prolonged, the platelet count falls to less than $10\,000/mm^3$ and the prothrombin time is greatly prolonged. Heparinization of the patient allows platelets and prothrombin to return to normal, but transfusion of platelets and other clotting factors may be necessary.

SYSTEMIC THROMBOEMBOLISM

The commonest cause of systemic embolism is paradoxical embolism from the systemic veins in patients with cyanotic congenital heart disease. In addition, embolism from the heart itself may occur in bacterial endocarditis, from a left atrial myxoma and from mural thrombi in primary myocardial disease. Any part of the systemic circulation may be affected by thrombosis or embolism but involvement of the cerebral circulation is much the most common. The risks are proportional both to the polycythaemia and to the degree of right-to-left shunting. Embolism is probably much more common than thrombosis *in situ* in the arterial tree but, apart from the more abrupt onset in patients with emboli, the symptoms are similar. Some idea of the degree of risk in cyanotic congenital heart disease is given by the fact that 22 per cent of children with transposition in one series developed cerebral thromboembolism whilst waiting an average of two years for definitive surgery (Parsons and co-workers, 1971).

CORTICAL THROMBOPHLEBITIS

Primary thrombophlebitis of cerebral veins accounts for a small percentage of patients with cerebral thombosis. It may be precipitated by infections or follow immunization procedures. Headache and vomiting occur initially and weakness or hemiplegia with drowsiness follow.

MESENTERIC ARTERY EMBOLISM

Mesenteric artery embolism is rare in infancy and childhood. Sudden and severe abdominal pain is usually the first symptom and intestinal ileus develops quickly. There may be melaena or frank blood passed per rectum. Treatment is difficult, but a conservative approach with intravenous replacement and anticoagulants is the first choice; resection of bowel (which needs to be extensive) is reserved for patients with perforation or with no evidence of recovery after several days. With or without resection, some degree of malabsorption is common in survivors.

MESENTERIC VENOUS THROMBOSIS

The onset of mesenteric venous thrombosis is less acute and pain is less severe but, clinically, differentiation from mesenteric arterial embolism is difficult. Conservative treatment usually results in eventual recovery.

RENAL EMBOLISM

Pain in the loin and haematuria are the usual symptoms in large renal emboli, but microscopic haematuria and hypertension may occur with repeated emboli.

RENAL VEIN THROMBOSIS

Renal vein thrombosis causes albuminuria and a nephrotic picture. The onset is insidious and with pre-existing heart failure diagnosis may be difficult. Anticoagulant therapy is logical.

CEREBRAL ABSCESS

Cerebral abscess is rare in children under 2 years of age (unlike cerebral thrombosis). Strangely enough, it is rarely associated with bacterial endocarditis even though there is a bacteraemia. Infection probably occurs in an area where there has been some previous local damage following thrombosis.

The symptoms are of malaise, fever and loss of appetite followed by headache and vomiting. There may be convulsions and visual defects. Usually pyrexia develops and headache persists. Papilloedema may be present. Hemiplegia or monoplegia may follow.

An electroencephalogram may help by localizing the lesion but if the diagnosis is still in doubt the patient should be referred to a neurologist for brain scan. The development of the CT scan has enabled abscess to be differentiated from infarct with a high degree of accuracy, and it should always be carried out if there is any doubt. Brain abscess is a treatable condition and delay in referral to a neurologist should be avoided. The abscess may rupture and cause meningitis if treatment is delayed.

Treatment

Small abscesses respond well to treatment with antibiotics but larger ones may need surgical drainage. The best results are obtained when diagnosis is made early and treatment given promptly, but the overall mortality rate is high—it was 40 per cent in patients with tetralogy of Fallot in Taussig's (1971) series.

INFECTIVE ENDOCARDITIS

When a child with congenital heart disease has a septicaemia from any cause, there is always a possibility that the endocardium will become infected. The lesions most likely to develop endocarditis are ventricular septal defect, patent ductus arteriosus, coarctation of the aorta and lesions of the mitral and aortic valves—particularly when the last-named has a bicuspid valve. Isolated pulmonary stenosis is relatively immune. Small defects are more likely to develop endocarditis than large ones. It never occurs in ostium secundum atrial septal defects and when it occurs in ostium primum defects, it is the abnormal cleft mitral valve which is affected and not the atrial septal defect. The infection often develops in areas where there has been damage by a jet of blood impinging on the endocardium, so that it occurs on the right ventricular wall in ventricular septal defects and in the pulmonary artery opposite a patent ductus arteriosus. Taussig (1971) found a remarkably high incidence of subacute bacterial endocarditis (14.3 per cent) in the longterm follow-up of 779 patients with tetralogy of Fallot. Gersony and Hayes (1977) in a series of 2420 patients with congenital heart disease found an incidence of 1.5 per thousand patient years for VSD, 1.8 for aortic stenosis and only 0.2 for pulmonary stenosis.

Aetiology

The disease can occur at any age but is rare below the age of 2 years. The source of infection is the mouth in about one-eighth of the cases, but the nose and tonsils may also be the site of entry.

Organisms

Streptococcus viridans is the commonest causative organism. Staphylococci are not common but are found particuarly after cardiac surgery when they may be penicillin-resistant strains. The pneumococcus, meningococcus, proteus, pyocyaneus, *Haemophilus influenzae* and *Brucella abortus* have all been reported. Rarely, *Rickettsia burneti* (Q fever) and fungi such as candida, monilia or aspergillus are the cause.

Clinical presentation

Clinical presentation may be acute or subacute in onset but the symptoms and signs are essentially the same. Staphylococcal infections tend to give an acute onset but nowadays the clinical picture is often not the classic one because the patient has already been given antibiotics before referral to hospital. The initial signs are those associated with the septicaemia. There is fever, malaise, lassitude, loss of appetite and pallor due to anaemia. Clubbing of the fingers and toes may develop, the spleen is enlarged and in some patients heart failure occurs.

Emboli from the site of the endocarditis cause splinter haemorrhages, haematuria and cerebral incidents with hemiplegia or meningitis. Osler's nodes are uncommon in childhood. When the lesion is on the right side of the heart, as in pulmonary stenosis and ventricular septal defect, embolization occurs to the lungs. This may cause pleuritic pain and a cough.

If the child has been seen prior to the endocarditis, there may be a change in the cardiac signs due to involvement of a valve cusp, as for example when aortic regurgitation develops on a bicuspid aortic valve.

Diagnosis

Infective endocarditis must always be suspected when there is unexplained fever in a child with congenital heart disease. The diagnosis becomes even more likely when there is an enlarged spleen, heart failure or evidence of embolization. The following tests should be carried out immediately.

(1) Blood cultures: Four cultures should be taken in the first 24 hours, then twice in the next 24 hours – a total of six cultures.

(2) Blood count: This usually shows a polymorphonuclear leuco-cytosis but occasionally there is neutropenia. Anaemia may be severe. Erythrocyte sedimentation rate is increased as a rule but may occasionally be normal.

(3) Urine: Microscopic examination must be carried out to look for red cells. If there is renal infection, albuminuria, casts and haematuria are found.

(4) Chest radiograph: This may show areas of pulmonary infarction.

(5) Four-hourly temperature recordings.

Ideally, it is best to know the organism involved and its sensitivity to antibiotics before beginning treatment, but positive blood cultures are not always obtained, particularly if antibiotics have been given before admission to hospital. A firm diagnosis can usually be made before the results of blood culture are available and it is often dangerous to wait for the results of these while the patient deteriorates and cardiac damage progresses. It is no light matter to embark on a six-week course of antibiotic therapy in a child, but it is preferable to withholding treatment while the child develops a cerebral embolus! The majority of patients with endocarditis can be cured today but good results depend on early diagnosis and early treatment. The motto must always be 'DO NOT DELAY'.

Treatment

Streptococcal infections

Bactericidal drugs must be used. Penicillin is bactericidal and is thought to penetrate the fibrin matrix around vegetations.

An intravenous drip of 5% dextrose should be set up and the penicillin given into this line.

6–10 million units/day in 6 divided doses is advised.

If the infection is severe up to

20 million units/day can be given and gentamycin added in a dose of 5 mg/kg per day 8-hourly intravenously.

Treatment should be continued for at least 6 weeks and blood cultures repeated 1 week after all treatment has been stopped.

Staphylococcal infections

The organisms are frequently penicillin-resistant and other drugs have to be used but they must be bactericidal. The combination of cloxacillin and gentamycin intraveneously is recommended as they act synergistically

Cloxacillin 250 mg/kg per day i.v. in 6 divided doses.
Gentamycin 5 mg/kg i.v. 8-hourly

If the organism is found, its sensitivity must be assessed and the serum level necessary to achieve suppression of growth determined. Blood must be taken from the patient to ensure that effective bacteriocidal concentrations are being achieved. Samples should be taken immediately before an intravenous dose is given and $\frac{1}{2}$–1 hour after the dose. There is no place for bacteriostatic drugs in the treatment of endocarditis—they must be *bactericidal*. High blood levels are necessary initially and intravenous therapy is first given. The choice of drugs given depends on the organism and its sensitivity. If the infection is severe it is always wise to give *two* antibiotics.

The oral route is *not* advised as there is such a variability of absorption.

Treatment of bacterial endocarditis due to *Streptococcus faecalis, Staphylococcus albus* and similar organisms is much less satisfactory (*S. albus* is particularly a problem following intracardiac surgery). No fixed programme is possible, but the principle is to use a 6-week course of the bactericidal antibiotic to which the organism is most sensitive *in vitro*. A useful test is to check the *in vitro* effect of the patient's serum during therapy on the organism which has been cultured. An eightfold dilution of serum should kill the organism.

During the course of therapy, treatment for heart failure may be necessary. Heart failure occurs because of either valve damage or the embolic myocarditis which occurs in advanced cases. In rare instances surgery may be required for mycotic aneurysms or for major emboli.

Usually the pyrexia ceases within a day or two of starting treatment. The teeth should be examined by a dentist, and radiographically. If septic foci are found these should be eliminated either during or after the course of penicillin under the cover of a different antibiotic (since mouth organisms will have become penicillin-resistant). A period of 7–10 days of observation should follow the course of treatment and then a further series of three blood cultures should be taken. If the patient remains afebrile 2 weeks after antibiotics have finished he can be sent home, but the parents should record his temperature twice daily for a further 2 weeks.

Patients who have had an attack of bacterial endocarditis are much more likely to have another, and the most stringent precautions are necessary. An attack of bacterial endocarditis may be an indication to close a ventricular septal defect which would not otherwise have required closure.

Prognosis

The cure rate for subacute bacterial endocarditis due to *Streptococcus viridans* and treated effectively soon after symptoms occur is near to 100 per cent. The success rate falls off sharply when there is another causative organism, when there is delay in diagnosis and when ineffective antibiotic treatment has been given before the diagnosis has been established. It is also lower when prosthetic materials have previously been used in an open-heart operation.

Prophylaxis

Prophylaxis is no longer necessary after successful surgery for the following conditions.

    patent ductus arteriosus
    atrial septal defect
    ventricular septal defect.
    pulmonary stenosis

It must however be given after surgery for:

    tetralogy of Fallot
    aortic stenosis
    transposition of the great arteries
    Blalock and Waterston's shunts
    coarctation of aorta
    ostium primum atrial septal defect
    any operation involving valve replacement or insertion of conduit.

It is necessary for all other congenital heart lesions which have not had operations except ostium secundum atrial septal defect.

Predisposing factors

In children, dental treatment, tonsillectomy and adenoidectomy are the commonest predisposing factors. Dental treatment is less commonly implicated in children than in adults, presumably because of a lower incidence of periodontal disease. Over a 25 year period at the Hospital for Sick Children, Toronto, there were 82 cases of endocarditis but only 4 of them followed dental extraction (Keith *et al.*, 1978). There is no evidence that the shedding of deciduous teeth is associated with bacteraemia, but bacteraemia may occur after any dental procedure.

Manipulative procedures or operations on the respiratory, genito-urinary and gastrointestinal tracts may be implicated. The present vogue for ear-piercing in children should be avoided in children at risk. Sometimes the predisposing factor is never found.

Basis for prophylaxis

Surprisingly little scientific work exists on the best means of preventing infective endocarditis. The regimes advised previously have been based on the work of Durack and Petersdorf (1973) in rabbits. They showed that bactericidal drugs must be used and that there should be adequate serum levels of antibiotic both at the time of the bacteraemia and for a critical period of 6–9 hours afterwards when surviving bacteria might settle on the damaged heart and multiply. Their experiments involved producing vegetations on aortic valves by inserting catheters and introducing large doses of streptococci intravenously. Treatment was aimed at sterilizing the blood over 24 hours. In practice this may be more difficult than eliminating the transient bacteraemia which occurs after dental treatment in man, so dosage regimes based on Durack's work are likely to give a wide margin of safety.

Streptococcus viridans is the commonest organism entering the bloodstream from the mouth and this and other organisms from the upper respiratory tract are usually penicillin-sensitive. In the recent past most paediatricians have followed the recommendations of the American Heart Association (1977) and have given an oral regime using phenoxymethylpenicillin (penicillin V) or a combined paren-teral and oral schedule. Unfortunately the absorption of oral penicillin V is unpredictable so an injection regime is preferable. Since most dentists do not give intramuscular injections and an injection is difficult to organize at the appropriate time, most children are given the oral regime despite doubt about its adequacy.

Shanson *et al.* (1978) have recently shown that in adults amoxycillin gives a higher and more sustained serum level than penicillin V and that a 3g oral dose of amoxycillin one hour before dental treatment gives serum concentrations well above the minimal bactericidal levels for at least 10 hours—thus covering the critical period after treatment (Shanson *et al.*, 1980). Studies on oral amoxycillin in children have confirmed the same satisfactory absorption as in adults (Deasy and Bourke, 1974).

Present recommendations

All children at risk should have a high standard of oral hygiene and regular dental supervision.

Oral amoxycillin using half the adult dose for children under ten years may be used for prophylaxis outside hospital when dental treatment is carried out without anaesthesia. If anaesthesia is required the patient should be referred to hospital and amoxycillin given parenterally.

All children at risk should be given a card to show to any doctor or dentist. A suitable format is:

'This child has a heart lesion and it is essential that he/she has prophylactic therapy against infective endocarditis before dental treatment, removal of tonsils or adenoids, or any procedure involving the upper respiratory tract. Outside hospital when anaesthesia is not required the following regime is recommended. Amoxycillin 3g orally one hour before treatment. The dose is halved for children under 10 years.

If an anaesthetic is required the patient should be referred to hospital and amoxycillin given by i.m. injection.

If the patient is sensitive to penicillin, erythromycin 1g orally one hour before treatment is advised, halving the dose for children under 10 years.'

In gastrointestinal and genito-urinary tract surgery, enterococci are frequently responsible for endocarditis and prophylactic therapy should be aimed at these organisms. The patient is usually in hospital and a combination of gentamicin 2 mg/kg i.m. and ampicillin 1g i.m. (half dose under 10 years) is a suitable combination.

Patients with prosthetic heart valves have a particularly high risk of developing endocarditis and the organism may have been acquired in hospital. There is less agreement about the best prophylaxis in this group (fortunately small in children) and they should be under observation in hospital. Ampicillin 1g i.m. and cloxacillin 1g i.m. (half dose for children under 10 years) before treatment and repeated 8 hourly for 2 doses should suffice.

ABNORMALITIES OF ACID–BASE BALANCE

The acid–base status of the blood and extracellular fluid are closely linked. Hydrogen ions diffuse freely into and out of the cells so that intra- and extracellular pH are similar, but the buffering systems inside and outside the cells are different. There are three variables: the carbon dioxide tension, pH and buffer concentrations. (In the blood, bicarbonate and proteins each normally make up about a half of the buffering capacity.) If any two of the variables are known it is possible to estimate the other. In practice one of two methods is used to define the acid–base state. In the first the pH and P_{CO_2} are measured and the bicarbonate, total buffer base and base deficit or excess are calculated, or read off a nomogram. In the second, the Astrup method, the pH of the blood is measured directly and the pH is also determined after equilibration with two gases of known P_{CO_2}. From this the P_{CO_2}, total buffer base and standard bicarbonate are estimated from the Siggaard-Andersen nomogram. Results are most reliable when arterial blood is used, but by warming the foot to ensure rapid circulation, 'arterialized' capillary blood can be obtained by heel puncture which has a pH and P_{CO_2} very similar to those of arterial blood.

Metabolic acidosis

Tissue oxygenation may be impaired either by a low arterial oxygen saturation, as in cyanotic congenital heart disease, or by a reduced blood flow, as occurs with myocardial failure or with obstruction to the left heart (aortic atresia). Anaerobic metabolism results in the accumulation of lactic acid in the tissues. To some extent the kindneys compensate by excreting hydrogen ions, but, particularly in the first few weeks of life when tubular function is poor, this is usually insufficient compensation and a progressive metabolic acidosis develops. This can be demonstrated by measuring the pH and bicarbonate of the blood. The pH may fall below 7.0 and the bicarbonate below 10 mmol/litre. A pH below 7.20 indicates a poor prognosis unless a palliative operation is performed.

The depressant effect of acidaemia on the myocardium is at first masked by stimulation of the sympathoadrenal system with release of catecholamines and these increase the contractile force of the ventricle. Finally, however, cardiovascular failure occurs in the presence of high catecholamines. The ventricular fibrillation threshold decreases in the presence of acidaemia.

The reduction in pH causes myocardial and central nervous system depression. The former is indicated by poor peripheral pulses and cold, blotchy extremities with poor return of capillary filling after pressure. Central nervous system depression manifests itself by absent or reduced spontaneous movements and diminished reflexes. Below a pH of 7.20 the respiratory centre is depressed, so that a respiratory element is added to the acidosis and respiratory effort becomes reduced and finally ceases.

Metabolic acidosis can be corrected temporarily by giving sodium bicarbonate. In mild cases it can be given orally but if the pH is below 7.2 intravenous therapy is indicated. Sodium bicarbonate is a hyperosmolar solution and its administration in the acidotic and hypoxic newborn infant will result in profound vasodilatation and pooling of blood in the skeletal muscle causing severe hypotension. A solution containing 5 mmol/10 ml (0.42 g/10 ml) of sodium bicarbonate should be used in the newborn and 50 mmol/50 ml (4.2 g/50 ml) in older children. 2 mmol/kg bodyweight should be given slowly and the pH measured again. Excessive sodium bicarbonate administration will produce hypernatraemia and intraventricular cerebral haemorrhage in the sick newborn. The calcium should be measured and any associated hypocalcaemia treated with calcium gluconate. Dextrose 5% should be given if there is hypoglycaemia.

The child's general condition will improve following correction of the acidosis but the acidosis recurs unless measures are taken to correct the underlying situation. Correction of the acidosis is only a means of buying time to allow cardiac catheterization or operation to take place.

Metabolic alkalosis

This rarely occurs after prolonged diuretic therapy. It may also be iatrogenic. It can be corrected by giving ammonium chloride orally.

Respiratory acidosis

Infants with reduced lung compliance due to high pulmonary blood flow or pulmonary venous congestion frequently have a mild or moderate respiratory acidosis, the P_{CO_2} rising as high as 70 mmHg. Usually there is nearly complete renal compensation with increased bicarbonate production and hydrogen ion excretion, so that the pH does not usually fall much below 7.32. Where there is superadded infection or pulmonary oedema the P_{CO_2} may rise much higher, sometimes over 100 mmHg, and, in an attempt to compensate, the bicarbonate may be increased to as high as 70 mmol/litre, with a corresponding reduction in chloride. (It should be noted that if the pH is not measured this is frequently reported erroneously as a metabolic alkalosis.) A P_{CO_2} over 80 mmHg which is not corrected promptly by diuretics in the case of pulmonary oedema or by suction and antibiotics in the case of infection is an indication for artificial ventilation pending operative intervention.

Respiratory alkalosis

A respiratory alkalosis of any degree rarely occurs naturally but may be produced by overenthusiastic artificial ventilation. The high pH may produce tetany of fits, and the kidneys excrete potassium ions in preference to hydrogen ions so that hypokalaemia results. The level of ventilation must be reduced or a 'dead space' added.

Cardiac arrest

Acid–base abnormalities must be corrected after an episode of acute cardiorespiratory failure. The administration of sodium bicarbonate is the same as described under metabolic acidosis.

BIBLIOGRAPHY AND REFERENCES

Thrombosis and embolism
Johnson, C. A., Abilgaard, C. F. and Schulman, I. (1968). Absence of coagulation abnormalities in children with cyanotic congenital heart disease. *Lancet* **2**, 660
Parsons, C. G., Astley, R., Burrows, F. G. O. and Singh, S. P. (1971) Transposition of great arteries. A study of 65 infants followed for 1 to 4 years after balloon septostomy. *Br. Heart J.* **33**, 725
Paul, M. H., Cirrimbhoy, Z., Miller, R. A. and Schulman, I. (1961). Thrombocytopenia in cyanotic congenital heart disease. *Circulation* **24**, 1013
Somerville, J., McDonald, L. and Edgill, M. (1965). Post-operative haemorrhage and related abnormalities of blood coagulation in cyanotic congenital heart disease. *Br. Heart J.* **27**, 440
Taussig, H. B. (1971). Long-term results of the Blalock–Taussig operation.' *Johns Hopkins med. J.* **129**, 243

Infective endocarditis
American Heart Association Committee Report. (1977). *Circulation* **56**, 139A
Barritt, D. W. and Gillespie, W. A. (1960). Subacute bacterial endocarditis. *Br. med. J.* **1**, 1235
Beeson, P. B. and Ridley, M. (Eds.) (1969). *Bacterial Endocarditis.* A symposium held at the Royal College of Physicians. London: Beecham Research Laboratories
Deasy, P. F. and Bourke, M. (1974). Trial of amoxycillin in paediatrics. *J. Irish med. Ass.* **67**, 463
Durack, D. T. and Petersdorf, R. G. (1973). Chemotherapy of experimental streptococcal endocarditis. 1. comparison of commonly recommended prophylactic regimes. *J. clin. Invest.* **52**, 592
Gersony, W. M. and Hayes, C. J. (1977). Bacterial endocarditis in patients with pulmonary stenosis, aortic stenosis and ventricular septal defect. *Circulation* **56**, Suppl. 1–84
Jawetze, E. (1962). Assay of antibacterial activity in serum. *Am. J. Dis. Child.* **103**, 81
Jordan, S. C. (1979). Dental treatment of children with heart disease. *Proc. Br. Paedodontic Soc.* **9**, 13
Keith, J. D., Rowe, R. D. and Vlad, P. (1978). *Heart Disease in Infancy and Childhood.* Third Edition. p. 239. New York: Macmillan

Report from the Joint Study on the Natural History of Congenital Heart Defects. (1977) *Circulation* **56**, 2, Supplement (1)

Shanson, D. C., Cannon, P. and Wilks, M. (1978). Amoxycillin compared with Penicillin V for prophylaxis of dental bacteraemia. *J. antimicrob. Chemother.* **4**, 43

Shanson, D. C., Ashford, R. F. U. and Singh, J. (1980). High-dose oral amoxycillin for preventing endocarditis. *Br. med. J.* **1**, 446

Abnormalities of acid–base balance

Kamath, V. R. and Jones, R. S. (1966). Acid–base abnormalities in infants with congenital heart disease. *Br. med. J.* **2**, 434

Sanyal, S. K., Ghosh, K., Bigram, R., Sarkar, D. and Madhavan, S. (1971). The biochemical aspects of congestive heart failure in children. *J. Pediat.* **79**, 250

Siggaard-Andersen, O. (1962). The pH–log P_{CO_2} blood acid–base nomogram revised. *Scand. J. clin. Lab. Invest.* **14**, 598

CHAPTER 17

Disorders of Cardiac Rhythm

Many disturbances of cardiac rhythm are of no functional significance but are problems in diagnosis when they are detected on
routine examination or when an electrocardiogram is performed for
some other reason. Serious cardiac dysrhythmias make up about 2
per cent of paediatric cardiological problems but the presentation is
often obscure, and in many cases the true diagnosis can only be
made by careful history taking, since physical examination and
special investigations may all be completely normal except during
the paroxysmal dysrhythmia. A typical case is a 7-year-old boy with
a long history of episodes of abdominal pain and vomiting diagnosed
after various investigations as psychosomatic. A prolonged attack
led to his admission as 'acute appendicitis' when he was found to
have tachycardia of 280/minute and the abdominal pain was
localized to the enlarged tender liver. His mother's first recorded
description of the attacks included the sentence: 'The attacks upset
him so much that I can see his heart beating nineteen to the dozen
through his clothes'.

In the majority of children we see with arrhythmias the heart is
structurally normal and the ECG may be normal or show some
abnormality of conduction, e.g. Wolff–Parkinson–White syndrome.
Arrhythmias may also occur in association with congenital heart
disease and the commonest are:—

    Atrioventricular discordance (L-transposition)
    Ebstein's anomaly of the tricuspid valve
    Cardiomyopathy
    Mitral valve prolapse.

Nowadays an increasing number of arrhythmias are seen after

surgery, particularly after Mustard's operation for transposition of the great arteries and after repair of tetralogy of Fallot. They may also be drug induced.

NORMAL ANATOMY AND PHYSIOLOGY OF THE CONDUCTING SYSTEM

The *sinoatrial node* lies at the junction of the superior vena cava and right atrium and consists of a small crescentic mass of specially differentiated cells which possess an enhanced power of rhythmic depolarization at a rate of up to 200/minute. The rate is influenced by the vagus (cardio-inhibiting) and sympathetic (cardio-stimulating) nerves. The impulse generated in the sinoatrial node spreads throughout both atria, causing depolarization and contraction of atrial muscle. Although there are 'preferential pathways' through the atria there is no specialized conducting tissue between the sinoatrial node and the *atrioventricular node*, which lies in the lower part of the right atrium, close to the tricuspid valve and coronary sinus. The atrioventricular node is histologically similar to the sinoatrial node but has two parts, the upper portion being functionally concerned with picking up the atrial depolarization and the lower portion in passing it on to the *atrioventricular bundle*, which passes through the fibrous ring separating the atrial and ventricular muscle. It then travels for a short distance in the membranous portion of the interventricular septum before dividing into right and left branches. Due to the presence of the fibrous atrioventricular ring, the atrioventricular bundle (bundle of His) is normally the *only path* by which impulses can pass between the atria and ventricles. The *right bundle branch* travels as a discrete bundle on the right ventricular aspect of the interventricular septum to the apex of the right ventricle where it divides into numerous small branches. The *left bundle branch* is a wide sheet of fibres which runs down the left ventricular aspect of the interventricular septum for a short distance before dividing into three sub-branches, the septal, anterior and inferior branches.

The atrioventricular node (and hence the ventricles) are normally controlled by the rate of the sinoatrial node; however, if the sinoatrial node ceases to function or becomes excessively slow, the intrinsic rhythmicity of the atrioventricular node takes over, but at a slower rate (normally about 50–60/minute in older children but as fast as 100/minute in infants). The rate is under the control of the vagus and sympathetic nerves but to a lesser extent than the sinoatrial node. If the atrioventricular node or bundle cease to conduct impulses the ventricles will produce their own idioventricular rate, usually about 30–50/minute. It is thought that this impulse is generated in the conducting tissue of the ventricles rather than in the ventricular muscle.

Investigation of arrhythmias

In the past decade new techniques have become available to investigate arrhythmias. One is continuous ambulatory 24-hour monitoring of the electrocardiogram and the other is intracardiac electrocardiograms with programmed intracardiac stimulation. Exercising testing is also of value.

All these tests are not always required but their use has increased our knowledge of arrhythmias and helped us to treat them, when necessary, in the best possible way.

Twenty-four-hour continuous ECG monitoring

In the past, diagnosis of arrhythmias in childhood was made from the resting ECG taken for short periods and often depended on chance recordings. Since 24-hour ECG monitoring on magnetic tapes became available, the type, frequency and duration of any arrhythmias can usually be determined, even in newborn infants. One chest electrode is placed on the upper part of the sternum and the other in the position of chest lead V4. They are fixed to the skin without any air trap, taped down and connected to a battery-operated miniature analogue tape recorder. The cassette is housed in a leather bag worn round the waist, or in babies it can lie on the mattress. The children or their parents keep a diary of their activities and if they have any unusual symptoms an 'alarm' button is pressed which marks the tape so that the record at that time can be correlated with the symptoms. For analysis an instrument is used which automatically detects changes in heart rate and rhythm from preset R.R. intervals. Printouts are made of any abnormalities and at 4-hourly intervals throughout the trace for 10-second periods even when no abnormalities are detected. The analyser is expensive but is usually available in special centres—the magnetic tapes can easily be sent to that centre for analysis. One of the problems of using these tapes is that they have been used to study the *abnormal* before the 24-hour records in *normal* healthy children have been analysed. Scott, Williams and Fiddler (1980) however have already studied 131 boys between the ages of 10 and 13 years. They showed that:

1. The maximal heart rates during the day ranged from 100 to 200 beats/minute and minimal rates from 45 to 80.
2. During sleep the maximal rates were 60–110 beats/minute and the minimal rates 30–70 beats/minute.
3. P waves changed in form during sleep in 15 per cent and in 5 per cent when awake. In 13 per cent the abnormal 'P' waves were associated with junctional rhythm.
4. First degree heart block occurred in 8 per cent.
5. Wenckebach phenomenon occurred in 10 per cent mostly at night when it was associated with slow heart rates.
6. Premature ventricular beats were always single and occurred in 26 per cent, mostly when awake but occasionally during sleep and during exercise. The number of premature beats was not greater than 4 in 24 hours except in two boys, one of whom had 35 premature beats and periods of coupling lasting for 9 seconds. The other had 27 premature beats in 24 hours.
7. Atrial premature beats occurred in 13 per cent; they were always single and occurred during sleep and when awake. They were never more frequent than 2 in 24 hours except in one boy who had two half-hour periods of coupling during sleep.
8. Complete sinoatrial block was seen in 8 per cent and never lasted for more than one cycle.

Intracardiac electrophysiology

This is an invasive study in which multipolar electrode catheters are passed into the heart usually via the femoral vein. A detailed sequence of cardiac activation can be made during sinus rhythm, paced atrial and ventricular rhythms or abnormal rhythms. It can be used to localize sites of conduction delay and block. A valuable application is to delineate tachycardia circuits. Paroxysmal atrial tachycardia can be induced and the effect of various drugs studied. Therapeutically it can be of great importance to know the exact mechanism underlying the tachycardia. The study can be done in infancy and childhood but is reserved for patients whose abnormal rhythm does not respond to standard methods of treatment.

Exercise testing

An ECG can be recorded after various measured amounts of exercise and the effect of exercise evaluated. Sometimes ectopic beats will disappear but sometimes exercise will induce some arrhythmia or aberrant conduction.

SINUS TACHYCARDIA

Infants and children have very variable pulse rates and under certain circumstances the sinoatrial node can produce a rate as high as 200/minute. Such conditions include physical exercise, anxiety and pyrexia and when the sinoatrial node is freed from the inhibitory influence of the vagus by atropine. Under these circumstances the condition is harmless and no treatment is needed. Rarely, excess adrenaline secretion in thyrotoxicosis or from phaeochromocytoma may produce a prolonged tachycardia and can then be treated with beta-adrenergic blocking drugs such as propranolol, until the underlying condition can be treated. Sinus tachycardia can be differentiated from paroxysmal supraventricular tachycardia by the fact that in the former the rate varies from minute to minute and can be slowed gradually by carotid sinus pressure or, if this fails, by intravenous Tensilon.

SINUS ARRHYTHMIA

Variation in sinus rate is usual in children and normally is related to respiration, the rate increasing on inspiration and slowing on expiration. (This variation is usually absent in patients with atrial septal defects.) Occasionally the variation is so great as to simulate intermittent atrioventricular block, but the relationship to respiration nearly always allows the distinction to be made clinically.

Sinus bradycardia

A slow rate is usual in athletic children and adolescents and is not associated with any symptoms and requires no treatment. If a child has attacks of loss of consciousness associated with bradycardia he should be investigated further (*see* Sinus node dysfunction, p. 304).

ATRIAL ARRHYTHMIAS

Atrial ectopic beats are not infrequently seen in newborn infants. They are usually not associated with symptoms and do not require treatment. Twenty-four-hour tapes can be used to ensure that there are no prolonged episodes of tachycardia. They are entirely benign.

PAROXYSMAL SUPRAVENTRICULAR TACHYCARDIA

This is the commonest arrhythmia in infancy and childhood. Approximately 70–80 per cent of patients subject to paroxysmal supraventricular tachycardia have normal hearts, the remainder have atrial septal defects, Ebstein's anomaly, mitral prolapse or disease of the cardiac muscle. Occasionally paroxysmal atrial tachycardia occurs *in utero* and causes immediate problems at birth. Radford *et al* (1976) reviewed 10 cases and concluded that cardioversion should be used promptly in severely ill patients or if they do not respond to digoxin. Fetal electrocardiography will also be of value in such cases. In those cases where the condition is diagnosed well before term digitalization of the mother has resulted in termination of the arrhythmia or slowing of the ventricular rate.

Pathophysiology

The majority of tachycardias in childhood are now thought to be due to re-entry tachycardias; the remainder are due to enhanced atrial or A-V nodal automaticity.

Four abnormal pathways have been described:

1. Wolff–Parkinson–White syndrome (WPW) in which the accessory pathway goes from the left atrium to the left ventricle (Type A) or in which the accessory pathway is from the right atrium to right ventricle (Type B). When the accessory pathways are being used, the ECG shows a very short P–R interval followed by a delta wave. The appearances in Type A may be mistaken for right bundle branch block and Type B mistaken for left bundle branch block (*Figure 17.3*). The conduction by the accessory route may be intermittent and at times the ECG is normal. When conduction occurs in a retrograde manner in the accessory pathway there is re-entry into the chamber of origin, a circus movement is set up and tachycardia results.
2. Lown–Ganong–Levine syndrome in which the accessory pathway bypasses the A–V node but the ventricular excitation is normal. The P–R interval is short on the ECG but there is no delta wave.
3. A type in which fibres bypass the lower part of the His bundle and enter the ventricular septum directly. This results in early and abnormal sequence of ventricular depolarization producing a delta wave, but the P–R interval is normal.
4. Intra A–V nodal pathway. The resting ECG is normal.

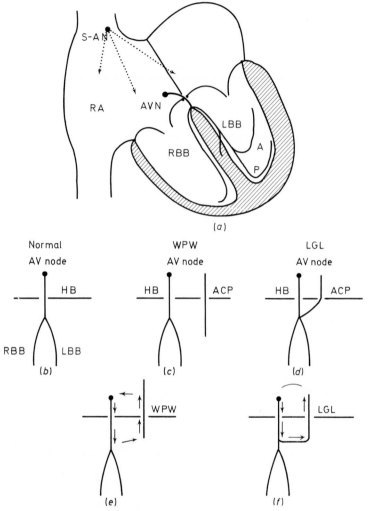

Figure 17.1. Normal conducting system of the heart (*a* and *b*) and the
genesis of atrial tachycardia. (*c*) In the Wolff–Parkinson–White
syndrome (WPW), in addition to the normal His bundle (HB) there is
an accessory conducting pathway (ACP) from the atria to the ventricles.
(*d*) In the Lown–Ganong–Levine syndrome (LGL) the accessory
conducting pathway joins the His bundle. (*e* and *f*) In either case a
circus movement, reactivating the atrioventricular node is set up by
retrograde conduction in the accessory pathway. S-A N: sinoatrial
node; RA: right atrium; AVN: atrioventricular node; RBB and LBB:
right and left bundle branches; A and P: anterior and posterior
divisions of the left bundle

Clinical presentation

Paroxysms tend to occur repeatedly over several months and then frequently subside spontaneously. It is not uncommon for attacks to occur in infancy and then stop, only to recur in teenage or adult life. In infancy, brief attacks are often detected because of pallor and rapid breathing ('white attacks') or they may produce vomiting. More prolonged attacks cause cardiac failure with cough and dyspnoea due to left heart failure, and vomiting and abdominal pain due to hepatic engorgement. Older children usually, but not invariably, complain of rapid heart beating and careful questioning reveals information that attacks start suddenly: 'My heart gives a sudden thump and off it goes'. The termination may be equally sudden, but since a sinus tachycardia may persist afterwards it is not always quite as abrupt subjectively. With rapid rates there is usually faintness on standing up, breathlessness and infrequently central chest pain. Occasionally, attacks may cause sudden loss of consciousness or a major fit due to cerebral anoxia. Polyuria often occurs following an attack and is an important diagnostic pointer.

Physical signs

During an attack the patient is pale, the pulse small in volume as well as rapid. The heart rate is absolutely regular, except when there is a changing degree of block, and frequently as high as 280/minute. If an attack at this high rate has lasted more than 20–30 minutes there will be evidence of excess catecholamine production (sweating and coldness of extremities) and the liver is enlarged.

Examination between attacks is completely normal unless there is underlying heart disease, but clinical examination needs to be careful in order to detect associated abnormalities such as Ebstein's anomaly or atrial septal defect.

Investigation

Chest radiographs may show slight or moderate cardiac enlargement and evidence of pulmonary oedema in or following a prolonged attack.

The electrocardiogram between attacks is normal (except in patients with underlying heart disease or with the Wolff–Parkinson–White syndrome, described on p. 298). Twenty four hour ECG tapes may show bursts of supraventricular tachycardia. Following attacks the T waves may be inverted and ST segments depressed for up to 24 hours. During attacks the electrocardiogram is characteristic and the following points are seen.

1. When P waves can be distinguished the atrial rate is completely regular at 240–300/minute (often slower in older children).
2. When there is 1:1 atrioventricular conduction, the ventricular rate is also completely regular and each QRS complex has the same temporal relationship to the preceding P wave—the P–R interval is constant. When there is 2:1 or a higher degree of block the relationship of QRS to the preceding P wave is also constant (*Figure 17.2*).
3. The QRS complexes always have an initial rapid component. They may be identical with the patient's normal QRS complexes but occasionally there is slurring of the terminal portion due to interventricular conduction delay.
4. Carotid sinus pressure may have no effect on the rate or produces a higher degree of block or causes return to sinus rhythm. A gradual slowing does not occur.

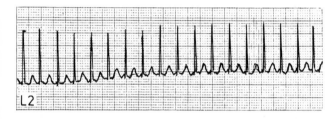

Figure 17.2. Supraventricular tachycardia

Treatment

Brief attacks with few or no symptoms require no treatment. A few patients are able to abort attacks by various manoeuvres which induce vagal stimulation, eyeball pressure, gagging, or the Valsalva manoeuvre. Carotid sinus massage will only occasionally cause reversion in a prolonged attack. Most older children find attacks revert spontaneously if they lie down for an hour or two.

Patients admitted to hospital in a prolonged attack can be treated either by electroversion or by drugs. Electroversion requires a synchronized 'defibrillator' (that is, one which can be set to deliver the direct current shock synchronous with the QRS complex to avoid the dangers of producing ventricular fibrillation) and can be performed under general anaesthesia or under sedation with intravenous diazepam. Usually sinus rhythm can be restored with a single shock varying from 5 joules (J) in an infant to 50 J in an adolescent (roughly 1J/kg). The method has the advantage of rapidity and a limited period of monitoring and is virtually always successful, although relapse may occur. Its disadvantages are the requirements for specialized equipment and experience, and for anaesthesia.

Drugs

Drug treatment to terminate an attack should always be given under continuous ECG monitoring. Digoxin is still a valuable and safe drug in infancy and should be given intramuscularly to produce a rapid effect using the schedule described in the section on heart failure (p. 264). It prolongs A-V node conduction and will cause interruption of the circus movement. In addition its inotropic effect is valuable if the child is in heart failure.

There is a tendency nowadays to use some of the newer drugs which act more quickly. It is important to use only one drug at a time; the combination of verapamil and a β-blocking drug such as propranolol, for example, may cause severe hypotension.

Verapamil

Verapamil intravenously should first be used.

> *Dose* Newborn: 0.75–1.0 mg.
> Infants and up to 5 years: 2–3 mg.
> 6–14 years: 3–5 mg.

The injection should be stopped when normal rhythm returns. The dose may be repeated after 10 minutes, but a close watch must be kept for signs of hypotension or diminished cardiac output.

Disopyramide

This is valuable in aborting an attack but should not be given until half an hour after verapamil. The dose is 2–5 mg/kg intravenously.

Propranolol

This is given intravenously in a dose of 0.1 mg/kg. It may be combined with digoxin but not with disopyramide or verapamil.

Suppression of attacks

If digoxin alone is not effective, propranolol should be added in a dose of 0.5–1.0 mg/kg orally daily in 3 divided doses. If this fails the propranolol should be stopped and disopyramide given instead in a dose of 5–10 mg/kg daily in 3 divided doses. Plasma levels must always be measured for safety. In resistant cases amiodarone has proved effective but it has unpleasant side-effects in the form of corneal opacities and the eyes must be carefully examined at intervals during its use. The dose is 10 mg/kg orally, daily, initially then reduced to 2–3 mg/kg daily, orally.

In patients who have recurrent attacks unresponsive to drug therapy, division of the accessory tracts surgically is possible, but would be the last resort in childhood and careful electrophysiological studies would be necessary first.

Prognosis

There is a low incidence of recurrence of attacks when the first one occurs before three months of age. Type A Wolff–Parkinson–White syndrome has a better prognosis than Type B. It has been suggested that accessory pathways cease to be used as the infant grows and may disappear. Nevertheless suppressive drug therapy should always be continued for at least six months.

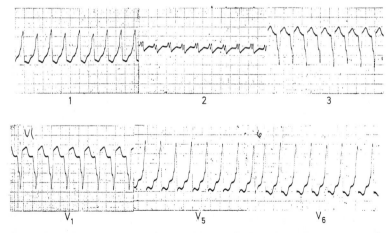

Figure 17.3. Pre-excitation (Wolff–Parkinson–White syndrome) Type B. A 2-year-old girl with Ebstein's anomaly. Note the slurred upstroke to the R waves.

Sinus node dysfunction

This is a condition in which the sinus node ceases to function and there is cardiac standstill for a few cycles after which a heart beat is initiated from an abnormal focus. Patients with this disorder frequently have syncope on exertion (Scott, Macartney and Deverall, 1976). The syndrome (also known as sick sinus syndrome) is often associated with bradycardia but at other times the patients may have tachycardia—the so-called 'brady-tachy syndrome'. Drugs which help the bradycardia may make the tachycardia worse so that drug therapy is difficult. Exercise tests may show periods of atrial arrest followed by an ectopic rhythm. The condition may be associated with sudden death and to avoid this in patients with repeated syncope, a pacemaker is required. The condition occurs after surgery for congenital heart disease (Radford and Izukawa, 1975).

ATRIAL FLUTTER AND FIBRILLATION

Both atrial flutter and fibrillation are rare in childhood and almost always occur in association with severe heart disease and high left or right atrial pressures (mitral valve disease, Ebstein's anomaly) or with myocardial disease such as acute rheumatic fever or cardiomyopathy. (They may also be provoked during cardiac catheterization.) Treatment is by digitalization, or by electroversion.

LOWN–GANONG–LEVINE SYNDROME

Atrial flutter and atrial fibrillation also occur in patients with an accessory conducting bundle from the atrium joining the bundle of His. The mechanism is similar to that of paroxysmal supraventricular tachycardia, the more rapid rhythm being due to the shorter pathway.

VENTRICULAR ARRHYTHMIAS

Ventricular ectopic beats

It is important to recognize that ventricular ectopic beats may occur in children whose hearts in every other respect are normal. Such ectopic beats usually occur singly, arise from the same focus and disappear on exercise. No treatment is required other than reassurance.

The situation is different if the ventricular ectopic beats:

are not abolished by exercise
are associated with heart disease
are multifocal
cause runs of coupling
are associated with a long Q–T interval on the ECG
are associated with bizarre QRS complexes on the ECG
occur more frequently than 2 at a time
cause syncope.

One must first make sure that the arrhythmia is primary and not secondary to hypoxia, acid–base disorder or electrolyte disturbance, particularly hypokalaemia, which may cause ectopic beats *per se* or as a result of potentiation of digitalis effects. (Hyperkalaemia occurs as a result of renal failure and the ECG shows tall T waves, atrial asystole and intraventricular block with wide QRS complexes). Drugs which cause ventricular extrasystoles include antidepressants, digitalis, and occasionally other antiarrhythmic drugs.

Investigation of malignant ventricular extrasystoles

These patients should have:

1. 24-hour ECG monitoring.
2. Exercise test.
3. Echocardiography.

If ventricular tachycardia, i.e. 3 or more successive extrasystoles with wide abnormal QRS complexes and a rate of 150–200/minute, is shown or the child is symptomatic with attacks of syncope, then full investigation by cardiac catheterization, angiography and electrophysiology should be undertaken. Although ventricular arrhythmias are rare in childhood, they can cause syncope and sudden death. If ventricular tachycardia is suspected the patient must be investigated further and the aetiology of the condition determined if possible. Coronary artery abnormalities are excluded by angiocardiography. Echocardiography helps to exclude tumours, prolapse of the mitral valve and cardiomyopathy which can be further defined by ventricular angiocardiography. Twenty four hour monitoring may show evidence of sinus node dysfunction. ECG may show a long Q–T interval which may be intermittent and in some of these patients syncope is provoked by exercise. Radford, Izukawa and Rowe (1977) investigated 8 children fully; only 1 patient was asymptomatic and the ventricular tachycardia was found by chance. Only 2 of these 8 cases were unexplained, the other 6 had some associated abnormality.

Treatment

Ventricular arrhythmias associated with prolapsing mitral valve are best treated by propranolol. Patients with prolonged Q–T interval may also respond to propranolol but if not they may be cured by left stellate ganglionectomy. Lignocaine 1–4 mg/kg as a bolus intravenously followed by the same dose as a slow infusion over 60 minutes is usually effective in controlling ventricular tachycardia. If syncope is associated with the sick sinus syndrome either because of sinus arrest or the ventricular tachycardia which may follow the sinus arrest, then a cardiac pacemaker is required.

Ventricular tachycardia associated with cyanotic congenital heart disease is probably caused by irritable foci in the myocardium secondary to ischaemia. They must be treated with propranolol or quinidine or a combination of both. Propranolol is again the drug of choice for ventricular tachycardias associated with hypertrophic obstructive cardiomyopathy.

Some patients may develop their ventricular tachycardia and syncope after exercise and in these patients a combination of propranolol and amiodarone is valuable (Julian, 1980) but the possibility of corneal opacities must be remembered when the latter drug is used.

The effects of treatment as well as relieving symptoms can also be monitored by 24-hour ECG.

Accidental ingestion of drugs by children

Digoxin

It is not uncommon nowadays for children to eat their grandparents' digoxin tablets. If vomiting can be induced to stop absorption, so much the better. If marked cardiac slowing occurs with heart block, cardiac pacing may be necessary. If potassium levels are low, potassium supplements should be provided (*see* p. 266). Potassium should not be given without measuring the serum level as hyperkalaemia frequently occurs in severe digoxin poisoning.

Tricyclic antidepressants

These drugs cause ventricular ectopic beats with wide QRS complexes and bradycardia when taken by children. The cardiac output falls and the child loses consciousness and there is severe acidosis. Correction of this and cardiac pacing are necessary if the tablets cannot be recovered by vomiting or stomach wash-out. Unfortunately if the myocardium is severely damaged the heart will not respond to pacing. The arrhythmias produced seem to be resistant to antiarrhythmic drugs.

Sudden infant death syndrome

The possibility of arrhythmias being associated with this syndrome has been raised. Shinebourne *et al.* (1977) have shown that apparently well babies have arrhythmias, some of which are associated with spells of apnoea. There is circumstantial evidence of a possible association of arrhythmias with sudden infant death syndrome but this has not so far been proved. Near-miss deaths have been known to be associated with arrhythmias (Keaton *et al.*, 1977).

Arrhythmias after surgery

Paediatricians must be informed about the possibility of arrhythmias after operations. Ventricular ectopic beats may occur after operation for ventricular septal defects and tetralogy of Fallot. They are sometimes induced by exercise. Their presence may precede episodes of ventricular tachycardia and sudden death and they must therefore be treated and suppressed—the drug of choice is propranolol. Although Mustard's operation produces very good results in the majority, some patients have symptomatic arrhythmias. The most serious is the sick sinus syndrome where there is sinus arrest and syncope. Other patients develop profound bradycardia resulting in dizziness or unconsciousness. Both conditions require cardiac pacemakers. Occasionally supraventricular tachycardia occurs—its treatment is the same for atrial tachycardias due to other causes. It is rare now to find atrial tachycardias after operation to close atrial septal defects; more care is now taken to avoid damage to the sinoatrial node. Atrial ectopic beats and atrial tachycardia occur infrequently and are treated in the same way as atrial tachycardias from other causes. Twenty four hour monitoring will show the frequency and duration of various arrhythmias, many of which are not associated with symptoms.

ATRIOVENTRICULAR BLOCK

Atrioventricular block is an interference with the normal conduction of impulses from the atria to the ventricles through the atrioventricular node. Three degrees of heart block are described.

(1) First degree block

This is essentially an electrocardiographic diagnosis. The P–R interval is longer than it should be for the patient's age and heart rate (*Figure 17.4a*). It may occur in normal hearts but is also found in rheumatic carditis, diphtheria and digitalis overdosage. The most common congenital heart lesions associated with first degree block are atrial septal defect, endocardial cushion defects, Ebstein's anomaly and L-transposition. The block itself does not cause any symptoms or require any treatment.

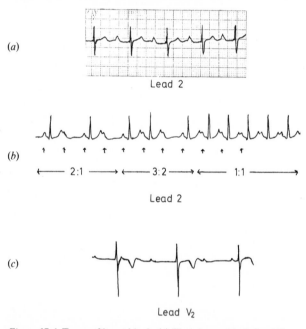

(a)

Lead 2

(b)

←—— 2:1 ——→ ←— 3:2 —→ ←—— 1:1 ——→

Lead 2

(c)

Lead V₂

Figure 17.4. Types of heart block. (*a*) First degree block (lead 2). The P–R interval is 0.3 seconds. (*b*) Second degree block (lead 2). Initially 2:1, then every third beat is dropped, and finally 1:1 conduction is restored. (*c*) Third degree or complete heart block (lead V₂). The atrial rate is 100/minute and the ventricular rate 44/minute. The QRS complexes are normal in morphology. This was a case of congenital heart block and the block is between the atria and the atrioventricular node

(2) Second degree block

In this type some of the atrial depolarization waves are not conducted to the ventricles. This may happen irregularly, or only every second or third atrial impulse is conducted to the ventricle, giving a so-called 2:1 or 3:1 heart block (*Figure 17.4b*). Sometimes there is progressive lengthening of the P–R interval until a beat is dropped—this is called the Wenckebach phenomenon. Second degree block is usually associated with heart disease of the same types as first degree block.

(3) Third degree block

The atria and ventricles beat quite independently of each other, the atrial rate being higher than the ventricular rate (*Figure 17.4c*). It is usually congenital. There may be no other congenital heart lesion or it may be associated with L-transposition of the great arteries, septal defects and aortic stenosis.

It may be diagnosed during late pregnancy when the obstetrician hears an unusually slow fetal heart rate. If however the slow rate is not observed until the patient is in labour, the child is often delivered by Caesarean section because fetal distress is suspected.

An interesting finding recently has been the occurrence of congenital heart block in infants of mothers who actually have systemic lupus erythematosis or who subsequently develop that condition (McCue *et al.*, 1977; Esscher and Scott, 1979).

In children the ventricular rate is higher than in adults with acquired heart block; it is usually in the region of 45–60/minute and may rise to 65–80/minute on exercise.

On examination, as well as the slow rate of the pulse, there is a full volume because of the increased stroke output. The heart is a little enlarged and the left ventricular beat is forceful. There are intermittently large 'a' waves (cannon waves) visible in the neck due to the right atrium contracting at times against a closed tricuspid valve. An ejection systolic murmur may be heard at the base—again due to the increased stroke output. Sounds due to atrial contraction may be heard and the first sound varies in intensity depending on the closeness of atrial contraction to ventricular contraction.

Prognosis

The majority of patients with congenital heart block lead normal lives without symptoms. They have a big stroke volume associated with the slow rate and are often athletic children. A few children however may have very slow ventricular rates below 50/minute and may have episodes of dizziness or syncope (Stokes–Adams attacks).

Twenty-four-hour ECG tapes often reveal very slow rates at times and the only way to relieve symptoms and avoid death is to insert a cardiac pacemaker. Heart block may follow operations for closure of ventricular septal defect and tetralogy of Fallot. If a patient has had transient heart block after surgery which subsequently reverts to sinus rhythm, there is a definite risk that that patient may subsequently develop permanent heart block and require a pacemaker. The likelihood of sudden death is greater following surgery than in congenital heart block and pacing is advised.

Forty per cent of patients with congenital heart block have congenital heart disease, most commonly ventricular inversion (L-transposition). There is a greater risk of death when heart block is found at an early age. Of 10 deaths in the series of Prinsky, Gillette and McNamara (1979) 6 were diagnosed before 1 month of age and 8 of the 10 had associated congenital heart disease. Additional neonatal risk factors are a falling or low ventricular rate, frequent ventricular ectopic beats and a prolonged Q–T interval.

Investigation

In patients who have stable congenital heart block without symptoms it is not usually necessary to carry out detailed investigation. In patients who have symptoms, or A-V block associated with a wide QRS complex it is often helpful to determine the site of the block by intracardiac recording of His bundle potentials. When first degree block is in the atrioventricular node (as in most congenital block) the interval A–H (atrial to His bundle interval) is prolonged.

Treatment

None is required if there are no symptoms but if dizziness or syncope are noted a pacemaker is advised. Ephedrine 1 mg/kg 6-hourly or saventrine (long-acting isoprenaline) are given temporarily until a pacemaker is inserted.

Artificial pacemakers

Over the last 10 years much technical work has been carried out on the development of reliable circuitry and batteries with lives of up to 15 years. At the same time, clinical experience in the indications for pacing and the methods employed has been considerable, although most of it has been in adult patients. The paediatrician and paediatric cardiologist have benefited from this experience resulting in an increased use of pacemakers in children.

Indications for pacing

With a few exceptions, pacemakers are required for rhythm disturbances producing excessively slow heart rates, and particularly those associated with the occurrence or risk of ventricular standstill.

Pacing methods

Most pacing wires are inserted transvenously (subclavian, cephalic or jugular veins) and the tip positioned in the right ventricle under X-ray control (endocardial pacing). The generator is then implanted in the pectoral region. When the presence of heart block is noted at the end of an operation it may be possible to suture permanent pacing wires to the epicardium and the generator is then implanted in the abdominal wall. When there is atrial disease, it may be better to pace the right atrium, although the technical problems are greater.

Types of pacemakers

All commonly used pacemakers now have some form of lithium battery which gives an expected life, according to size and current drain, of 7–15 years. With endocardial systems the need in a growing child to replace the endocardial wire after a period of a few years makes it rather pointless to use the longest life pacemakers, particularly as they are physically larger than those with a life of 7–10 years. Various electronic circuits are used to provide varieties of pacemaker function, but only a few are commonly used.

1. Ventricular inhibited pacemakers are 'shut off' when the patient's heart rate is higher than that of the pacemaker, thus avoiding competition between pacemaker and the patient's own rhythm.
2. Programmable ventricular pacemakers can be altered by an external device to change the pacing rate or strength of the stimulus. The increased rates available may be useful in children, and by setting the strength of the stimulus just above the minimum required, excessive drain on the battery can be avoided.
3. Atrial pacemakers are similar to ventricular pacemakers but need more sensitive circuitry to detect spontaneous atrial activity to enable them to switch off when the patient's own atrial rate is high enough.

4. Atrioventricular sequential pacemakers require a connection both to the right atrium and right ventricle. They pick up the atrial activity and generate a corresponding impulse to stimulate the ventricle so that they allow the ventricular rate to vary with exercise in a more physiological way. They are mainly used in complete atrioventricular block, but also have a regular standby mode if atrial activity ceases. Their technical problems largely outweigh the theoretical advantages.
5. Specialized pacemakers used to interrupt tachycardias are mainly used for paroxysmal supraventricular tachycardia, which is sensed by the pacemaker and leads to a short series of impulses being delivered to the atrium, which usually abolishes the tachycardia.

Complications of pacemakers

Infection occurs in about 5–7 per cent of all insertions or replacements, and usually requires removal of the system and reinsertion of a new one. Premature battery failure normally produces a distinct slowing of stimulus rate for some weeks before final failure, allowing a new unit to be substituted. Pacemaker generator failure due to component failure is rare with modern circuitry, but may cause slowing of pacing rate or, rarely, a speeding up. During, and immediately following insertion, ventricular ectopics and, rarely, ventricular fibrillation may occur, but these usually settle within hours or days. Wire dislodgement or breakage due to stretching from growth of the child is a real problem and frequently requires the introduction of a new system well before the generator battery fails.

Pacemaker clinics

Because of all these potential problems patients require regular follow-up at clinics where the rhythm and various pacemaker parameters can be checked. In places where patients live a long way from such a clinic it may be possible to make these checks using a special transducer with a telephone link to the pacing centre.

BIBLIOGRAPHY

Canent, R. V., Spach, M. S., Morris, J. J. and London, W. L. (1964). Recurrent ventricular tachycardia in an infant. *Pediatrics, Springfield* **33**, 926
Esscher, E. and Scott, J. S. (1979). Congenital heart block and maternal systemic lupus erythematosus. *Br. med. J.* **1**, 1235–1238
Fryda, R. J., Kaplan, S. and Helmsworth, J. A. (1971). Postoperative complete heart block in children. *Br. Heart J.* **33**, 456

Glenn, W. W. L., de Leuchtenberg, N., von Keekeren, D. W., Sato, G., Holcombe, W. G. and Palsson, K. (1969). Heart block in children. Treatment with a radio-frequency pacemaker. *J. thorac. cardiovasc. Surg.* **58**, 545

Hurwitz, R. A., Riemenschneider, T. A. and Moss, A. J. (1968). Chronic postoperative heart block in children. *Am. J. Cardiol.* **21**, 185

Keaton, B. R., Southall, E., Rutter, N., Anderson, R. H., Shinebourne, E. A. and Southall, D. P. (1977). Cardiac conduction disorders in six infants with near-miss sudden infant deaths. *Br. med. J.* **2**, 600–603

Lev, M., Silverman, J., Fitzmaurice, F. M., Paul, M. H., Cassell, D. E. and Miller, A. (1971). Lack of connection between the atria and more peripheral conduction system in congenital atrioventricular block. *Am. J. Cardiol.* **27**, 481

McCue, C. M., Mantakas, M. E., Tingelstad, J. B. and Ruddy, S. (1977). Congenital heart block in newborns of mothers with connective tissue disease. *Circulation* **56**, 82–89

Prinsky, W. W., Gillette, P. C. and McNamara, D. G. (1979). Diagnosis and management of congenital complete atrioventricular block. *Paediat. Cardiol.* **1**, 1. Abstract p. 93

Radford, D. J., Izakawa, R. and Rowe, R. D. (1977). Evaluation of children with ventricular arrhythmias. *Archs. Dis. Childh.* **52**, 345–353

Radford, D. J., Izakawa, T. and Rowe, R. D. (1976). Congenital paroxysmal atrial tachycardia. *Archs. Dis. Childh.* **51**, 613–617

Radford, D. J. and Izakawa, R. (1975). Sick sinus syndrome –symptomatic cases in children. *Archs. Dis. Childh.* **50**, 879–885

Rowlands, D. J., Howitt, G. and Markman, P. (1965). Propranolol in disturbances of cardiac rhythm. *Br. med. J.* **1**, 891

Scott, Olive, Williams, G. J. and Fiddler, G. I. (1980). Results of 24-hour ambulatory monitoring of the electrocardiogram in 131 healthy boys age 10–13 years. *Br. Heart J.* **44.3**, 304–308

Stock, J. P. P. (1969). *Diagnosis and Treatment of Cardiac Arrhythmias.* London: Butterworths

CHAPTER 18

Rheumatic Fever and Chorea

Rheumatic fever was always commonest in children living in poor communities with poor social conditions. Its incidence has fallen over the last 30 years so that it is now a rarity in paediatric wards in the Western world. Not only has the incidence fallen sharply but also the frequency of cardiac involvement and of recurrence is now less. Perry (1969) found that 80 per cent of children with acute rheumatic fever seen prior to 1939 had evidence of carditis, 55 per cent had recurrences and 71 per cent were left with evidence of valvular disease. Between 1955 and 1962 only 55 per cent had carditis, 9 per cent had recurrences and 18 per cent had permanent valvular damage.

There is little doubt that the decline in rheumatic fever is associated with socio-economic development. It began in the last century and most of the decline was achieved before prophylaxis with penicillin began (Strasser, 1978). It is difficult to assess the impact that penicillin prophylaxis has had on the incidence. The disease is still prevalent however in the less wealthy developing countries in other parts of the world. Surprisingly, when the causes of death in the age group 15–24 years were analysed in six European countries, rheumatic heart disease and rheumatic fever ranked between second and fourth commonest (Strasser, 1978). In the world as a whole, the incidence varies from 0.06/1000 (Nashville, USA) to 11/1000 in Delhi (Padmavati *et al.*, 1980). Shaper (1972) has emphasized that the occurrence of rheumatic fever in underdeveloped countries relates less to climate than to the ecology of rheumatic fever, including poverty, crowding, very poor housing and grossly inadequate health services. Climate is just one variable in which high temperatures favour the spread of pharyngeal streptococci. In other words he supports the old adage that rheumatic fever is a disease of the poor. Furthermore, the severity of the disease in such areas may well be related to the high rates of recurrent infections associated with inadequate medical care.

AETIOLOGY

The disease is closely related to infection with group A streptococci. Kaplan (1969) reviewed the evidence and proposed the hypothesis that antibodies to the streptococcus cross-react with heart muscle in subjects whose own heart antigens resemble those of the streptococcus, causing an autoimmune reaction. In many patients a similar cross-reaction occurs with synovial tissue to produce arthritis, or with brain tissue causing chorea.

PATHOLOGY

Involvement of the heart leads to a pancarditis. In the myocardium round cell infiltration, muscle swelling and necrosis occur. The Aschoff bodies are the scars left by areas of inflammation. The pericardium shows swelling, infiltration and fibrinous exudate. The endocardium, including the valves (which are normally virtually avascular), becomes hyperaemic, oedematous and infiltrated. Adhesion of cusps leads to stenosis of the valves, and scarring and retraction to regurgitation. These changes continue after the acute stage has declined.

CLINICAL PRESENTATION

The condition is rare before the age of 3 years and symptoms occur between 10 and 21 days after a streptococcal infection, usually a sore throat. The onset is insidious and arthritis is usually the first manifestation; the large joints are affected and the pain moves from one joint to another. The child is pale and often sweats freely and is pyrexial. The joints are swollen and warm, and movement is painful. The severity of the arthritis bears no relation to the severity of the carditis and indeed about 15 per cent of patients have carditis without any joint manifestations. They present with fever, cough and dyspnoea. Skin rashes often occur, particularly erythema marginatum and occasionally erythema nodosum. About 10 per cent of patients have rheumatic nodules, either over the occiput or on the extensor surfaces of elbows, wrists and fingers.

In patients with arthritis it may be difficult to be certain whether there is cardiac involvement and the following points are helpful.

1. *Heart murmur*. A blowing, high-pitched systolic murmur is heard at the cardiac apex and is conducted to the axilla and back. It is evidence of mitral insufficiency due to dilatation of the mitral valve ring. A mid-diastolic mitral murmur may be heard when the regurgitation is marked and is due to an increased flow through the mitral valve secondary to the mitral regurgitation. Aortic incompetence may occur and causes a high-pitched diastolic murmur immediately after the second sound. It is best heard down the left sternal edge when the patient sits up, leans forward and holds his breath in expiration.
2. *Cardiac enlargement*. Increasing size of the heart is good evidence of carditis and this may be detected clinically or radiographically. It is important, however, to make sure that the radiograph is a good inspiratory one with correct tube distance, otherwise apparent enlargement may be misinterpreted.
3. *Pericarditis*. A pericardial friction rub is evidence of cardiac involvement.
4. *Heart failure* occurs in severe cases and is often preceded by vomiting and abdominal pain.

Investigations show a raised erythrocyte sedimentation rate and a leucocytosis but these are non-specific. A rising antistreptolysin O titre is good evidence of previous streptococcal infection even when the organism cannot be cultured. The absence of a rising titre, however, does not rule out streptococcal infection because a few organisms do not produce streptolysin or antibiotics may have suppressed the antistreptolysin O response. The presence of C-reactive protein in the serum of patients with rheumatic fever indicates a pathological state and suggests rheumatic activity. C-reactive protein is not present in normal blood but may be present in acute nephritis, malignant tumours and rheumatoid arthritis as well as rheumatic fever. Prolongation of the P–R interval (greater than 0.2 seconds) on the electrocardiogram is good evidence of rheumatic infection. Flattening of T waves, Q–T prolongation and ventricular ectopic beats are less specific. Typical changes of pericarditis may be seen. Jones (1944) enumerated the various criteria necessary to diagnose rheumatic fever. These were modified by the American Heart Association in 1955.

Rheumatic infection tends to recur and a previous history of rheumatic fever makes symptoms, which may be equivocal, more likely to be due to rheumatic infection.

Chorea may occur many weeks after an acute streptococcal infection. It is more common in females and there are changes of mood followed by purposeless movements and inability to sustain muscular contraction.

TREATMENT

Patients should be confined to bed but enforced immobility, which used to be advised, is unnecessary.

Adequate antibiotic therapy should be given to eradicate the streptococcal infection. Intramuscular penicillin should be used initially and throat swabs taken to make sure that the organism is no longer present. Benzathine penicillin G 600 000–1 200 000 units is given once intramuscularly or oral treatment with 250–500 mg penicillin at 8-hourly intervals is given for 10 days. If the patient is sensitive to penicillin, erythromycin should be used. Salicylates are specific in relieving the joint pains and this is a good diagnostic test. A dose of 120 mg/kg per day is given up to a maximum of 8g/day. The full dose should be continued for two weeks and then halved until the signs of rheumatic activity have disappeared. If the dose is too great, salicylism will occur; tinnitus, deafness, vomiting, hyperpnoea and headache should be looked for when salicylates are being given so that if necessary the drug can be withdrawn or the dose reduced.

There is no conclusive evidence that any drugs, salicylates, cortisone or ACTH influence the longterm course of the disease. Some workers believe that steroids should be given when carditis is present but there is insufficient evidence to support this. When there are acute, life-threatening complications of heart failure or complete heart block, steroids may induce a temporary remission although a 'spring-back' usually occurs following their withdrawal.

In general, surgery should be avoided in childhood because of the presence of rheumatic activity in the heart. There are now reports, however, of valve replacement in children who were unresponsive to conservative therapy. Simcha et al. (1980) report valve replacement in 14 children aged 9–16 years in whom there were no operative deaths. Girdwood et al. (1980) report 62 children aged less than 15 years who had valve replacement with 5 hospital deaths and 10 late deaths, 8 of whom had grossly dilated left ventricles at autopsy and abundant Aschoff nodes.

PREVENTION

Rheumatic fever can be prevented if an infection with Group AB-haemolytic Streptococcus is diagnosed early and adequately treated. The B-haemolytic Streptococcus is unlikely ever to be eradicated because it is so prevalent and there are high carrier rates. If recurrences however can be prevented in susceptible individuals then the secondary effects of the disease on the heart will be lessened. Supervision is essential to ensure that prophylactic penicillin continues to be taken. Also the relatives of children who have had rheumatic fever should be closely watched, as children having oral penicillin for prevention may have masked infections which may spread to their siblings.

The control of rheumatic fever in developing countries is difficult. The cost of its prevention has to be assessed with other priorities; there may be a scarcity of trained personnel and scattered populations making surveillance impossible. It is hoped that there will be a decline in the disease with improved socio-economic conditions but meanwhile Streptococcal infections must be controlled. This may be accomplished by—

1. Early and adequate treatment of streptococcal infections when they occur.
2. Prevention of repeated streptococcal infections.

Treatment of streptococcal infection

This must be given early and adequately. It is wise to give crystalline penicillin by injection for 48 hours and then follow this with oral treatment for 8 days to ensure that the infection is completely eradicated. Alternatively an injection of a long-lasting penicillin such as Benzathine Penicillin G may be used. If the patient is sensitive to penicillin, Cephalexin should be used.

Prevention of repeated streptococcal infections

The Rheumatic Fever Committee of the Council on Rheumatic Fever and Congenital Heart Disease of the American Heart Association (1971) recommends the following programme.

Prophylaxis should be continued indefinitely

  1. Benzathine Penicillin G i.m. is best
     Dosage: 1 200 000 units/month
  or 2. Penicillin G orally
     Dosage: 200 000 units b.d. $\frac{1}{2}$ hour before a meal
  or 3. Sulphadiazine
     Dosage: 1 g/day if the patient is over 60 lb weight
            0.5 g/day if the patient is under 60 lb weight
  or 4. If the patient is sensitive to penicillin and sulphadiazine
     use erythromycin 250 mg b.d.

Tetracyclines should not be used because there is a high prevalence of strains resistant to this antibiotic.

CONVALESCENCE

As the disease has become less severe and cardiac involvement less common the restrictions enforced in previous years have been generally relaxed. If there has been no clinical or electrocardiographic evidence of cardiac involvement the patient is allowed up one week after arthritis has disappeared. If carditis is suspected bed rest is usually continued until the sedimentation rate has returned to near normal levels (below 20 mm) although sometimes a compromise has to be reached when the sedimentation rate stays high but the patient is well. Return to school can be allowed from 2 to 4 weeks later, but organized games are advised against for six months if there has been evidence of carditis.

Continued follow-up is important for two reasons: firstly to ensure that prophylactic penicillin is taken regularly and secondly to detect evidence of established rheumatic valvular disease. Mild mitral regurgitation particularly may only become apparent when the patient increases his activities. Increasing signs of valve damage or persistent or increasing heart size in radiography should be regarded as evidence of active rheumatism.

If there has been evidence of carditis, even though the heart is subsequently normal clinically, there is a risk of bacterial endocarditis and antibiotic prophylaxis is indicated for at least two years if the patient requires dental extractions. Since the patient will already be taking penicillin, another antibiotic must be used. The best choice at the moment is cephaloridine or erythromycin. Purely bacteriostatic antibiotics, such as tetracycline, are useless.

BIBLIOGRAPHY AND REFERENCES

Jones, T. D. (1944). The diagnosis of rheumatic fever. *J. Am. med. Ass.* **126**, 481

Kaplan, M. E. (1969). The cross-reaction of group A streptococci with heart tissue and its relation to induced autoimmunity in rheumatic fever. *Bull. rheum. Dis.* **19**, 560

Padmavati, S., Sreshta, N. K., Vijayan, N. K. and Gupta, V. K. (1980). Secondary prophylaxis of rheumatic heart disease in Delhi. Abstract. World Congress on Paediatric Cardiology

Perry, C. B. (1969). The natural history of acute rheumatism. *Ann. rheum. Dis.* **28**, 471

Prevention of rheumatic fever. A statement prepared by the Rheumatic Fever Committee of the Council on Rheumatic Fever and Congenital Heart Disease of the American Heart Association (1971). *Circulation* **43**, 983

Shaper, A. G. (1972). Cardiovascular disease in the tropics. *Br. med. J.* **3**, 683

Strasser, T. (1978). Rheumatic fever and rheumatic heart disease in the 1970s. *W.H.O. Chronicle* **32**, 18–25

CHAPTER 19

Myocardial and Pericardial Disease

ENDOMYOCARDIAL DISEASES

There is a group of diseases in which the heart muscle or the endocardium is abnormal. The diseases are often ill-defined, the diagnosis during life is uncertain and the aetiology of the conditions is often obscure. They are:

1. Congestive cardiomyopathy (non-obstructive)
2. Endocardial fibroelastosis
3. Myocarditis

Congestive cardiomyopathy

A small number of infants and children presenting with cardiac failure are shown by investigations to have no gross structural abnormality of the heart and the failure is attributed to myocardial disease, for which there is no extrinsic cause. In a small proportion the disease is familial. The majority of these patients are first seen in infancy because of breathlessness. Examination reveals evidence of right heart failure, enlargement of the left ventricle and a loud gallop rhythm (third heart sound). Often there is an apical pansystolic murmur due to functional mitral regurgitation.

Investigations

Chest radiographs show a greatly enlarged heart (*Figure 19.1a*) with a sharp outline (due to diminished movement). The lung vessels are

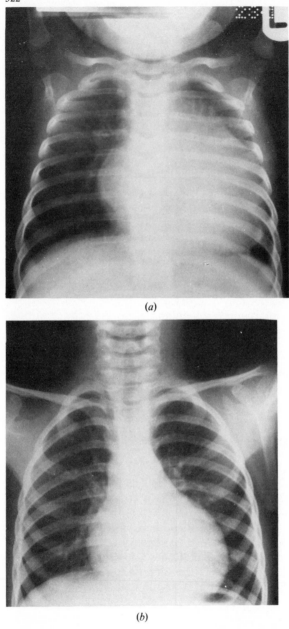

(a)

(b)

Figure 19.1. Endocardial fibroelastosis. There is marked cardiac
enlargement at 10 months (*a*) and decrease in heart size by 3 years (*b*)

normal or show pulmonary venous congestion. Electrocardiograms show the picture of advanced left ventricular hypertrophy, often with exceptionally deep Q waves in leads 3, V_5 and V_6. Nearly always the T waves are inverted in left ventricular leads (*Figure 19.2*).

Cardiac catheterization is seldom required since the clinical picture, chest radiographs and electrocardiograms usually indicate the diagnosis. (In early infancy it may be difficult to distinguish the condition from an anomalous coronary artery.) If catheterization is carried out, it indicates an elevated left atrial pressure with mild pulmonary hypertension, and angiography shows a large, poorly contracting left ventricle.

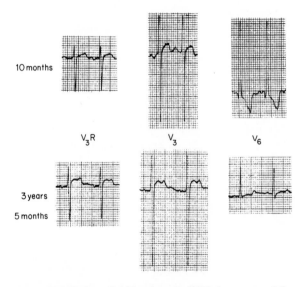

Figure 19.2. Endocardial fibroelastosis. ECG shows severe left ventricular hypertrophy in 10-month-old child (upper trace) and slight left ventricular hypertrophy by 3 years (lower trace)—the T waves are now upright

Treatment and prognosis

Digoxin and diuretics are required to control the cardiac failure. Although the majority of patients have a slow downhill course a few, particularly those in whom the disease appears within the first few months of life, ultimately improve. It is possible that the latter are in fact examples of intrauterine myocarditis.

Primary endocardial fibroelastosis

Primary endocardial fibroelastosis (EFE) is the commonest condition in the group of endomyocardial diseases and it usually presents in the first two years of life with heart failure and cardiomegaly. There are often no cardiac murmurs and no evidence of associated congenital heart defects.

The cause is unknown but some believe it is secondary to infection of the myocardium. A relationship between mumps virus and primary endocardial fibroelastosis was postulated by Noren, Adams and Anderson (1963) but has not been confirmed.

The disease affects mainly the left ventricle and, less often, the left atrium. There is a thick, smooth, glistening, white endocardium. The aortic and mitral valves are often involved and mitral and aortic incompetence or stenosis result. Edwards (1960) classified primary endocardial fibroelastosis into two groups, according to whether the left ventricle was dilated or contracted. The dilated type is by far the most common; the left ventricle has a large volume and the myocardium is hypertrophied. In the contracted type the left ventricle is normal or reduced in size and the endocardium markedly thickened.

It is thought that the rigid endocardium prevents normal left ventricular function as regards both its ability to fill in diastole and its contractility.

Clinical presentation

Tachypnoea may be noted from birth; heart failure usually develops sometime before 2 years of age and is often precipitated by a chest infection. Recurrent chest infections and pneumonia are common. The heart is enlarged with the apex beat displaced to the anterior axillary line. Cardiac murmurs are absent but sometimes a systolic murmur due to mitral regurgitation occurs. A loud gallop rhythm, due to rapid ventricular filling in early diastole, is almost invariable.

Investigation

The findings from radiology, electrocardiography and at cardiac catheterization are essentially the same as those in congestive cardiomyopathy.

Differential diagnosis

It is often difficult to differentiate from myocarditis but if the electrocardiogram shows the typical changes of left ventricular hypertrophy and there is mitral regurgitation, then the most probable diagnosis is endocardial fibroelastosis or cardiomyopathy.

Treatment

There is no doubt that digitalization is the best form of treatment. It often produces a marked improvement and should be continued even if the patient's symptoms disappear. Diuretics may also be required. Chest infections must be promptly and enthusiastically treated, otherwise the child will deteriorate rapidly.

Natural history

Severe cases die within months of the disease presenting, despite treatment. Others follow a more chronic course with periods of deterioration following chest infections but gradually improvement occurs and they can be maintained in a stable state for many years, although deterioration may still occur later. A few show marked improvement following digitalization and the heart decreases in size and the electrocardiogram returns to normal. (*Figures 19.1 and 19.2.*)

It will be seen that the conditions described as congestive cardiomyopathy and primary (dilated) endocardial fibroelastosis are clinically virtually indistinguishable, the differentiation being made only at autopsy. Indeed, some authorities believe that the two conditions are aetiologically not distinct and that endocardial fibroelastosis is simply a reaction to disordered myocardial functions. We have seen families where several members have died from cardiac failure in early childhood and at autopsy some have had endocardial fibroelastosis and some simply congestive cardiomyopathy.

Secondary endocardial fibroelastosis

Lesions which cause obstruction to the left heart (coarctation and aortic stenosis) frequently show some degree of endocardial fibroelastosis and some patients, particularly those with coarctation of the aorta, have abnormal myocardial function as shown by an unusual degree of cardiac enlargement which is not reversed by operation. Patients with hypoplasia of the left heart due to coarctation, aortic atresia or severe aortic stenosis usually show endocardial fibroelastosis, sometimes described as the contracted type. A few patients with ventricular septal defects also have myocardial disease with or without endocardial fibroelastosis and are more ill and have larger hearts than those with uncomplicated ventricular septal defects. When myocardial disease is associated with an atrial septal defect the raised left atrial pressure increases the left-to-right shunting and severe heart failure occurs. Indeed, when heart failure is diagnosed in childhood or infancy as due to an atrial septal defect it is likely that there is an associated obstructive lesion or myocardial disease on the left side of the heart.

Right heart endocardial fibroelastosis

The occurrence of endocardial fibroelastosis in the right side is seen in association with pulmonary atresia and hypoplastic right ventricle and with Ebstein's anomaly of the tricuspid valve, when both atrium and ventricle are involved.

Myocarditis

Inflammation of the heart muscle occurs in a number of conditions, some of which are associated with known infective agents, some associated with systemic diseases, while yet others have an unknown aetiology.

Virus myocarditis

The most common known aetiological agent is the Coxsackie virus, types B1–5 in infants and A4 and A5 in adolescents. Children have pyrexia, upper respiratory tract and gastrointestinal symptoms and then develop breathlessness and signs of congestive heart failure. Sudden death has also been reported. Infants usually present with vomiting and lethargy. The heart sounds are often faint and a third heart sound is usual. Electrocardiograms show small voltage QRS complexes, a prolonged Q–T interval, flat T waves and rhythm disturbances including ventricular extrasystoles, supraventricular and ventricular tachycardias and occasionally heart block. Chest radiographs show a moderate increase in heart size and pulmonary venous congestion or oedema. Treatment with digoxin and diuretics usually controls the condition and most patients recover after a few weeks, but a few (particularly infants under the age of 6 months) die in the acute stage or develop chronic heart failure and die early. The main difficulty in diagnosis is in distinguishing the condition from cardiomyopathy or endocardial fibroelastosis, but in myocarditis gross cardiac enlargement is rare and the electrocardiogram does not show the pattern of left ventricular hypertrophy.

Postinfluenzal myocarditis has been reported and is probably common in a mild form. It may be an auto-immune response rather than a true invasion of the tissues with virus, and beneficial results have been reported from corticosteroid therapy. Other viruses reported as causative agents include cytomegalovirus, rubella virus, adenovirus, herpesvirus and the virus of vaccinia. Cardiac involvement has recently been reported in viral hepatitis.

Endomyocardial fibrosis

A condition in which there is overgrowth of the endocardium with fibrous tissue has been described extensively from Central and East Africa. Its epidemiology is such as to suggest that the cause is an infective agent moderated by racial and environmental conditions. An acute phase with fever, lassitude and evidence of myocarditis is followed by a chronic phase with severe heart failure, usually mainly or entirely right sided, with evidence of tricuspid regurgitation. In patients coming to autopsy the apex of the right ventricle is obliterated by dense fibrous tissue which grows on to the chordae tendineae, causing shortening and eventually affecting the valve cusps. Similar less severe lesions are seen in the left ventricle.

Treatment with diuretics produces some improvement but most patients remain severely disabled and eventually die from right heart failure.

HYPERTROPHIC OBSTRUCTIVE CARDIOMYOPATHY (HOCM)

Hypertrophic obstructive cardiomyopathy is a disease of children, adolescents and young adults which has been described under various names, starting as 'asymmetric cardiac hypertrophy', first diagnosed at autopsy in patients dying suddenly without previous symptoms of heart disease.

Incidence and aetiology

Although rare, recognition of the condition has led to the diagnosis being made in a greater number of patients. It is now known that the condition is passed on with a Mendelian dominant form of inheritance with incomplete penetrance. The evidence for this comes from echocardiographic studies on relatives of patients with the clinical condition, in which 50 per cent were shown to have an interventricular septum 30 per cent or more thicker than the left ventricular free wall (Clark *et al.*, 1973). One or other parent, where both could be tested, showed such a thickening. In most cases these relatives had no clinical or ECG abnormalities but a small proportion had clinical features to suggest HOCM. In our experience the condition is seen commonly in patients with the Ulrich–Noonan syndrome. Lentiginosis is another associated condition. The cause of the abnormality is unknown. Theories included a hamartomatous overgrowth of muscle, increased sensitivity to sympathetic stimulation and abnormal distribution of muscle bundles increasing the work of the ventricle and producing secondary hypertrophy. An alternative theory is that the muscle fibres are initially normal but that the septum has an abnormal curvature in its long axis, convex towards the left ventricle which results in longitudinal and circumferential fibres acting against each other when they contract, so that the septum hypertrophies from excessive tension built up by isometric contraction.

Pathology and pathophysiology

The abnormality affects primarily the left ventricle but sometimes both ventricles are involved. There is an enormous overgrowth of left ventricular muscle. The whole ventricle, including the papillary muscles, is involved but the hypertrophy is most obvious in the upper part of the septum where it produces a large bulge below the aortic valve (*see Figure 7.1*, p. 112). The principal feature is excessively rapid contraction of ventricular muscle, so that the ventricle empties almost completely into the aorta in the first third or half of systole. Thereafter the hypertrophied septum comes into apposition with the anterior leaflet of the mitral valve, preventing further ejection, and the pressure in the proximal part of the ventricle may then rise above that in the aorta, producing a gradient of up to 100 mmHg (*see Figure 7.3*, p. 117). Excessive contraction of papillary muscles may hold the mitral valve open and produce regurgitation. In addition, the greatly hypertrophied muscle is distended with difficulty in diastole, so that, particularly on exercise, the left atrial pressure rises.

Clinical presentation

Many children are referred because of a systolic murmur and are asymptomatic. Breathlessness, ischaemic cardiac pain and syncope are common in adolescence and adult life. Sudden death occurs in this condition in about 15 per cent of patients who have been previously diagnosed, but a similar number of patients come to autopsy having died suddenly, not always upon exertion, when the disease has not been suspected in life. Supraventricular and ventricular tachycardias, and ventricular extrasystoles are experienced by a few.

The clinical signs are characteristic and in many cases allow a diagnosis to be made. The pulse is unusually jerky, due to rapid ventricular ejection, and may give a double spike. The left ventricle is forceful and usually shows a double impulse. Forceful atrial contraction may produce a palpable fourth heart sound so that the impulse becomes triple. An early systolic murmur at the left sternal edge is conducted into the aortic area. Aortic closure is delayed so that splitting of the second heart sound becomes absent or reversed. About one-quarter of patients have an apical systolic murmur due to mitral regurgitation.

Radiology and electrocardiography

Chest radiographs in the early stages may be normal, but later the left ventricle is enlarged and in symptomatic patients the left atrium is prominent. Pulmonary venous congestion and frank oedema occur as the disease progresses. The electrocardiogram is usually abnormal. Most patients, even without symptoms, show advanced left ventricular hypertrophy but about 20 per cent show abnormal Q waves in many leads, simulating infarction but probably due to the septal hypertrophy (*Figure 19.3*).

Echocardiography

The diagnosis can nearly always be established by echocardiography, which is more reliable than cardiac catheterization. The most constant finding is gross thickening of the interventricular septum— often to twice or more the normal for age. The left ventricular free wall is also thickened but to a lesser degree. The mitral valve echo shows a characteristic pattern of apparent systolic anterior movement of the mitral valve (*Figure 19.4*). In fact this echo has been

330

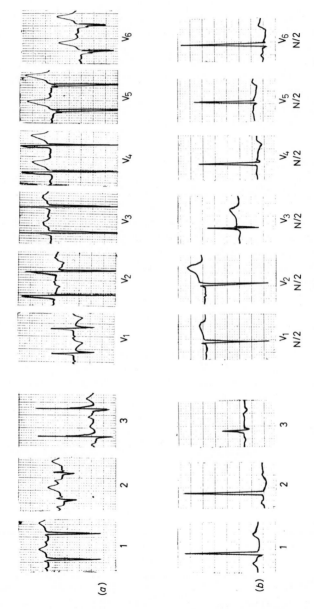

Figure 19.3. The electrocardiogram in hypertrophic obstructive cardiomyopathy. (*a*) From a 3-month-old boy, showing Q waves in leads 2, 3, and V$_{5-6}$. (*b*) From a 12-year-old girl, showing marked left ventricular hypertrophy. Note that leads V$_{1-5}$ are recorded at half sensitivity

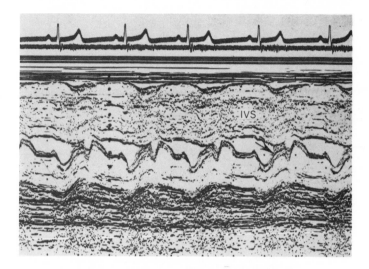

Figure 19.4. Echocardiogram of 7-year-old boy with hypertrophic
obstructive cardiomyopathy. Note the greatly thickened interventricular septum – 4.5 cm-(IVS) and apparent systolic anterior movement
of mitral valve due to hypertrophied papillary muscle

shown by two-dimensional studies to be due to greatly hypertrophied
papillary muscles. Because the ejection from the left ventricle is
completed early in systole the aortic valve cusps show premature
closure, although this is a less rapid movement than is seen in
discrete subaortic stenosis.

Investigation

Right heart catheterization usually reveals little except some
elevation of pulmonary wedge pressure, but a gradient may occur
between the inflow and outflow portions of the right ventricle.
Retrograde catheterization of the left ventricle reveals a gradient
between the body and outflow portion of the ventricle in about 50
per cent of patients (*see Figure 7.3*) and this may be provoked or
increased by isoprenaline* and reduced or abolished by propranolol.
Left ventricular angiography demonstrates the thick-walled ventricle, the small ventricular cavity in systole and the functional
obstruction produced by the hypertrophied septum (*Figure 19.5*).

* The increase in gradient is not a specific test for HOCM as it also occurs in
valvular aortic stenosis.

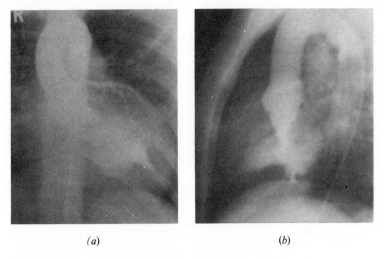

(a)   (b)

Figure 19.5. Left ventricular angiograms from a 15-year-old girl with hypertrophic obstructive cardiomyopathy. (*a*) Anteroposterior and (*b*) lateral views. Note the extreme thickness of the left ventricular muscle and, in the lateral view, how the bulging, hypertrophied ventricular septum anteriorly and the mitral valve posteriorly constrict the outflow

Treatment

Asymptomatic children require no treatment but athletics and competitive games are advised against. It may be that the beta-sympathetic blocking drugs will improve survival in the absence of symptoms but this has yet to be proved. Patients who have symptoms of chest pain, dyspnoea or arrhythmias should be treated with propranolol in the first instance. An alternative drug is the calcium antagonist verapamil. Surgical resection of hypertrophied muscle has helped patients with large gradients whose symptoms are not relieved by medical therapy.

Prognosis

Although the disease ultimately proves fatal in the vast majority of patients, the interval from discovery until death is often measured in decades, especially in asymptomatic patients. We feel that parents and patients should be told that follow-up is required as symptoms can be treated if they occur but that a gloomy prognosis should not be given and the question of sudden death should not be raised.

CARDIAC TUMOURS

Primary cardiac tumours are rare, but four types have been described.

Rhabdomyomas

Rhabdomyomas (tumours of cardiac muscle) present with systolic murmurs due to obstruction to right or left ventricular outflow. They can be demonstrated by angiography; removal using cardiopulmonary bypass is possible. They are particularly associated with epiloia.

Fibromas

Fibromas present in a similar way to rhabdomyomas but may also give rise to ventricular tachycardia. Surgical removal has been reported.

Teratomas

Teratomas are usually outward growing and produce cystic tumours within the pericardium. Cardiac compression or unexplained cardiomegaly are the presenting features. Operation is possible without cardiopulmonary bypass and is usually successful.

Myxomas

Myxomas occur most commonly in the left atrium, attached to the interatrial septum. Rarely, they are found in the ventricles or right atrium. They produce systemic effects, malaise, weight loss and low grade fever with high sedimentation rate and abnormal serum proteins, and also give rise to emboli, as well as producing local effects. Left atrial myxomas may simulate mitral stenosis and the combination of mitral murmurs (frequently variable) and low grade fever suggests rheumatic carditis. The systemic emboli raise the possibility of bacterial endocarditis. Diagnosis is usually by angiography (injecting contrast material into the pulmonary artery and opacifying the left atrium after passage through the lungs) but may also be made by ultrasound.

Right sided myxomas usually produce embolic pulmonary hypertension.

Surgical removal, using cardiopulmonary bypass, is indicated urgently as soon as the diagnosis is made since the risks of catastrophic embolism are high and the possibility exists of the tumour completely obstructing the circulation. Regrowth has only occasionally been reported.

PERICARDIAL DISEASES

Acute pericarditis

Bacterial infection of the pericardial cavity occurs occasionally by spread from the lungs, or as a result of septicaemia – particularly with staphylococci, less often with pneumococci or other organisms. Tuberculous pericarditis may present as an acute infection. Virus

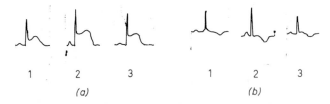

Figure 19.6. Electrocardiogram in pericarditis. (*a*) Acute stage. (*b*) Subacute stage. Note that in the acute stage there is ST elevation in all the standard leads

pericarditis, due mainly to Coxsackie B virus, is probably the commonest form of so-called benign acute pericarditis. The disease is rare in infants and young children but occurs in adolescents, sometimes in mild epidemics. There is usually a prodromal period with malaise and fever, and the presenting symptom of the pericarditis is central chest pain which may be constant or accentuated by changes in posture, respiration or coughing. It is sometimes felt mainly in the epigastrium. The characteristic sign is the pericardial rub, and the electrocardiogram shows changes illustrated in *Figure 19.6.*

Despite the term 'benign', serious complications occur in half the patients. Atrial and ventricular tachycardias occur and tamponade may develop. Relapses after weeks or months are not uncommon.

Rest and mild analgesics are all that is required in mild cases. Corticosteroids will suppress the disease but make relapse rather more common.

Apart from virus infection, pericarditis may occur in rheumatoid disease, disseminated lupus erythematosus and leukaemic infiltration of the heart.

Pericardial effusion

Small effusions within the pericardial cavity are common in patients with cardiac failure, and a small serous effusion frequently occurs in acute pericarditis. An effusion large enough to cause interference with cardiac function is rare in childhood but may occur in the course of benign pericarditis, as a complication of rheumatoid disease, following cardiac surgery (postpericardiotomy syndrome) and in malignant diseases, including leukaemia. A syndrome of chronic pericardial effusion with constriction, possibly postviral, has been reported (Jordan and Haycock, 1979).

Presentation

The clinical picture varies according to the rapidity with which the effusion gathers. With rapid accumulation of fluid, children experience dyspnoea, cough and abdominal pain due to hepatic engorgement. With subacute effusions symptoms are more vague and consist of tiredness, mild breathlessness and swelling of the abdomen due to ascites. Physical signs are characteristic. The pulse has a small volume and is reduced or disappears on inspiration. The venous pressure is often so high that the upper limit of filling is above the angle of the jaw; the liver is enlarged. The cardiac impulse is impalpable, cardiac dullness is increased and the heart sounds are very soft.

The chest radiograph shows enlargement of the cardiac silhouette which is sharply defined and in children and infants it is often possible, especially on screening, to see the heart as a separate shadow within (*Figure 19.7*). The electrocardiogram shows low voltage complexes and usually widespread T wave inversion. Ultrasonic scans produce diagnostic reflections showing the effusion separating the pericardium from the cardiac surface. Angiocardiography is rarely necessary but shows the heart chambers to be small and abnormally far inside the cardiac shadow. Albuminuria, severe enough to simulate the nephrotic syndrome, and malabsorption, have been reported as complications.

Treatment

Digitalis is contra-indicated, because slowing of the heart rate reduces cardiac output when the stroke volume is fixed. Diuretics should be given with caution as too great a reduction in venous pressure may further lower the cardiac output. Aspiration of the effusion is indicated if there is rapid accumulation or very high venous pressure, and is carried out either in the fourth left interspace inside the midclavicular line (through the portion of the pericardium not covered by lung) or from below, immediately lateral to the xiphisternum. Facilities for monitoring and electroversion should be available because ventricular fibrillation is a complication of pericardial aspiration. If the fluid reaccumulates, partial pericardiectomy is indicated.

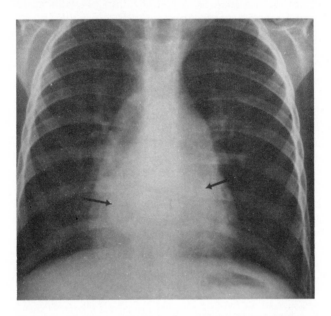

Figure 19.7. Pericardial effusion with constriction. There is a slight increase in the size of the cardiac shadow and a faint inner shadow due to the heart within the effusion. In this case there is little enlargement of the cardiac shadow because the pericardium was thickened and causing constriction

Constrictive pericarditis

Tuberculosis is still the commonest cause of constrictive pericarditis in children in most countries, but occasional cases complicating rheumatoid disease or other collagen diseases are seen. Constriction due to a combination of effusion and pericardial thickening is seen in rheumatoid disease.

Presentation

Lassitude, abdominal pain and swelling of the abdomen are usual, while breathlessness and oedema are uncommon. There is sometimes atrial fibrillation, especially in older children; the pulse is of small volume and shows a reduction in volume on inspiration. The jugular venous pressure is high and shows a rapid descent at the beginning of ventricular diastole. Coincident with this there is a clearly audible early diastolic sound, often as loud as the heart sounds, due to rapid filling of the ventricle. There is no murmur. The liver is enlarged and ascites is frequently present.

Investigations

Chest radiographs show the heart to be normal or small in size, except where there is an associated effusion, and screening shows poor pulsation. Pericardial calcification occurs in about half of tuberculous cases. The electrocardiogram shows widespread T wave inversion.

Treatment

As with pericardial effusion, digitalis is contra-indicated and diuretics must be used with care. Pericardiectomy is indicated if the venous pressure is more than slightly raised but should otherwise be avoided if there is evidence of tuberculous activity since reconstriction may occur. Antituberculous therapy is indicated if there is any reason to suspect active infection.

BIBLIOGRAPHY AND REFERENCES

Endomyocardial diseases
Ainger, L. E. (1964). Acute aseptic myocarditis: cortico steroid therapy. *J. Pediat.* **64**, 716
Edwards, J. E. (1960). Congenital malformations. Malformations of endocardium and pericardium. In *Pathology of the Heart*, 2nd edition, p. 417. Ed. S. E. Gould, Springfield, Illinois: Charles C. Thomas
Grist, N. R. and Bell, E. J. (1969) Coxsackie virus and the heart. *Am. Heart J.* **77**, 295
Harris, L. C., Rodin, A. E. and Nghiem, Q. X. (1968). Idiopathic non-obstructive cardiomyopathy in children. *Am. J. Cardiol.* **21**, 153
Hastrecter, A. R. (1968) Endocardial fibroelastosis. In *Heart Disease in Infants, Children, and Adolescents*. Eds A. J. Moss and F. H. Adams, Baltimore, Md: Williams and Wilkins
Kibrick, S. (1966). In *Year Book of Paediatrics 1965–6*, p. 262. Chicago: Year Book Medical Publishers

Noren, G. R., Adams, P. Jr. and Anderson, R. C. (1963). Positive skin reactivity to mumps viral antigen in endocardial fibroelastosis. *J. Pediat.* **62**, 604

Rosenberg, H. S. and McNamara, D. G. (1964). Acute myocarditis in infancy and childhood. *Prog. cardiovasc. Dis.* **7**, 179

Endomyocardial fibrosis

Abrahams, D. G. (1962). Endomyocardial fibrosis of the right ventricle. *Q. Jl Med.* **31**, 1

D'Arbela, P. G., Mutazindwa, T., Patel, A. K. and Somers, K. (1972). Survival after first presentation with endomyocardial fibrosis. *Br. Heart J.* **34**, 403

Parry, E. H. O. (1964). Endomyocardial fibrosis. In *Cardiomyopathies*, Ciba Symposium. London: Churchill; Boston, Mass.: Little, Brown

Shillingford, J. P. and Somers, K. (1960). Clinical and haemodynamic patterns in endomyocardial fibrosis. *Br. Heart J.* **22**, 546

Hypertrophic cardiomyopathy

Clark, C. E., Henry, W. L. and Epstein, S. E. (1973). Familial prevalence and genetic transmission of idiopathic hypertrophic subaortic stenosis. *New Engl. J. Med.* **289**, 709

Hopf, R., Kober, G., Bussmann, W. D., Keller, M. and Petersen, Y. (1980). Treatment of hypertrophic obstructive cardiomyopathy with verapamil. *Br. Heart J.* **42**, 35

Rossen, R. M., Goodman, D. J., Ingham, R. E. and Popp, R. L. (1974). Echocardiographic criteria in the diagnosis of idiopathic hypertrophic subaortic stenosis. *Circulation* **50**, 747

Shand, D. G., Sell, C. G. and Oates, J. A. (1971). Hypertrophic obstructive cardiomyopathy in an infant. Propranolol therapy for 3 years. *New Engl. J. Med.* **285**, 843

Swan, D. A., Bell, B., Oakley, C. M. and Goodwin, J. (1971). Analysis of symptomatic course and prognosis and treatment of hypertrophic obstructive cardiomyopathy. *Br. Heart J.* **33**, 671

Cardiac tumours

Simcha, A., Wells, B. G., Tynan, M. J. and Waterston, D. J. (1971). Primary cardiac tumours in childhood. *Archs Dis. Childh.* **46**, 508

Van der Hanwaert, L. G. (1971). Cardiac tumours in infancy and childhood. *Br. Heart J.* **33**, 125

Pericardial diseases

Cayler, G. G., Taybi, H., Riley, H. D. Jr. and Simon, J. L. (1963). Pericarditis with effusion in infants and children. *J. Pediat.* **63**, 264

Jordan S. C. and Haycock, G. B. (1979). Chronic pericardial constriction with effusion in childhood. *Archs Dis. Childh.* **54**, 11

Plouth, W. H. Jr., Waldman, R. A., Wachner, R. A., Braunwald, N. and Braunwald, E. (1964). Protein losing enteropathy secondary to constrictive pericarditis in children. *Pediatrics, Springfield* **34**, 634

Simcha, A. and Taylor, J. F. N. (1971). Constrictive pericarditis in childhood. *Archs Dis. Childh.* **46**, 515

CHAPTER 20

The Heart in Systemic Disease

SYSTEMIC HYPERTENSION IN INFANTS AND CHILDREN

Measurement of the blood pressure should be part of the routine examination of every child. Details of accurate measurement are given on page 21.

The Brompton study has shown that on the second day of life the mean systolic pressure is 70 mmHg and then rises gradually over the next six weeks to a level of 93 mmHg. Thereafter the pressure remains remarkably level at 95 mmHg until two years of age. Other studies from Miami, Muscatine and Rochester in the USA show that this level is maintained until the age of six years after which it begins to rise gradually again to reach levels of 125 mmHg by 16 years of age.

The definition of hypertension must be related to age. A systolic pressure greater than 115 mmHg is hypertension in a child between 6 weeks and 6 years, whereas 150 mmHg is hypertension in a boy of 16 years.

The National Heart, Lung and Blood Institute task force on blood pressure (1977) gives percentile charts for systolic and diastolic pressures for girls and boys. Under the age of puberty there is little difference between the sexes, but by the age of 18 years the 95th percentile in boys is about 10 mmHg higher than in girls. Under the age of 6 years the blood pressure remained more or less level at 78–113 systolic and 48–79 diastolic (5th phase) for 5th to 95th percentiles. Thereafter the systolic pressure rose linearly to 18 years, but the diastolic pressure plateaued over the age of 12. The figures at 18 years were $\dfrac{102-145}{63-95}$ for girls and $\dfrac{105-155}{60-95}$ for boys.

Hypertension most commonly occurs in association with glomerulonephritis and with coarctation of the aorta but other causes are listed below.

Renal	Acute glomerulonephritis
	Chronic glomerulonephritis
	Chronic pyelonephritis
	Polycystic kidneys
	Wilm's tumour
	Hypoplastic kidney
	Collagen diseases such as polyarteritis nodosa and systemic lupus erythematosus
Vascular	Coarctation of the aorta
	Abnormalities of the renal artery
	Thrombosis of the renal artery or vein
Endocrine	Phaeochromocytoma
	Neuroblastoma
	Adrenogenital syndrome
	Cushing's disease
	Primary aldosteronism
Drugs	Cortisone ACTH
	Antidepressants

Clinical presentation

Hypertension may be discovered on routine examination and be symptomless. When symptoms occur they are essentially due to complications of the disease. Headache and vomiting, the most constant symptoms, are due to cerebral oedema and raised intracranial pressure, which may also cause fits, hemiplegia, ophthalmoplegia, visual defects and clouding of consciousness. Breathlessness on exertion and cough or breathlessness at night are due to left ventricular failure. Nocturia and polyuria or oliguria are due to renal involvement. Cerebral or subarrachnoid haemorrhage may occur catastrophically, as may dissecting aneurysm of the aorta.

Examination of the ocular fundi is important prognostically. The first signs are narrowing and irregularity of the arterioles with decreased arteriovenous diameter ratio. Haemorrhages, exudates and papilloedema indicate a poor prognosis, likely to be measured in weeks or months.

The cardiac impulse will usually show some degree of left ventricular enlargement and either the third or the fourth heart sound is accentuated. The former sound suggests left ventricular failure and the latter left atrial hypertrophy occurring when the disease has been present for several months at least. Normal splitting of the second heart sound is lost in the presence of left ventricular failure and may be replaced by 'reversed' splitting—left ventricular ejection may delay aortic closure beyond pulmonary closure so that splitting is heard on expiration.

Examination of the abdomen should include palpation of kidney size and gentle palpation for the presence of suprarenal or other tumour. (Pressure on a phaeochromocytoma may precipitate a hypertensive episode.) Auscultation over the kidneys both at the front and at the back should be performed. A single arterial stenosis frequently causes a bruit.

After physical examination the patient's urine should be examined. Acute nephritis may present with hypertension rather than oliguria and haematuria, but examination of the urine for albumen, red cells and casts will confirm the diagnosis. In chronic glomerulonephritis and chronic pyelonephritis (particularly if there has been no acute episode) hypertension is frequently the finding which leads to the detection of the disease, and in renovascular disease hypertension is virtually the only indication. Hypertension may occur in polycystic renal disease before there is obvious renal involvement and in childhood and adolescence is frequently asymptomatic.

Systemic hypertension complicating intracranial lesions usually only occurs when there is raised intracranial pressure and other symptoms will precede it, but difficulties may arise in differentiating this situation from cerebral symptoms of encephalopathy resulting from severe hypertension.

An adrenalin- or noradrenalin-secreting adrenal medullary tumour (phaeochromocytoma) may present with fixed or spasmodic hypertension. In the latter instance, hypertensive attacks may be accompanied by pallor, sweating, tachycardia, chest pain, abdominal pain and headache. Older children complain of a feeling of tension or anxiety and there may be diarrhoea and vomiting. Differentiation of these symptoms from functional disturbances is made by the absence of precipitating emotional cause and the intense sweating. About 20 per cent of the tumours occur outside the adrenal glands, in proximity to the aorta, bladder, heart or base of the skull. Hyperglycaemia and glycosuria occur when the tumour secretes a high proportion of adrenalin.

The features of Cushing's syndrome are obvious and hypertension is mild. Cohn's syndrome is excessively rare and hypertension is again mild. The diagnosis is usually suspected from the low serum potassium (below 3.0 mmol/litre) and raised sodium (over 143 mmol/litre).

Investigation

Hypertension in the presence of symptoms or of advanced retinopathy should be regarded as a medical emergency and investigation planned and started at once. Since essential hypertension is uncommon and the prognosis poor unless a treatable condition is detected, no effort should be spared to find a cause.

Urine examination

Proteinuria and small numbers of red cells may result from renal damage due to the hypertension as well as from intrinsic renal disease. Heavy proteinuria with cellular and granular casts favour chronic glomerulonephritis. Numerous white cells, pus cells and bacteria suggest chronic pyelonephritis, but even in their absence the urine should be cultured. In addition a 24-hour collection of urine for catecholamine estimation should be made as soon as possible since treatment (particularly with methyldopa) interferes with the test. Different measurements are used in some centres but the most widely used estimation is that of vanillyl mandelic acid (VMA). In the presence of a phaeochromocytoma the results are usually excessively high but since catecholamine excretion may be irregular two or more estimations may be required.

Rogitine test

Hypertension due to excessive catecholamine excretion responds rapidly to the intravenous injection of phentolamine mesylate (Rogitine) 0.1 mg/kg intravenously. A fall of systolic pressure of 40 or more mmHg or of 20 mmHg in the diastolic pressure is considered a positive result.

Electrocardiography

Even when the hypertension is of recent origin the electrocardiogram usually shows an increase in R wave voltage in left ventricular leads, and when left ventricular failure occurs as a complication there is ST segment depression or, less frequently, T wave inversion in these leads.

Chest radiography

Chest radiography is useful in determining heart size and indicating pulmonary venous hypertension.

Blood urea

Blood urea estimation is useful as a prognostic guide. In severe hypertension the blood urea is often slightly or moderately raised, but a value over 120 mg/100 ml (20 mmol/l) is suggestive of primary renal disease.

Blood electrolytes

A low serum potassium (under 3.2 mmol/l) and a raised serum sodium are suggestive of hyperaldosteronism, but may occur as a secondary finding in renal hypertension. Aldosterone antagonists (spironolactone) correct both the electrolyte abnormalities and the hypertension in primary aldosteronism, but have no effect on the hypertension of secondary aldosteronism.

Corticosteroid estimations

Corticosteroid estimations in urine and blood are only indicated where there are clinical findings suggestive of Cushing's syndrome.

Intravenous pyelography

Intravenous pyelography is probably still the most useful specialized renal investigation (high dose infusion pyelography is used when renal function is poor). It may show obvious structural defects, such as hydronephrosis, polycystic kidneys or absence of function on one side, but, provided early films are taken, the size of the kidneys can be determined and the thickness of the renal cortex estimated. Unilateral renal artery stenosis produces a characteristic triad of delayed excretion, higher density (due to increased water reabsorption) and a smaller capacity renal pelvis compared with the normal side.

Aortography

Aortography is probably justified in all cases even when the pyelogram is normal. Renal artery stenosis is demonstrated and, in addition, a phaeochromocytoma in or near the suprarenals is demonstrated by a 'blush' of increased vessels. Some care is required in interpreting apparent arterial stenoses when these are mild, since they may not be functionally important.

Adrenal and renal vein catheterization

Adrenal and renal vein catheterization is sometimes employed to obtain samples for estimation of catecholamine and of renin, respectively, but these techniques are not at the moment standard and adrenal vein catheterization is virtually impossible in small children. An adrenal venogram may be the best angiographic method of demonstrating a suprarenal cortical tumour.

Renography

The renogram is the pattern of excretion of radioactive substances, usually ^{131}I Hippuran, by the kidney. Counters are placed over both kidneys and counting performed following intravenous injection of the tracer. There is normally a rapid increase in counting rate to a maximum at about 5 minutes and then a gradual decay over 30–40 minutes. Renal artery stenosis produces a delayed peak and a slow fall.

Scintillation renography

Scintillation renography is performed using a gamma camera or similar scanning device over the renal area following the injection of a tracer (technetium-99) which is taken up in the renal tubules. Functional defects (for example, tumours, cysts or areas served by an obstructed arterial branch) give a lower count than the normal kidney.

Renal biopsy

Renal biopsy is probably the most sensitive way of detecting glomerulonephritis and may also be helpful in detecting systemic diseases such as disseminated lupus erythematosus. In many cases it will be necessary to biopsy both kidneys, particularly if nephrectomy is contemplated.

Treatment

Where a definite underlying cause is found, this clearly needs to be dealt with. Nephrectomy is indicated in strictly unilateral pyelonephritis with a shrunken kidney and in unilateral renal artery stenosis when this is not amenable to repair or bypass. If no treatable cause is found, the hypertension has to be controlled with drugs.

Drugs

The beta-blocking drugs such as propranolol and the centrally acting drug methyldopa are the most commonly used main drugs. Thiazide diuretics are useful adjuvant therapy and the vasodilator drugs hydrallazine and prazosin are used in patients resistant to other forms of therapy and those with poor renal function, since they increase renal blood flow.

Propranolol is given in a dose of about 0.5–1 mg/kg three times daily initially, and the dose increased if necessary. Serious side-effects are few in children, but cold hands and irritability are reported by a few patients. If adequate control is not obtained with doses of about 2 mg/kg three times daily, with or without a thiazide diuretic, methyldopa or hydrallazine should be used in addition.

Methyldopa is started in a dose of about 20 mg/kg per day, given in three or four doses and increased every two to three days. If response is inadequate a small dose of thiazide diuretic or propranolol can be added. Methyldopa frequently causes drowsiness, nasal congestion and postural hypotension.

Methyldopa worsens hypertension due to phaeochromocytoma and in this situation the alpha-sympathetic blocking drugs—phentolamine and phenoxybenzamine—should be used, coupled with a beta-receptor blocker such as propranolol. A rise in pressure in a patient with hypertension being treated with methyldopa should arouse a strong suspicion of phaeochromocytoma.

Hydrallazine is given in a dose of 0.5 mg/kg three times daily. Higher doses can be used, but they may produce a high output state (which can be controlled with a beta-blocker) and a lupus erythematosus-like syndrome.

Hypertensive crises such as encephalopathy are best treated initially with intravenous frusemide 10–40 mg followed by intravenous methyldopa 10 mg/kg every 6 hours. The fall in pressure is slightly less dramatic but easier to handle than that produced by intravenous ganglion-blocking drugs. Sodium nitroprusside given as a slow intravenous drip has also been used, starting with about 0.5–1 μg/kg per minute.

Prognosis

When a correctable lesion, such as phaeochromocytoma or unilateral renal disease, is detected and removed prior to the development of complications the prognosis is excellent. If delay occurs, hypertensive changes in the kidneys may result in the postoperative blood pressure not returning to normal. In hypertension complicating advanced bilateral renal disease or systemic disease the hypertension can usually be controlled and the prognosis is that of the underlying disease. Where no underlying cause can be found, adequate control of blood pressure is achieved in about half the patients in childhood and the disease is arrested. In the other half there is progression at a rate inversely proportional to the degree of control and the patient succumbs from renal failure, cerebral haemorrhage or cardiac failure in decreasing order of frequency. The spectrum is too wide for survival figures to have much meaning.

HYPERKINETIC CIRCULATORY STATES

There is a group of conditions in which the cardiac output is increased by a tachycardia and a raised venous filling pressure. There is dilatation of the skin and muscle vessels. The arterial pulse is collapsing and capillary pulsation may be seen. In children, anaemia is the commonest and most important cause of such a high cardiac output, but it may also occur in association with arteriovenous aneurysms and shunts, and in thyrotoxicosis.

Anaemia

Heart failure does not usually occur until the haemoglobin in the blood falls below 6.0 grams per cent (g/100 ml), but in children who already have heart failure due to a congenital heart lesion, a milder degree of anaemia may make the heart failure worse and such children improve considerably when the anaemia is corrected.

In severe chronic anaemia from any cause the circulation is hyperkinetic. The patient has bounding pulses with a high pulse pressure and warm extremities. The heart is increased in size with a forceful left ventricle and the neck veins are distended. A basal ejection systolic murmur due to an increased flow through the pulmonary and aortic valves is heard. Congestive heart failure may follow with oedema and enlargement of the liver.

The cause of the anaemia should be determined first, but if it is causing heart failure, blood transfusion is usually necessary. A transfusion of packed red cells (20 ml/kg) should be given over a period of 8 hours. Intravenous frusemide should be given at the start of the transfusion and the patient carefully observed. If there is any evidence of pulmonary oedema developing (as shown by a rise in respiratory rate, cough or restlessness) then a further dose of frusemide should be given. Further transfusion of the same amount of blood may be given over the next 8 hours if indicated.

Arteriovenous aneurysm

In a congenital cirsoid aneurysm, arteries and veins are in direct communication with one another. An impressive continuous machinery murmur may be heard over the aneurysm and will disappear if the arteries supplying it can be compressed. When the aneurysm is in the cerebral circulation a murmur can be heard by listening over the eyeball or over the skull. If the aneurysm is in a limb, the affected limb will be larger and the skin feel warmer than the normal one. When the aneurysm is large, all the pulses are collapsing, the heart is enlarged and a systolic ejection murmur is audible at the base of the heart. Heart failure may occur and it is important to appreciate that there is an extracardiac cause for the heart failure in these patients, otherwise unnecessary cardiac investigations may be carried out. The heart failure resolves when the aneurysm has been treated.

Hyperthyroidism

Hyperthyroidism is rare in childhood. There is a high cardiac output with tachycardia, bounding pulses and an increased pulse pressure. The heart gradually enlarges and a systolic murmur is audible at the cardiac apex or in the pulmonary area.

The thyrotoxicosis should be controlled by drug therapy and the cardiac state then improves. If heart failure is present when the patient is first seen, then digoxin should also be given to control this. Newborn infants of mothers with thyrotoxicosis may develop heart failure and require treatment with digoxin as well as drugs to control the hyperthyroidism.

HYPOTHYROIDISM

Cretinism and juvenile hypothyroidism are both rare. In the cretin, symptoms begin after the second week of life, the infant feeds poorly, is inactive and constipated and later appears apathetic. As the child grows it is noticed that the eyelids are prominent, the tongue is large and the skin dry and wrinkled. In the older child with juvenile myxoedema there is apathy, dullness and growth retardation. The skin is dry and there is an increase in subcutaneous fat.

There may be no cardiac symptoms but the heart action is quiet and slow. In severe cases heart failure occurs. The radiograph shows a normal or slightly enlarged heart. The electrocardiogram shows distinctive changes (*Figure 20.1*). There is slow sinus rhythm, the P–R interval is often prolonged, QRS complexes are of low voltage and the T waves are flattened or inverted. The Q–T interval is prolonged. The electrocardiogram is of value in making the diagnosis; if it is normal, cretinism or myxoedema are unlikely. After treatment with thyroid, the electrocardiogram returns to

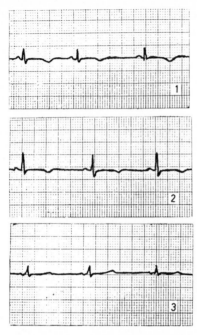

Figure 20.1. Hypothyroidism. Electrocardiogram of an 8-year-old girl. There is slow sinus rhythm (56 per minute in lead 2), inverted T waves and a prolonged (0.5 second) Q–T interval

normal and changes in the electrocardiogram may be used to assess the adequacy of the dose of thyroid being given.

INFANTILE HYPERCALCAEMIA AND THE HEART

The association of severe infantile hypercalcaemia with a curious facies and with cardiac murmurs was reported by Schlesinger, Butler and Black in 1952. About ten years later reports began to appear (Beuren and co-workers, 1964) of an apparently unrelated syndrome of curious facial appearance and supra-aortic stenosis, sometimes occurring in families. The identity of these two syndromes was established by Black and Bonham Carter (1963) who discovered that patients who had originally been seen in infancy with severe hypercalcaemia were presenting later with signs of aortic stenosis. Soon, other cardiac abnormalities were added to the syndrome. The relationship to infantile hypercalcaemia was originally explained by postulating that the hypercalcaemia caused the deposition of calcium in the supra-aortic region which caused fibrosis and stenosis. However, more than half the patients with supra-aortic stenosis give no history to suggest infantile hypercalcaemia. The possibility of there being fetal hypercalcaemia has also been explored, but there is no proof of this theory. It is probably best to consider the facies, the hypercalcaemia and the cardiac abnormalities as variable parts of a somewhat loosely connected syndrome, the possible components of which are given in *Table 20.1*.

TABLE 20.1
The hypercalcaemic syndrome

Genetic aspects	Family history in about 25 per cent
Facies	Epicanthic folds
	Hypertelorism
	Snub nose
	Carp mouth
	Low-set ears
Dental	Hypoplastic primary dentition
	Serrated secondary dentition
	Missing first premolars
Neurological	Mental retardation
	Ataxia
	Personality defect
Hypercalcaemia	Clinical
	Biochemical
	Latent
Cardiac	Supra-aortic stenosis
	Aortic valve stenosis
	Peripheral pulmonary artery stenoses
	Coarctation of aorta
	Atrial septal defect
	Peripheral arterial stenoses
	Ventricular septal defect
	Hypertension

Supra-aortic stenosis

Although a few isolated cases have been reported, most patients with supra-aortic stenosis have some of the features of the hypercalcaemic syndrome. Symptoms are unusual in early childhood but breathlessness, pain and syncope on effort occur as with aortic valve stenosis, and the physical signs are similar except that an ejection click is not heard (*see* p. 113).

Peripheral pulmonary artery stenosis

Peripheral pulmonary artery stenosis is usually detected on routine examination and symptoms are unusual. As well as occurring as part of the hypercalcaemic syndrome, it may occur in congenital rubella and in association with other cardiac lesions, particularly Fallot's tetralogy. Characteristically, the lesions are multiple and give rise to a loud murmur heard over the lungs which is mainly systolic but extends into diastole. When the stenosis is severe there is right ventricular hypertrophy and the pulmonary element of the second heart sound is loud, unless the stenosis is near the pulmonary valve

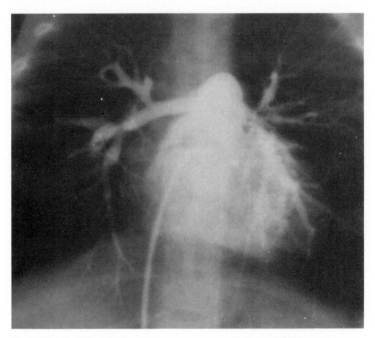

Figure 20.2. Peripheral pulmonary artery stenoses. Patient with severe infantile hypercalcaemia and typical facies. There are narrowings on the origins of all branches of the right pulmonary artery, with poststenotic dilation. Coarctation was also present

when the second sound is quiet (due to the small amount of blood between the pulmonary valve and the stenosis).

Chest radiographs may show poststenotic dilatation or variation in vascularity in different parts of the lungs. Electrocardiograms show mild or moderate right ventricular hypertrophy. Gradients of from 10 to 80 mmHg may be recorded across the stenoses, and the lesions are shown by angiography (*Figure 20.2*). Owing to the multiplicity of lesions, surgical treatment is not possible. Serial studies have shown that the lesions do not tend to progress.

GLYCOGEN STORAGE DISEASE AFFECTING THE HEART

Glycogen storage disease affecting the heart is a rare metabolic disorder, the cause of which is unknown. Large amounts of glycogen are deposited in the muscle cells of the heart. Symptoms usually develop soon after birth. The infants feed poorly and develop tachycardia with rapid respirations followed later by cardiac failure. They have a broad forehead, a broad bridge of the nose and a protruding tongue. Their muscles are weak and they often lie in the 'frog leg' position. There is marked enlargement of the heart and murmurs may or may not be present but are of no help in diagnosis.

A mild and self-limiting variety may be seen in infants of diabetic mothers.

Investigation

The electrocardiogram shows a normal axis, a short P–R interval and either left or combined ventricular hypertrophy. The radiograph shows generalized cardiac enlargement and the lung fields may show pulmonary congestion.

Muscle biopsy confirms the diagnosis by showing more than 1 per cent glycogen net weight. The increased glycogen storage can also be seen in the muscle.

Prognosis

It is rare for anyone to survive the first year of life.

Treatment

Treatment is supportive only. Digoxin and diuretics will help in most cases but if obstruction of the left ventricle is demonstrated, digoxin should not be used.

FRIEDREICH'S ATAXIA

Friedreich's ataxia is a rare, familial, inherited disease in which there is degeneration of the posterior columns and the spinocerebellar and pyramidal tracts of the spinal cord.

Symptoms are usually present by 10 years of age. The gait is broad based, there is inco-ordination of movement and speech is impaired. Knee and ankle jerks are lost and there is loss of vibration and position sense but pain and temperature sensation remain.

Cardiac abnormalities are present in the majority of patients. The heart is normal in size or moderately enlarged and there may be no murmurs or soft systolic murmurs which are of no help in diagnosis. The electrocardiogram shows inverted T waves in leads AVF, V_5 and V_6. Dysrhythmias are common as the condition progresses. Patients may die from heart failure in adult life or suddenly, presumably from dysrhythmias. The cause of death is usually cardiac.

Treatment

There is no specific treatment and the heart failure and dysrhythmias should be treated in the usual way.

TURNER'S SYNDROME

Patients with Turner's syndrome are short of stature, have webbing of the neck, a low hairline, cubitus valgus, a broad chest with wide apart nipples and sexual infantilism. Pitting oedema of the hands and feet is often present in infancy and then gradually disappears. Chromosomal studies have shown that there is a deficiency of an X chromosome.

Coarctation of the aorta is the commonest cardiovascular lesion but aortic stenosis is also frequently found. Ventricular septal defect has also been observed.

The management of the cardiac lesions is the same as in normal patients.

NOONAN'S SYNDROME

Children with the facial and skeletal characteristics of Turner's syndrome but with normal chromosomes (Noonan or Ulrich syndrome) have a high incidence of heart disease of which pulmonary stenosis, infundibular stenosis and hypertrophic cardiomyopathy are the commonest. One curious feature of the patients with pulmonary stenosis is the appearance of left axis deviation in the electrocardiogram.

LENTIGINOSIS

A high incidence of hypertrophic cardiomyopathy has been reported. There appears to be some overlap with Noonan's syndrome as some of the reported cases have had similar skeletal abnormalities. Cardiac tumours, including myxoma, have also been reported.

GARGOYLISM

Gargoylism is an inherited disorder of connective tissue in which the mucopolysaccharide metabolism is abnormal.

The facies are grotesque, the head is large with hypertelorism and the nasal bridge is depressed. The mouth is held open and the tongue protrudes. There is kyphosis and a broad chest. The hands are held in a claw-like position. Corneal opacities may be present.

The cardiac disorders involve the valves of the heart and the coronary arteries. The valves have shiny nodules along their free margins and the chordae tendineae are shortened. This results in valvular incompetence. The mitral and tricuspid valves are most commonly affected. There is thickening of the intima of the coronary arteries, causing narrowing.

MARFAN'S SYNDROME

Marfan's syndrome is an inherited disorder in which the dominant gene is transmitted by either sex. There is a widespread disorder of connective tissue, the exact nature of which is not understood.

Severe cases may be suspected at birth, the infant being particularly long and thin with poor musculature. The child is slow to thrive and is easily tired and complains of vague pains in the limbs. The pubis-to-sole measurement is greater than the pubis-to-vertex measurement. The arm span is greater than the height. There is hypermobility of the joints. The palate is high and arched, the skull is dolichocephalic and there is pectus excavatum. The eyesight is poor, there being a high degree of myopia associated with dislocation of the lenses.

About half the patients have some cardiac abnormality. There is degeneration of the media of the aorta which results in aneurysmal dilatation. Less frequently the pulmonary artery is affected. The aortic ring is dilated and aortic incompetence develops, often of a severe degree. There may also be dilatation of the mitral ring with mitral incompetence, or the mitral valve may be floppy with redundant cusps.

Radiology will demonstrate dilatation of the ascending aorta when there is aneurysm formation. The electrocardiogram shows evidence of left ventricular hypertrophy when there is aortic or mitral incompetence.

Many patients die in infancy from infections. Later in life, death is due to heart failure or rupture or dissection of an aortic aneurysm.

Treatment is largely supportive. Surgery has been carried out in efforts to prevent aortic rupture but the widespread abnormality of the tissues makes it difficult and hazardous.

BIBLIOGRAPHY AND REFERENCES

Systemic hypertension in infants and children

Loggie, J. M. H. (1969a). Hypertension in children and adolescents. I: causes and diagnostic studies. *J. Pediat.* **74**, 331

Loggie, J. M. H. (1969b). Hypertension in children and adolescents. II: drug therapy. *J. Pediat.* **74**, 640

Londe, S. (1966). Blood pressure in children as determined under office conditions. *Clin. Pediat.* **5**, 71

Moss, A. J. and Adams, F. H. (1962). *Problems of Blood Pressure in Childhood.* Springfield, Illinois: Charles C. Thomas

Nadas, A. S. (1963). *Pediatric Cardiology*, 2nd ed., p. 773. Philadelphia and London: W. B. Saunders

National Heart, Lung and Blood Institute (1977). Task force on blood pressure control in children. *Pediatrics* **59**, 797.

Hypercalcaemia syndrome

Barold, S. S., Linhart, J. W. and Samet, P. (1968). Coarctation of the aorta with unusual facies and mental retardation. *Ann. intern. Med.* **69**, 103

Beuren, A. J., Schulze, C., Eberle, P., Hamjanz, D. and Apetz, J. (1964). Syndrome of supravalvular aortic stenosis, peripheral pulmonary artery stenosis, mental retardation and similar facial appearances. *Am. J. Cardiol.* **13**, 471

Black, J. A. and Bonham Carter, R. E. (1963). Association between aortic stenosis and facies of severe infantile hypercalcaemia. *Lancet* **2, 745**

Hartmann, A. F., Elliott, L. P and Goldring, D. (1965). The course of peripheral pulmonary artery stenosis in children. *J. Pediat.* **73**, 212

Joseph, M. C. (1964). Sequelae of infantile hypercalcaemia. *Develop. Med. child Neurol.* **6**, 419

McDonald, A. H., Gerlis, L. M. and Somerville, J. (1969). Familial arteriopathy with associated pulmonary and systemic arterial stenoses. *Br. Heart J.* **31**, 375

Schlesinger, B. E., Butler, N. R. and Black, N. A. (1952). Chronic hypercalcaemia with osteosclerosis, renal failure and retardation. *Helv. paediat. Acta* **7**, 335

Friedreich's ataxia

Hewer, R. L. (1969). The heart in Friedreich's ataxia. *Br. Heart J.* **31**, 5

Gargoylism

Krovetz, L. J., Lorincz, A. E. and Scheibler, G. L. (1965). Cardiovascular manifestations of the Hurler syndrome. Hemodynamic and angiographic observations in 15 patients. *Circulation* **31**, 132

Noonan's syndrome

Siggers, D. C. and Polani, P. E. (1972). Congenital heart disease in male and female subjects with somatic features of Turner's syndrome and normal sex chromosomes (Ulrich and related syndromes). *Br. Heart J.* **34**, 41

Lentiginosis

Somerville, J. and Bonham Carter, R. E. (1972). The heart in lentiginosis. *Br. Heart J.* **34**, 58

CHAPTER 21

Social Problems of Congenital Heart Disease

Over the last ten years the management of heart disease in children has become much more scientific, the diagnostic tests are more sophisticated and surgical treatment has advanced greatly. Much work, expense and discussion are involved in deciding the best way to treat the heart defects which are present. It is important nevertheless not to neglect other aspects of child care and to remember the problems of the whole family when a child has congenital heart disease.

THE CHILD'S FAMILY

Adequate time must be given to explain the child's heart condition to the parents, who are usually shocked when they first learn that a heart defect is present and often do not understand or remember the first explanation which the doctor gives. He must be prepared to repeat it all a second or third time and allow the parents to ask any questions which have occurred to them. It is important that the family doctor, paediatrician and paediatric cardiologist all speak in the same terms to the parents, otherwise they will become confused and worried. A 'hole in the heart', a 'leak between the two sides' and 'a gap in the heart muscle', three terms used to explain a ventricular septal defect, may not be realized by the parents to refer to the same abnormality. Family doctors, paediatricians and cardiologists should therefore inform each other exactly what they have told the mother and father.

Parents always try to find some explanation for the heart disease and there must be some discussion about the possible causes. It is important to tell them that very often we do not know the cause, but that it is not their fault. A mother will so often remember something that has happened during her pregnancy and blame herself for the child's illness. Fears like this can only be allayed by frank and open discussion. Apley, Barbour and Westmacott (1967) have shown that it is much more common for both parents to attend the out-patient clinic when the child has heart disease than when there are other disorders of childhood.

The risks to further pregnancies should be indicated to both parents so that they are aware there is a good chance that a subsequent child will be normal.

When the child is severely handicapped, there is a great strain on the parents, particularly the mother. Their lives are restricted, their sleep frequently disturbed and they have to try to meet the demands of other healthy siblings. The family needs all the support that can be given from relatives, social workers and doctors to avoid total disruption of family life. Fortunately, now that more heart lesions can be helped by surgery these problems are usually temporary and one sees the benefits that successful surgery brings, not only to the child but also to his parents and brothers and sisters.

THE CHILD

Exercise restriction

Many children with heart disease may be allowed to lead a normal life and the doctor must make sure that such children are not overprotected. Parents must be assured that exercise will not damage the child's heart and shorten his life. Mild lesions are compatible with a normal exercise tolerance and in moderate and severe lesions the child may be allowed to join in physical activities and he will limit his own exercise. Children with the same heart lesion will vary in their activities just like normal children and this must be recognized.

The exceptions to this advice are lesions which may be associated with sudden death on exertion. These are aortic stenosis, obstructive cardiomyopathy, prolonged QT interval syndrome (p. 305), sinus node dysfunction (p. 304). Nowadays such patients are recognized and treated when possible but in patients with aortic stenosis, for example, the lesion is progressive and symptoms may occur while the child is waiting for surgery.

Education

Sometimes parents reject a handicapped child and he then receives inadequate care. It is important to appreciate the reasons for lack of care and deal with them sympathetically.

Whenever possible the child should attend an ordinary school, but there must be clear instructions to the teaching staff regarding physical activity. It is now the aim to correct heart lesions before the child starts school whenever possible so that he can then integrate like a normal child. Often children with symptoms are well enough to attend ordinary schools if transport is provided to and from school to relieve them of a tiring journey.

Parents and teachers are naturally concerned about the effect cyanosis may have on the child's development and the fear that he may be permanently mentally retarded. It must be stressed that delay in walking and motor development is associated with the tiredness, cyanosis and breathlessness, but they must be reassured that the child can be allowed to take part in physical activities and that this will not damage his heart or brain. Although there is a wide variation in the range of intelligence in children with congenital heart disease the mean I.Q. falls within the normal range (Linde *et al.*, 1967). The slowness in development is often associated with tiredness and an inability to explore and learn in the normal way. Following successful surgery that child will catch up physically and mentally.

If the child is too blue or breathless to enjoy an ordinary school, then he may be happier and less frustrated at a school for handicapped children. In rare instances home teaching is required because the child is not well enough to travel. In country areas there may not be a suitable school near enough for the child and in such cases home teaching is preferable to enforced residence at a school for the handicapped. It is our view that residential accommodation should be reserved for children whose parents are unable to care for them adequately at home. It is bad enough for a child to have symptoms from congenital heart disease without also being deprived of the love and care of his parents against their will.

Immunization

Clinic doctors and general practitioners often refuse to immunize children with congenital heart disease. In fact, there are no contra-indications to carrying out immunization procedures in the usual way. Children with increased pulmonary blood flow are at risk from intercurrent chest infections associated with measles and whooping cough and measures to prevent these illnesses are advised.

Admission to hospital

When it is necessary for a child to be admitted to hospital there must be a full discussion with the parents and they must know what is going to happen. Uncertainty causes unnecessary worry and can be avoided. If a child is going to be admitted, the parents should be given some idea of the time of admission and reassured if there is no urgency about admission—otherwise they will be worried by delay. When there are waiting lists it is preferable to go on seeing the patient at out-patient clinics so that he is under regular supervision.

The mother should come into hospital with the child if possible, or be allowed to stay with him all day. Many children who are admitted for investigation will have to enter hospital again for an operation and it is important that any undue upset is avoided. A little thought and organization can avoid upsetting the child. For example, blood for haemoglobin estimation and cross-matching can be taken at the time of cardiac catheterization, so avoiding venepuncture. Many children come for admission a second time with more confidence and if possible should be admitted to the same ward with the same nursing staff.

Investigation

The necessity for invasive investigations must be clearly described to the parents and the risks outlined. The risk in the newborn infant is 2 per cent if hypoplastic left heart is excluded and in older children is less than 0.5 per cent.

Operation

When operation is advised, the necessity for it and its risks must be fully explained to the parents. In particular, they must be told the prognosis if operation is not carried out. Both parents should be in agreement about consent for operation and be given adequate time to make their decision. We are often faced with recommending an operation when the child is symptom-free because the risks of surgery before secondary complications occur are much lower. The parents must be made aware of this in case their child is the one in a hundred who does not survive the operation.

Parents should be shown the intensive care ward and when it is expected that the child will require a ventilator, the parents should be told in advance. If they expect to see intravenous infusions and chest drains some of the shock of the intensive care ward will be prevented. The period when the child is in the intensive care ward is often more traumatic for the parents than the child.

The age of operation is important. Children below the age of about 8 years are less likely to worry about death and accept operation more readily than older children. As the child approaches his teens he is more aware of the magnitude of a heart operation and much more frightened. It is better whenever possible to operate early, before school age, making sure that the child has full support from his parents while he is in hospital.

Liaison with all personnel caring for the child

Parents, general practitioners, paediatricians, school medical officers, nurses, teachers and social workers are all concerned with the welfare of a child with congenital heart disease and it is important that all of them are aware of the best way of treating a particular child. They should know the results of investigations and when operation is required and be advised about the child's activities at all times. It is not easy to keep everyone in the picture, but if conflicting opinions are given to parents, unnecessary anxiety results and it is often the child who suffers. It is often valuable for the doctor to have the teacher's report about a child's behaviour or symptoms. Some parents minimize a child's symptoms while others will magnify them and an independent opinion often helps in deciding about surgery.

Self-help for children and parents

As with many handicaps, parents frequently have a sense of isolation and helplessness which can be improved by meeting parents of children with similar problems. Many cardiac centres have such groups associated with them and they may also be able to give practical help with problems such as 'babysitting'.

Pregnancy and contraception

Since pregnancy is now commoner at a younger age, advice must be given to patients. Patients who have had defects such as ventricular septal defects, atrial septal defects and patent ductus closed, tolerate pregnancy normally. The milder defects do not cause problems. The main hazard is the presence of pulmonary vascular disease and uncorrectable cyanotic congenital heart disease. The mortality in pulmonary vascular disease is in the region of 50 per cent (McCaffrey and Dunn, 1964). Oral contraceptives are contra-indicated because of risks of thromboembolism, hypertension and fluid retention. Intrauterine devices may cause bacteraemia. Tubal ligation is the most effective method for preventing pregnancy in older women with inoperable heart disease, but there are great ethical problems to be considered before it can be advised in a teenage girl. If pregnancy does occur, early therapeutic abortion should be advised.

CONGENITAL HEART DISEASE AND ASSOCIATED HANDICAPS

About 12–15 per cent of children with congenital heart disease will have other congenital abnormalities. Many of these are minor or easily correctable, but a small proportion of children are handicapped both by their heart disease and by their other lesions. Mental retardation is a particular problem. Cardiologists are frequently asked to see retarded children, including those with Down's syndrome, whose parents believe that a heart operation will help or cure the retardation. Occasionally this idea has been suggested by a medical attendant but more commonly it results from the parents' conscious or unconscious rationalization of the situation: 'If the blood supply to the brain could be improved he would be all right' or 'If he were able to do more physically this would stimulate the brain to grow' or even 'Anything is worth trying'. When the cardiac defect is not causing significant symptoms there is clearly no indication for operation, but the decision whether to offer operation to a retarded child with, for example, severe cyanosis or cyanotic attacks due to Fallot's tetralogy, is an extremely difficult one. If symptoms are preventing the child from attending a training centre it is reasonable to attempt to improve them, but it is important that the parents realize that the operation, if successful, will not have any dramatic effect on the child's rate of learning.

BIBLIOGRAPHY AND REFERENCES

Apley, J., Barbour, R. F. and Westmacott, I. (1967). Impact of congenital heart disease on the family: preliminary report. *Br. med. J.* **1**, 103
Linde, L. M., Adams, F. H. and Rozansky, G. I. (1971). Physical and emotional aspects of congenital heart disease in children. *Am. J. Cardiol.* **27**, 712
Linde, L., Rasof, B. and Dunn, O. J. (1967). Mental development in congenital heart disease. *J. Pediat.* **71**, 198

Index

Pulmonary venous congestion, 26
in infants, 245
Pulmonary venous connection, absence
of, 211
Pulmonary venous connection, partial,
233
with ASD, 94
Pulmonary venous connection, total
anomalous, 203
obstructed, 205, 207
to coronary sinus, 211
to left innominate vein, 207
Purpura, mechanical, 240
Pyelography, intravenous, in systemic
hypertension, 343

QRS axis, 33, 34–35
QRS complex, 31–32
Q–T interval, 38–39
Q waves, 31

Racial cyanosis in newborn, 240
Radiology, 22–29
abdominal viscera, 28
barium swallow, 29
bronchial arteries, 26
fluoroscopy, 28
heart shape and size, 22–26
of newborn, 245
pulmonary venous congestion, 26
skeletal structure, 28
after surgery, 58–59
thymic enlargement, 27, 28
vascularity of the lungs, 26
Rashkind septostomy, 191–193, 194, 195
Rastelli operation in transposition of the
great arteries, 195–197, 200, 201
Renal biopsy, 344
Renal causes of hypertension, 340
Renal embolism, 281
Renal vein
catheterization, 343, 344
thrombosis, 281
Renography in systemic hypertension,
344
Respiratory distress syndrome, 240
Respiratory obstruction, heart failure
due to, 274
Rhabdomyoma, cardiac, 333
Rheumatic fever, 314–319
aetiology, 315
clinical presentation, 315–317

Rheumatic fever (cont.)
convalescence, 319
pathology, 315
prevention, 318–319
treatment, 317
Ribs, radiographic examination, 28
Rogitine test for hypertension due to
excessive catecholamine, 342
Rubella
congenital, 349, 350
in pregnancy, 6
pulmonary artery stenosis in, 152

Schistosomiasis as cause of pulmonary
hypertension, 272
Scimitar syndrome, 233–234
Scintillation renography, 344
Sedation of infants, 45
Sepsis in newborn, 241
Septostomy, balloon, 191–193, 194, 195
Sick sinus syndrome, 304
Sinoatrial block, 297
Sinoatrial node, 294
Sinus arrhythmia, 297
Sinus bradycardia, 297
Sinus node
dysfunction, 304
effects of surgery, 59
Sinus tachycardia, 297
Sinus venosus defect, 94
Situs inversus, 215, 216
Situs solitus, 215, 216
Skeletal structure, radiographic exami-
nation, 28
Smoking, in pregnancy, 6
Social problems of congenital heart dis-
ease, 355–360
Sounds, normal and abnormal heart, 15–
16, 262–263 (See also Murmurs,
heart)
Spleen
absence, 217, 226
multiple, 217, 226
Squatting, in tetralogy of Fallot, 161–163
Staphylococcal infections, treatment,
284–285
Starling's 'law of the heart', 14
Starr–Edwards prosthetic valve, 118
Stokes–Adams attacks, 309
Streptococcal infections
and infective endocarditis, 287
and rheumatic fever, 318–319
treatment, 284